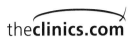

theclinics.com

UROLOGIC CLINICS
OF NORTH AMERICA

Sexual Medicine: State of the Art

GUEST EDITOR
Allen D. Seftel, MD

CONSULTING EDITOR
Martin I. Resnick, MD

November 2007 • Volume 34 • Number 4

SAUNDERS

An Imprint of Elsevier, Inc.
PHILADELPHIA   LONDON   TORONTO   MONTREAL   SYDNEY   TOKYO

W.B. SAUNDERS COMPANY

A Division of Elsevier Inc.

1600 John F. Kennedy Boulevard • Suite 1800 • Philadelphia, Pennsylvania 19103-2899

http://www.theclinics.com

UROLOGIC CLINICS OF NORTH AMERICA
November 2007
Editor: Kerry Holland

Volume 34, Number 4
ISSN 0094-0143
ISBN-13: 978-1-4160-5280-7
ISBN-10: 1-4160-5280-1

Urologic Clinics of North America (ISSN 0094-0143) is published quarterly by Elsevier Inc., 360 Park Avenue South, New York, NY 10010-1710. Months of issue are February, May, August, and November. Business and Editorial Offices: 1600 John F. Kennedy Blvd., Suite 1800, Philadelphia, PA 19103-2899. Customer Service Office: 6277 Sea Harbor Drive, Orlando, FL 32887-4800. Periodicals postage paid at New York, NY and additional mailing offices. Subscription prices are $249.00 per year (US individuals), $394.00 per year (US institutions), $285.00 per year (Canadian individuals), $472.00 per year (Canadian institutions), $333.00 per year (foreign individuals), and $472.00 per year (foreign institutions). Foreign air speed delivery is included in all *Clinics* subscription prices. All prices are subject to change without notice. **POSTMASTER:** Send address changes to *Urologic Clinics of North America*, Elsevier Periodicals Customer Service, 6277 Sea Harbor Drive, Orlando, FL 32887-4800. **Customer Service: 1-800-654-2452 (US). From outside the US, call 1-407-345-4000.**

Urologic Clinics of North America is covered in *Index Medicus, Excerpta Medica, Current Contents/ Clinical Medicine, Science Citation Index,* and *ISI/BIOMED.*

Printed in the United States of America.

CONSULTING EDITOR

MARTIN I. RESNICK, MD,[†] Lester Persky Professor and Chairman, Department of Urology, Case Medical Center, Cleveland, Ohio

GUEST EDITOR

ALLEN D. SEFTEL, MD, Professor of Urology, Case Medical Center; Attending Physician, University Hospitals of Cleveland; and Chief of Urology, Louis Stokes Cleveland VA Medical Center, Cleveland, Ohio

CONTRIBUTORS

STANLEY E. ALTHOF, PhD, Executive Director, Center for Marital and Sexual Health of South Florida, West Palm Beach, Florida; Professor of Psychology, Case Western Reserve University School of Medicine, Cleveland, Ohio; and Voluntary Professor, University of Miami School of Medicine, Miami, Florida

TRINITY J. BIVALACQUA, MD, PhD, Resident in Urology, Department of Urology, The James Buchanan Brady Urological Institute, Johns Hopkins Medical Institutions, Baltimore, Maryland

ARTHUR L. BURNETT, MD, Professor of Urology, Department of Urology, The James Buchanan Brady Urological Institute, Johns Hopkins Medical Institutions, Baltimore, Maryland

CULLEY C. CARSON III, MD, Rhodes Distinguished Professor and Chief of Urology, Department of Surgery, University of North Carolina, Chapel Hill, North Carolina

GERARD D. HENRY, MD, Staff Urologist, Regional Urology, Shreveport, Louisiana

JEFFREY W. JANATA, PhD, Associate Professor, Departments of Reproductive Biology and Psychiatry, University Hospitals Case Medical Center, Case Western Reserve University School of Medicine, Cleveland, Ohio

MOHIT KHERA, MD, Assistant Professor, Scott Department of Urology, Division of Male Reproductive Medicine and Surgery, Baylor College of Medicine, Houston, Texas

SHERYL A. KINGSBERG, PhD, Associate Professor, Departments of Reproductive Biology and Psychiatry, University Hospitals Case Medical Center, Case Western Reserve University School of Medicine, Cleveland, Ohio

ROBERT A. KLONER, MD, PhD, Director of Research, Heart Institute, Good Samaritan Hospital, Cardiovascular Division, Keck School of Medicine at the University of Southern California, Los Angeles, California

ASHAY KPARKER, MD, Department of Urology, University of Illinois at Chicago, Chicago, Illinois

LAURENCE A. LEVINE, MD, Professor of Urology, Department of Urology, Rush University Medical Center, Chicago, Illinois

LARRY I. LIPSHULTZ, MD, Professor, Scott Department of Urology; Lester and Sue Smith Chair in Reproductive Medicine; and Chief, Division of Male Reproductive Medicine and Surgery, Baylor College of Medicine, Houston, Texas

[†] Deceased

ANTOINE MAKHLOUF, MD, PhD, Department of Urology Surgery, University of Minnesota, Minneapolis, Minnesota

ARNOLD MELMAN, MD, Professor and Chairman, Department of Urology, Albert Einstein College of Medicine, Bronx, New York

MARTIN M. MINER, MD, Clinical Associate Professor, Division of Biology and Medicine, Department of Family Medicine, Warren Alpert Medical School of Brown University, Providence, Rhode Island

ABRAHAM MORGENTALER, MD, FACS, Director, Men's Health Boston; and Associate Clinical Professor of Surgery (Urology), Harvard Medical School, Boston, Massachusetts

CRAIG S. NIEDERBERGER, MD, Department of Urology, University of Illinois at Chicago, Chicago, Illinois

GEETU PAHLAJANI, MD, Cleveland Clinic Foundation, Glickman Urological and Kidney Institute, Prostate Center, Cleveland, Ohio

ROBERT TAYLOR SEGRAVES, MD, PhD, Chairperson of Psychiatry, MetroHealth Medical Center; and Professor of Psychiatry, Case School of Medicine, Cleveland, Ohio

ALLEN D. SEFTEL, MD, Professor of Urology, Case Medical Center; Attending Physician, University Hospitals of Cleveland; and Chief of Urology, Louis Stokes Cleveland VA Medical Center, Cleveland, Ohio

TARA SYMONDS, PhD, Global Outcomes Research, Pfizer Ltd., Kent, United Kingdom

FREDERICK L. TAYLOR, MD, Resident in Urology, Department of Urology, Rush University Medical Center, Chicago, Illinois

MARCEL D. WALDINGER, MD, PhD, Department of Psychiatry and Neurosexology, HagaHospital Leyenburg, The Hague; and Section of Psychopharmacology, Department of Pharmaceutical Sciences, Utrecht University, Utrecht, The Netherlands

STEVEN K. WILSON, MD, FACS, Professor of Urology, University of Arkansas for Medical Sciences, Little Rock, Arkansas

CRAIG D. ZIPPE, MD, Cleveland Clinic Foundation, Glickman Urological and Kidney Institute, Prostate Center, Cleveland, Ohio

CONTENTS

Historically, the office visit for a man complaining of sexual dysfunction focused on erectile dysfunction (ED). Over the past several years, epidemiologic studies and novel data have mandated that the clinician redirect this office visit. The office visit has now expanded into a variety of other areas, including premature ejaculation, libido, and hypogonadism as well as a cardiovascular assessment in light of the data suggesting that ED may be a sentinel sign of cardiovascular disease. This article provides the rationale for this global assessment paradigm.

The development of pharmacologic therapy for erectile dysfunction (ED) has been possible because of incremental growth in our understanding of the physiology of normal erections and the complex pathophysiology of ED. Although the oral phosphodiesterase type 5 (PDE5) inhibitors have provided safe, effective treatment of ED for some men, a large proportion of men who have ED do not respond to PDE5 inhibitors or become less responsive or less satisfied as the duration of therapy increases. Also, men who are receiving organic nitrates and nitrates, such as amyl nitrate, cannot take PDE5 inhibitors because of nitrate interactions. The current options for treatment beyond PDE5 inhibitors are invasive, unappealing to some patients, and sometimes ineffective. The search for other options by which ED can be treated has branched out and now encompasses centrally acting mechanisms that control erectile function. Drugs available in Europe include apomorphine. This article focuses on the mechanism of centrally acting agents and reviews clinical data on potential new centrally acting drugs for men who have ED.

Despite the increased popular attention that sexual dysfunction has received in the recent past, more often than not physicians and their patients remain avoidant of the topic in clinical visits. The patient hesitancy in this dynamic suggests that clinicians can best serve their patients by routinely initiating discussions about sexual function during clinical visits. In this article, we provide an overview of the female sexual dysfunctions and address screening and treatment options.

With three effective and safe phosphodiesterase type 5 (PDE5) inhibitors, the clinician now has multiple choices in the treatment of patients who have erectile dysfunction of all severities and etiologies. Based on pharmacokinetics, pharmacodynamics, efficacy, and safety, each of these agents can be used. Because no well-controlled head-to-head selection or patient preference studies are available, each clinician must choose an agent based on the profile of the patient, his tolerance, risk factors, and side effects. This discussion summarizes some of the current data on PDE5 inhibitors and their efficacy, safety, and use in other conditions.

Peyronie's disease is a psychologically and physically devastating disorder that is manifest by a fibrous inelastic scar of the tunica albuginea, resulting in palpable penile scar in the flaccid condition and causing penile deformity, including penile curvature, hinging, narrowing, shortening, and painful erections. Peyronie's disease remains a considerable therapeutic dilemma even to today's practicing physicians.

Throughout history, many attempts to correct erectile dysfunction (ED) have been recorded. For the last 35 years, intracavernosal inflatable prostheses have been used, and these devices have undergone almost constant enhancement. The three-piece inflatable penile prosthesis has the highest patient satisfaction rates and lowest mechanical revision rates of almost any medically implanted device.

Hypogonadism is highly prevalent in older men and men who have prostate cancer. The symptoms of hypogonadism, such as depression, decreased libido, erectile dysfunction, and decreased bone mineral density, can significantly impair a man's quality of life. Moreover, we know that testosterone plays an important role in erectile preservation and in the growth and function of cavernosal and penile nerves. There are compelling data to suggest that testosterone replacement therapy (TRT) in normal and high-risk men does not increase the risk for prostate cancer. In the few studies of men treated with TRT after a radical prostatectomy, there have been no biochemical recurrences. Based on these data, it is difficult to justify withholding TRT following a radical prostatectomy. If we do not lower the testosterone levels of eugonadal men after a radical prostatectomy, how can we justify not replacing testosterone levels in hypogonadal men to make them eugonadal following a radical prostatectomy?

similar efficacy for the daily treatment with the serotonergic antidepressants paroxetine hemihydrate, clomipramine, sertraline, and fluoxetine, with paroxetine hemihydrate exerting the strongest effect on ejaculation. On-demand treatment with SSRIs generally exerts much less ejaculation delay than daily SSRI treatment. Other on-demand treatment options are the topical use of anesthetics, tramadol, and phosphodiesterase type 5 inhibitors. Caution is needed with tramadol with regard to its potential addictive properties. There is insufficient evidence for the ejaculation delaying effects of phosphodiesterase type 5 inhibitors and intracavernous injection of vasoactive drugs.

GOAL STATEMENT

The goal of *Urologic Clinics of North America* is to keep practicing urologists and urology residents up to date with current clinical practice in urology by providing timely articles reviewing the state of the art in patient care.

ACCREDITATION

The *Urologic Clinics of North America* is planned and implemented in accordance with the Essential Areas and Policies of the Accreditation Council for Continuing Medical Education (ACCME) through the joint sponsorship of the University of Virginia School of Medicine and Elsevier. The University of Virginia School of Medicine is accredited by the ACCME to provide continuing medical education for physicians.

The University of Virginia School of Medicine designates this educational activity for a maximum of *15 AMA PRA Category 1 Credits™*. Physicians should only claim credit commensurate with the extent of their participation in the activity.

The American Medical Association has determined that physicians not licensed in the US who participate in this CME activity are eligible for *15 AMA PRA Category 1 Credits™*.

Credit can be earned by reading the text material, taking the CME examination online at http://www.theclinics.com/home/cme, and completing the evaluation. After taking the test, you will be required to review any and all incorrect answers. Following completion of the test and evaluation, your credit will be awarded and you may print your certificate.

FACULTY DISCLOSURE/CONFLICT OF INTEREST

The University of Virginia School of Medicine, as an ACCME accredited provider, endorses and strives to comply with the Accreditation Council for Continuing Medical Education (ACCME) Standards of Commercial Support, Commonwealth of Virginia statutes, University of Virginia policies and procedures, and associated federal and private regulations and guidelines on the need for disclosure and monitoring of proprietary and financial interests that may affect the scientific integrity and balance of content delivered in continuing medical education activities under our auspices.

The University of Virginia School of Medicine requires that all CME activities accredited through this institution be developed independently and be scientifically rigorous, balanced and objective in the presentation/discussion of its content, theories and practices.

All authors/editors participating in an accredited CME activity are expected to disclose to the readers relevant financial relationships with commercial entities occurring within the past 12 months (such as grants or research support, employee, consultant, stock holder, member of speakers bureau, etc.). The University of Virginia School of Medicine will employ appropriate mechanisms to resolve potential conflicts of interest to maintain the standards of fair and balanced education to the reader. Questions about specific strategies can be directed to the Office of Continuing Medical Education, University of Virginia School of Medicine, Charlottesville, Virginia.

The authors/editors listed below have identified no professional or financial affiliations for themselves or their spouse/partner:
Trinity J. Bivalacqua, MD, PhD; Kerry K. Holland (Acquisitions Editor); Jeffrey W. Janata, PhD; Ashay Kparker, MD; Geetu Pahlajani, MD; Robert Taylor Segraves, MD, PhD; Frederick L. Taylor, MD; and, Marcel D. Waldinger, MD, PhD.

The authors/editors listed below identified the following professional or financial affiliations for themselves or their spouse/partner:
Stanley E. Althof, PhD is a consultant and serves on the Advisory Board for Plethora and is a consultant, serves on the Speaker's Bureau and Advisory Board for Johnson & Johnson, King/Palitan, and Lilly.
Arthur L. Burnett, MD serves on the Speaker's Bureau for Pfizer and Lilly.
Culley C. Carson, III, MD is a consultant and serves on the Speaker's Bureau and Advisory Board for Pfizer, Lilly, and GSK.
Gerald D. Henry, MD is on the Speaker's Bureau for Pfizer, American Medical Systems, Coloplast, and Lilly.
Mohit Khera, MD is employed by Solvay and Pfizer and serves on the Speaker's Bureau for Vivus.
Sheryl A. Kingsberg, PhD is an independent contractor and consultant for Procter & Gamble, serves on the Speaker's Bureau and Advisory Committee for Eli Lilly, is an independent contractor for Boehringer-Ingelheim, and is a consultant for Johnson & Johnson.
Robert A. Kloner, MD, PhD is a consultant and serves on the Speaker's Bureau and Advisory Board for Pfizer and Lilly, and is a consultant for King.
Laurence A. Levine, MD is a consultant and serves on the Speaker's Bureau and Advisory Board for Pfizer and Auxilium, serves on the Speaker's Bureau and Advisory Board for Lilly, is a consultant and serves on the Speaker's Bureau for Coloplast, and is an independent contractor and serves on the Advisory Board for FS Physiomed.
Larry I. Lipschultz, MD is a consultant, serves on the speaker's bureau, and is on the advisory committee/board for Auxilium and Pfizer; and, is on the speaker's bureau for Solvay.
Antoine A. Makhlouf, MD, PhD is on the Speaker's Bureau for Pfizer and is a consultant for TIMM medical.
Arnold Melman, MD owns stock in, is a patent holder for, and is a directing member of Ion Channel Innovations.
Martin M. Miner, MD is a consultant for GSK, Auxilium Pharmaceuticals, and King Pharmaceuticals.
Abraham Morgentaler, MD, FACS is a lecturer for Auxilium, is a lecturer and investigator for Solvay, and is a lecturer, investigator, and serves on the Advisory Committee for Indevus.
Craig S. Niederberger, MD is a consultant for the Federal Trade Commission, and conducts a clinical trial for Medicis.
Allen D. Setfel, MD (Guest Editor) is a consultant for Pfizer, Lilly, Indevus, Auxilium, and Solvay.
Tara Symonds, PhD is employed by and owns stock in Pfizer Ltd.
Steven K. Wilson, MD, FACS is a consultant for, owns stock in, and is a patent holder for American Medical Systems.
Craig D. Zippe, MD serves on the Speaker's Bureau for Pfizer, Inc

Disclosure of Discussion of non-FDA approved uses for pharmaceutical products and/or medical devices:
The University of Virginia School of Medicine, as an ACCME provider, requires that all faculty presenters identify and disclose any "off label" uses for pharmaceutical and medical device products. The University of Virginia School of Medicine recommends that each physician fully review all the available data on new products or procedures prior to instituting them with patients.

TO ENROLL

To enroll in the Urologic Clinics of North America Continuing Medical Education program, call customer service at 1-800-654-2452 or visit us online at www.theclinics.com/home/cme. The CME program is available to subscribers for an additional fee of $195.00.

FORTHCOMING ISSUES

RECENT ISSUES

ELSEVIER
SAUNDERS

Urol Clin N Am 34 (2007) xi

UROLOGIC
CLINICS
of North America

Dedication

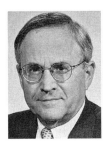

Martin I. Resnick, MD

"No person was ever honored for what he received. Honor has been the reward for what he gave."

Calvin Coolidge 1872–1933,
Thirtieth President of the United States

This issue of the *Urologic Clinics of North America* is dedicated to the late Martin I. Resnick, MD. Marty was the Lester Persky Professor of Urology and Chairman of the Department of Urology, Case Medical Center, Cleveland, Ohio, serving in that capacity for more than 25 years. Marty also was the former Secretary of the American Urological Association, past President of the American Urological Association, and most recently, editor of the *Journal of Urology*. He devoted many hours to the continued success of the *Urologic Clinics of North America* through suggestion of topics and editing of specific editions with boundless enthusiasm.

Marty was a leader, a pioneer, a friend, a mentor, and most importantly, a role model for academic success. His departure leaves a tremendous void in my life as well as in the urologic community at large.

Marty, it has been an honor!

Allen D. Seftel, MD
Department of Urology
Case Medical Center
11100 Euclid Avenue
Cleveland, OH 44106-5046, USA

E-mail address: allen.seftel@case.edu

ELSEVIER
SAUNDERS

Urol Clin N Am 34 (2007) xiii–xiv

UROLOGIC
CLINICS
of North America

Preface

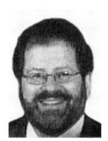

Allen D. Seftel, MD
Guest Editor

Sexual medicine remains a dynamic, evolving enterprise. To the novice, the field would seem rather superficial; the more sophisticated clinician will recognize the complex nature of the discipline. It is clear that many new concepts continue to evolve, and confusion often confronts the treating clinician.

This issue of the *Urologic Clinics of North America* has been prepared to assist the clinician in understanding the newer concepts that surround male sexual dysfunction and allow the clinician to feel comfortable in treating men and women with a variety of sexual complaints.

The articles include topics in office evaluation; treatment of erectile dysfunction with phosphodiesertase type 5 inhibitors; treatment of hypogonadism with testosterone; treatment of premature ejaculation with an assortment of drugs and possibly adjuvant psychotherapy; penile rehabilitation after prostatectomy; insertion of a penile prosthesis; treatment of priapism; and treatment of Peyronie's disease, among others. I am grateful to the many authors who contributed to this issue. They are to be congratulated.

I dedicate this issue of the *Urologic Clinics of North America* to the late Martin I. Resnick, MD. Marty was the Lester Persky Professor of Urology and Chairman of the Department of Urology, Case Medical Center, Cleveland, Ohio, serving in that capacity for over 25 years. Marty was also the former Secretary of the American Urological Association, past President of the American Urological Association, and most recently, editor of the *Journal of Urology*. Marty was an avid supporter of the *Urologic Clinics of North America* and devoted many hours to its continued success through suggestion of topics and editing of specific editions with boundless enthusiasm.

Early on, Marty recognized the importance of sexual medicine in urology. He also recognized that sexual dysfunction required a multidisciplinary, team approach. Joining with members of our psychiatry department, Marty spearheaded the development of a joint sexual medicine venture that was a model for others to follow. This combined clinic led to many important publications and became recognized nationally and internationally [1–3].

Marty was a leader, a pioneer, a friend, a mentor, and, most importantly, a role model for academic success. His departure leaves a tremendous void in my life as well in the urologic community at large. Marty, it has been an honor.

Allen D. Seftel, MD
*Department of Urology
Case Medical Center
11100 Euclid Avenue
Cleveland, OH 44106-5046, USA*

E-mail address: allen.seftel@case.edu

0094-0143/07/$ - see front matter © 2007 Elsevier Inc. All rights reserved.
doi:10.1016/j.ucl.2007.08.010

References

[1] Bodner DR, Lindan R, Leffler E, et al. The application of intracavernous injection of vasoactive medications for erection in men with spinal cord injury. J Urol 1987;138:310–1.

[2] Levine SB, Althof SE, Turner LA, et al. Side effects of self-administration of intracavernous papaverine and phentolamine for the treatment of impotence. J Urol 1989;141:54–7.

[3] Turner LA, Althof SE, Levine SB, et al. External vacuum devices in the treatment of erectile dysfunction: a one-year study of sexual and psychosocial impact. J Sex Marital Ther 1991;17:81–93.

ELSEVIER
SAUNDERS

Urol Clin N Am 34 (2007) 463–482

UROLOGIC
CLINICS
of North America

Office Evaluation of Male Sexual Dysfunction

Allen D. Seftel, MD[a,*], Martin M. Miner, MD[b],
Robert A. Kloner, MD, PhD[c], Stanley E. Althof, PhD[a,d]

[a]Department of Urology, Case Medical Center, Cleveland, OH, USA
[b]Department of Family Medicine, Brown University, Providence, RI, USA
[c]Heart Institute, Good Samaritan Hospital, Cardiovascular Division, Keck School of Medicine at the
University of Southern California, Los Angeles, CA, USA
[d]Center for Marital and Sexual Health of South Florida, West Palm Beach, FL, USA

Erectile dysfunction

Epidemiology of erectile dysfunction

Definition

For years, the terms *impotence* and *erectile dysfunction* (ED) had been used interchangeably to denote the inability of a man to achieve or maintain erection sufficient to permit satisfactory sexual intercourse [1]. Social scientists objected to the impotence label, because of its pejorative implications and lack of precision [2]. A National Institutes of Health (NIH) Consensus Development Conference [3] advocated that the term *erectile dysfunction* be used in place of the term *impotence*. ED or impotence was now defined as "the inability of the male to achieve an erect penis as part of the overall multifaceted process of male sexual function." This definition de-emphasizes intercourse as the sine qua non of sexual life and gives equal importance to other aspects of male sexual behavior.

The *Diagnostic and Statistical Manual of Mental Disorders, Fourth Edition–Text Revision* (DSM-IV-TR), the American Psychiatric Association's nomenclature manual, offers the following diagnostic criterion set for Male Erectile Disorder (302.72):

A. There is a persistent or recurrent inability to attain or to maintain until completion of the sexual activity an adequate erection.

B. The disturbance causes marked distress or interpersonal difficulty.
C. The ED is not better accounted for by another axis I disorder (other than a sexual dysfunction) and is not exclusively attributable to the direct physiologic effects of a substance (eg, drug of abuse, medication) or a general medical condition.

The DSM-IV-TR also asks the clinician to make three additional specifications:

1. Lifelong versus acquired
2. Generalized versus situational
3. Attributable to medical factors, psychologic factors, or combined factors

The definition offered by the NIH consensus panel is used most commonly for daily and practical application, although clinicians still think of ED as the inability to maintain or sustain an erection during coitus. The NIH definition allows for a broader interpretation of ED, allowing the clinician and patient greater latitude in the diagnosis and treatment of this disease entity.

Erectile dysfunction prevalence and medical risk factors

It is estimated that at least 10 to 20 million American men have ED [4,5]. Laumann and colleagues [5] have shown that the prevalence of male sexual dysfunction approaches 31% in a population survey of approximately 1400 men aged 18 to 59 years—the National Health and Social Life Survey. Hypogonadism (5%), ED (5%), and

* Corresponding author.
E-mail addresses: allen.seftel@case.edu (A.D. Seftel); allen.seftel@uhhospitals.org (A.D. Seftel).

premature ejaculation (PE; 21%) were the three most common male sexual dysfunctions noted.

The Massachusetts Male Aging Study [4], a large epidemiologic study, asked men between the ages of 40 and 70 years to categorize their erectile function as completely, moderately, minimally, or not impotent. Fifty-two percent of the sample reported some degree of ED. This study demonstrated that ED is an age-dependent disorder: "between the ages of 40-70 years the probability of complete impotence tripled from 5.1% to 15%, moderate impotence doubled from 17% to 34% while the probability of minimal impotence remained constant at 17%." By the age of 70 years, only 32% of the sample portrayed themselves as free of ED. Finally, cigarette smoking increased the probability of total ED in men who had treated heart disease, hypertension, or untreated arthritis. It similarly increased the probability for men on cardiac, antihypertensive, or vasodilator medications.

After the data were adjusted for age, men treated for diabetes (28%), heart disease (39%), and hypertension (15%) had significantly higher probabilities for ED than the sample as a whole (9.6%). Men with untreated ulcer (18%), arthritis (15%), and allergy (12%) were also significantly more likely to develop ED. Although ED was not associated with total serum cholesterol, the probability of dysfunction varied inversely with high-density lipoprotein cholesterol.

Certain classes of medication were related to increased probability for total ED. The percentage of men with complete dysfunction taking hypoglycemic agents (26%), antihypertensives (14%), vasodilators (36%), and cardiac drugs (28%) was significantly higher than the sample as a whole (9.6%).

Other epidemiologic data look at the ED phenomenon from a global perspective. Masumori and colleagues [6] compared age-related prevalence of ED among 289 Japanese men and 2115 American men (the latter group were from the Olmsted County study). Results from both groups indicated an age-related decline in erectile function, sexual libido, and sexual satisfaction. In particular, 71% of Japanese men aged 70 to 79 years reported having erections only "a little of the time or less" when sexually stimulated, and 80% perceived sexual drive once or less during the past month. Marumo and colleagues [7] reported a similar increase in the prevalence of ED among 2311 Japanese men between 23 and 79 years of age.

More recent data added greater depth to the US national estimates of ED. The National Health and Nutrition Examination Survey (NHANES), conducted by the National Center for Health Statistics, collected data by household interview supplemented by medical examination. The sample design was a stratified, multistage, probability sample of clusters of persons representing the civilian noninstitutionalized population; African Americans and Mexican Americans were oversampled. The NHANES used a four-stage probability design. First, counties (or groups of counties) are sampled as primary sampling units, then segments (clusters of blocks) within counties, and then households within segments; finally, individuals within households were sampled. The sample size for the entire survey for the 2-year period was 11,039, with a response rate of 71.1% for men aged 20 years and older. Data include medical histories in which specific queries are made regarding sexual function. The assessment of erectile function was based on respondent answers to one survey item (KIQ400). In men 20 years of age and older, ED affected almost one in five respondents. Hispanic men were more likely to report ED (odds ratio [OR] = 1.89), after controlling for other factors. The prevalence of ED increased dramatically with advanced age; 77.5% of men aged 75 years and older were affected. In addition, there were several modifiable risk factors that were independently associated with ED, including diabetes mellitus (DM; OR = 2.69), obesity (OR = 1.60), current smoking (OR = 1.74), and hypertension (OR = 1.56) [8].

Data specific to ED and related diseases have emerged recently and serve to support the relation between ED and cardiovascular disease (CVD). Seftel and colleagues [9] quantified the prevalence of diagnosed hypertension, hyperlipidemia, DM, and depression in male health plan members (United States) with ED, using a nationally representative managed care claims database that covered 51 health plans with 28 million lives for 1995 through 2002. Based on 272,325 identified patients who had ED, population and age-specific prevalence rates were calculated for the same period. Crude population prevalence rates in this study population were 41.6% for hypertension, 42.4% for hyperlipidemia, 20.2% for DM, 11.1% for depression, 23.9% for hypertension and hyperlipidemia, 12.8% for hypertension and DM, and 11.5% for hyperlipidemia and depression. The crude age-specific prevalence rates varied across age groups significantly for hypertension (4.5%–68.4%), hyperlipidemia (3.9%–52.3%), and DM (2.8%–28.7%) and significantly less for depression (5.8%–15.0%). Region-adjusted population prevalence rates were 41.2% for hypertension, 41.8% for hyperlipidemia, 19.7% for DM, and 11.9% for depression. Of 87,163 patients who had ED, 32% had no comorbid diagnosis of hypertension, hyperlipidemia, DM, or depression. These data suggested and confirmed that hypertension, hyperlipidemia, DM, and depression were prevalent in patients who had ED. This evidence supported the proposition that ED shares common risk factors with these four concurrent conditions. Therefore, as a pathophysiologic event, ED could be viewed as a potential observable marker for these concurrent diseases.

Esposito and colleagues [10] determined the effect of weight loss and increased physical activity on erectile and endothelial function in obese men. They conducted a randomized single-blind trial of 110 obese men (body mass index ≥ 30) aged 35 to 55 years, without diabetes, hypertension, or hyperlipidemia, who had ED that was determined by having a score of 21 or less on the International Index of Erectile Function (IIEF). The study was conducted from October 2000 to October 2003 at a university hospital in Italy. The 55 men randomly assigned to the intervention group received detailed advice about how to achieve a loss of 10% or more in their total body weight by reducing caloric intake and increasing their level of physical activity. Men in the control group (n = 55) were given general information about healthy food choices and exercise.

After 2 years, body mass index decreased more in the intervention group (from a mean [SD] of 36.9 [2.5] to 31.2 [2.1]) than in the control group (from 36.4 [2.3] to 35.7 [2.5]; $P<.001$), as did serum concentrations of interleukin 6 ($P = .03$) and C-reactive protein ($P = .02$). The mean (SD) level of physical activity increased more in the intervention group (from 48 [10] to 195 [36] min/wk; $P<.001$) than in the control group (from 51 [9] to 84 [28] min/wk; $P<.001$). The mean (SD) IIEF score improved in the intervention group (from 13.9 [4.0] to 17 [5]; $P<.001$) but remained stable in the control group (from 13.5 [4.0] to 13.6 [4.1]; $P = .89$). Seventeen men in the intervention group and 3 in the control group ($P = .001$) reported an IIEF score of 22 or higher. In multivariate analyses, changes in body mass index ($P = .02$), physical activity ($P = .02$), and C-reactive protein ($P = .03$) were independently associated with changes in IIEF score. The study concluded that lifestyle changes were associated with improvement in sexual function in approximately one third of obese men with ED at baseline.

If these clinical associations are valid, one could argue that there should be mechanistic data supporting these concepts. Eaton and colleagues [11] evaluated the cross-sectional association between the degree of ED and levels of atherosclerotic biomarkers. As part of an ongoing epidemiologic study, a subcohort of 988 US male health professionals between the ages 46 and 81 years had atherosclerotic biomarkers measured from blood collected in 1994 through 1995. In 2000, these same men had been retrospectively asked about erectile function in 1995 and in 2000. Biennial questionnaires since 1986 assessed medical conditions, medications, smoking, physical activity, body mass index, and alcohol intake. The retrospective assessment of erectile function in 2000 in these 988 men was as follows: very good (28.2%), good (25.1%), fair (19.2%), poor (13.6%), and very poor (13.9%). Men with poor to very poor erectile function compared with men with good and very good erectile function had 2.9 the odds of having elevated factor VII levels ($P = .03$), 1.9 times the odds of having elevated vascular cell adhesion molecule ($P = .13$), 2.0 times the odds of having elevated intracellular adhesion molecule ($P = .06$), and 2.1 times the odds of having elevated total cholesterol/high-density lipoprotein ratio ($P = .02$) comparing the top to bottom quintiles for each atherosclerotic biomarker after multivariate adjustment. Lipoprotein(a), homocysteine, interleukin-6, tumor necrosis factor receptor, C-reactive protein, and fibrinogen were not associated with the degree of erectile function after adjustment. They concluded that selected biomarkers for endothelial function, thrombosis, and dyslipidemia but not for inflammation were associated with the degree of ED in this cross-sectional analysis.

Important epidemiologic data have suggested that ED may be an early marker for CVD. Min and colleagues [12] studied 221 men referred for stress myocardial perfusion single-photon emission CT (MPS), which is commonly used to diagnose and stratify CVD. They found that 55% of the patients had ED and that these men exhibited more severe coronary heart disease (MPS summed stress score >8) (43% versus 17%; $P<.001$) and left ventricular dysfunction (left ventricular ejection fraction <50%) (24% versus 11%; $P =$ .01) than those without ED. These data suggested that ED was associated as an independent predictor of more severe coronary artery disease (CAD) and high-risk MPS findings.

Further data support the ED-cardiovascular paradigm. A sample of nearly 4000 Canadian men [13], aged 40 to 88 years, seen by primary care clinicians reported ED with the use of the IIEF. The presence of CVD or DM increased the probability of ED, and among those individuals without CVD or DM, the calculated 10-year Framingham coronary risk and fasting glucose level increase were independently associated with ED. ED was also independently associated with undiagnosed hyperglycemia (OR = 1.46), impaired fasting glucose (OR = 1.26), and the metabolic syndrome (OR = 1.45).

A prospective analysis by Thompson [14] of the nearly 9500 men randomly assigned to the placebo arm of the Prostate Cancer Prevention Trial (PCPT) revealed that men with ED are at significantly greater risk ($P<.001$) for having a cardiovascular event (angina, myocardial infarction [MI], or stroke) than those without ED. Furthermore, the findings indicate that the relation between incident ED (the first report of ED of any grade) and CVD is comparable to that associated with current smoking, family history of MI, or hyperlipidemia. Subsequent to the Thompson analysis and lending further support to the idea of ED as a precursor of CVD, Montorsi and colleagues [15] investigated 285 patients who had CAD. A key finding is that nearly all patients who developed CAD symptoms experienced ED symptoms first, on average, 3 years beforehand.

The studies noted here suggest that a presentation of ED should trigger an assessment of cardiovascular risk factors and, if appropriate, vigorous intervention. The Second Princeton Consensus Conference on sexual dysfunction and cardiac risk and a follow-up report recommend screening men with ED of uncertain etiology for vascular disease and abnormal metabolic parameters, including glucose, lipids, and blood pressure. It was stressed that men with ED and no cardiac disease should be considered at risk for CVD until proved otherwise [16].

The impact of ED frequently extends beyond a man's physical function; it can have a psychologic effect on a man and his partner, producing bother. Consequently, the emotional toll that ED can have on men and their partners should be considered in the diagnosis and management of ED. A global survey of 13,618 men from 29 countries found that 13% to 28% have ED [17], and a survey of 1481 men in The Netherlands [18] found that, of those with ED, 67% were bothered by it and 85% wanted help for their condition. Left untreated, the emotional bother associated with ED can have a significant impact on important psychosocial factors, including self-esteem and confidence, and can damage personal relationships [19–21] In their Consensus Development Panel on Impotence, the NIH recommended that studies continue to investigate the social and psychologic effects of ED in patients and their partners [3] There are few data on the effect of ED and its treatment on bother associated with ED, however. This may be attributable, in part, to the absence of data from an instrument designed to assess the bother or distress that is specific to ED.

Summary and recommendations

ED is common throughout the world, increases in prevalence with aging, is bothersome, and is a future marker for CVD. ED is associated with hypertension, diabetes, depression, hyperlipidemia, smoking [22,23], sedentary lifestyle [23], and obesity. Thus, the man presenting to the clinician complaining of ED should have these areas addressed. In addition to defining and characterizing the specific sexual complaint, a brief cardiovascular assessment of risk factors, including smoking, lifestyle and exercise, diet, blood pressure, lipids, weight, and distress, should all be part of the initial evaluation. A World Health Organization (WHO) consensus panel has deliberated and agreed that these recommendations are reasonable [24].

Hypogonadism

Epidemiology of hypogonadism

The Hypogonadism in Males (HIM) study estimated the prevalence of hypogonadism (total testosterone [TT] < 300 ng/dL) in men aged 45 years or older visiting primary care practices in the United States. A blood sample was obtained between 8:00 AM and noon and assayed for TT, free testosterone (FT), and bioavailable testosterone (BAT). Common symptoms of hypogonadism, comorbid conditions, demographics, and reason for visit were recorded. Of 2162 patients, 836 were hypogonadal, with 80 receiving testosterone. The crude prevalence rate of hypogonadism was 38.7%. Similar trends were observed for FT and BAT [25].

A recent review of this topic sheds light on the epidemiology of hypogonadism [26]. In healthy young eugonadal men, serum testosterone levels range from 300 to 1050 ng/dL, but they decline with advancing age, particularly after 50 years [27–29]. Using a serum testosterone level of 325 ng/dL, the Baltimore Longitudinal Study of Aging (BLSA) reported that approximately 12%, 20%, 30%, and 50% of men in their 50s, 60s, 70s, and 80s, respectively, are hypogonadal.

Longitudinal and cross-sectional studies have demonstrated annual testosterone decrements of 0.5% to 2% with advancing age [26–31]. The rate of decline in serum testosterone in men seems to largely depend on their age at study entry. In the BLSA, the average decline was 3.2 ng/dL per year among men aged 53 years at entry. Conversely, the New Mexico Aging Process Study of men aged 66 to 80 years at entry showed a decrease in serum testosterone of 110 ng/dL every 10 years. Although serum testosterone levels are generally measured in the morning when at peak, this circadian rhythm is often abolished in elderly men [32].

Definition of hypogonadism

The US Food and Drug Administration (FDA) has accepted a TT level of 300 ng/dL as the lower limit of normal for serum testosterone levels. Others have challenged this level, citing a variety of reasons as to why a level of 300 ng/dL is not a true reflection of hypogonadism. Reasons include a lack of age-specific norms, a lack of evidence that 300 ng/dL is a proper number, and a lack of symptoms reflecting what the testosterone level represents. Clinicians have gravitated to the term *late-onset hypogonadism* (LOH) to suggest that an older group of men might be a more appropriate group of individuals on whom we should focus with respect to testosterone deficiency. An international consensus statement (appearing in three or four journals simultaneously) [34] has been published, which has offered the following guidance:

1. Definition of LOH: a clinical and biochemical syndrome associated with advancing age and characterized by typical symptoms and a deficiency in serum testosterone levels. It may result in significant detriment in the quality of life and adversely affect the function of multiple organ systems.

2. LOH is a syndrome characterized primarily by the following:
   A. The easily recognized features of diminished sexual desire (libido) and erectile quality and frequency, particularly nocturnal erections
   B. Changes in mood with concomitant decreases in intellectual activity, cognitive functions, spatial orientation ability, fatigue, depressed mood, and irritability
   C. Sleep disturbances
   D. Decrease in lean body mass with associated diminution in muscle volume and strength
   E. Increase in visceral fat
   F. Decrease in body hair and skin alterations
   G. Decreased bone mineral density resulting in osteopenia, osteoporosis, and increased risk for bone fractures

3. In patients at risk for or suspected of hypogonadism in general and LOH in particular, a thorough physical and biochemical workup is mandatory and the following biochemical investigations should especially be done:
   A. A serum sample for TT determination and sex hormone-binding globulin (SHBG) should be obtained between 07:00 AM and 11:00 AM. The most widely accepted parameters to establish the presence of hypogonadism are the measurement of TT and FT, which are calculated from measured TT and SHBG or measured by a reliable FT dialysis method.
   B. There are no generally accepted lower limits of normal, and it is unclear whether geographically different thresholds depend on ethnic differences or on the physician's perception. There is, however, general agreement that TT greater than 12 nmol/L (346 ng/dL) or FT greater than 250 pmol/L (72 pg/mL) does not require substitution. Similarly, based on the data of younger men, there is consensus that serum TT levels less than 8 nmol/L (231 ng/dL) or FT less than 180 pmol/L (52 pg/mL) requires substitution. Because symptoms of testosterone deficiency become manifest between 12 and 8 nmol/L, trials of treatment can be considered in those patients in whom alternative causes of these symptoms have been excluded. (Because there are variations in the reagents and normal ranges among

laboratories, the cutoff values given for serum testosterone and FT may have to be adjusted depending on the reference values given by each laboratory).

C. Salivary testosterone has been shown to be a reliable substitute for FT measurements but cannot be recommended at this time because the methodology has not been standardized and adult male ranges are not available in most hospital or reference laboratories.

D. If testosterone levels are less than or at the lower limit of the accepted normal adult male values, it is recommended to perform a second determination, together with assessment of serum luteinizing hormone and prolactin.

4. A clear indication based on a clinical picture, together with biochemical evidence of low serum testosterone, should exist before the initiation of testosterone substitution.

The Endocrine Society has recently published its set of guidelines, entitled "Testosterone Therapy in Adult Men with Androgen Deficiency Syndromes: An Endocrine Society Clinical Practice Guideline" [33].

The Endocrine Society recommends making a diagnosis of androgen deficiency only in men with consistent symptoms and signs and unequivocally low serum testosterone levels. The authors suggest the measurement of morning TT level by a reliable assay as the initial diagnostic test. The authors recommend confirmation of the diagnosis by repeating the measurement of morning TT and, in some patients, by measurement of the FT or BAT level, using accurate assays. The authors recommend testosterone therapy for symptomatic men with androgen deficiency, who have low testosterone levels, to induce and maintain secondary sex characteristics and to improve their sexual function, sense of well-being, muscle mass and strength, and bone mineral density. The authors recommend against starting testosterone therapy in patients who have breast or prostate cancer, a palpable prostate nodule, or induration or prostate-specific antigen (PSA) greater than 3 ng/mL without further urologic evaluation, erythrocytosis (hematocrit $> 50\%$), hyperviscosity, untreated obstructive sleep apnea, severe lower urinary tract symptoms (LUTSs) with an International Prostate Symptom Score (IPSS) greater than 19, or class III or IV heart failure.

When testosterone therapy is instituted, the authors suggest aiming at achieving testosterone levels during treatment in the midnormal range with any of the approved formulations, chosen on the basis of the patient's preference, consideration of pharmacokinetics, treatment burden, and cost. Men receiving testosterone therapy should be monitored using a standardized plan.

In an insightful comment on the Endocrine Society guidelines, Shames and colleagues [34] of the FDA state that testosterone products are approved by the FDA as replacement therapy for men with classic androgen deficiency (ie, men with extremely low serum testosterone concentrations generally associated with specific medical disorders). The current authors refer to this condition as classic hypogonadism. Many prescribers, however, advocate administration of testosterone to older men with an array of signs and symptoms, many of which may be related to normal aging, and a "low" serum testosterone concentration based on normative values for young men. For the purposes of this review, the authors refer to this condition by its most popularly accepted name, andropause.

Further, Shames and colleagues [34] state:

In 2002, the National Institute of Aging and the National Cancer Institute asked the Institute of Medicine (IOM) to conduct a review of the current state of knowledge of the potential risks and benefits of testosterone therapy in older men and to make research recommendations regarding clinical trials. The IOM's report was published in 2004 and concluded in its executive summary that as the FDA-approved treatment for male hypogonadism, testosterone therapy has been found to be effective in ameliorating a number of symptoms in markedly hypogonadal males. Researchers have carefully explored the benefits of testosterone therapy, particularly placebo-controlled randomized trials, in the population of middle aged or older men who do not meet all the clinical diagnostic criteria for hypogonadism but who may have testosterone levels in the low range for young adult males and show one or more symptoms that are common to both aging and hypogonadism. The IOM further concluded that assessments of risks and benefits have been limited and uncertainties remain about the value of this therapy in older men.

Finally, Shames and colleagues [34] conclude:

We support the right of individual physicians to treat patients based on their own knowledge or advice from known experts in the field.

However, patients should be able to choose therapies based on accurate and evidence-based medical information and consultation with well-informed health care providers. Clinical guidelines and patient guides should be based on solid clinical evidence and must convey this information clearly and accurately to physicians and patients.

Summary and recommendations

Hypogonadism is a controversial topic, as can be seen here. One can easily recognize the cautionary stance provided by the FDA in the comments offered by Shames and colleagues [34]. Thus, it remains unclear as to the most appropriate testosterone level that allows for the bona fide diagnosis of hypogonadism. It also seems reasonable that irrespective of the testosterone level that is chosen by the clinician for the diagnosis of hypogonadism, certain hypogonadism-associated symptoms should be sought out and detailed in the patient record. For those clinicians unfamiliar with these symptoms, the questionnaires outlined in this article should suffice. Caution must be the guide here, as we make slow and steady progress. The recommendations noted in the two guidelines outlined previously should suffice for guidance.

Newer concepts

Low levels of testosterone, hypogonadism, have several features in common with the metabolic syndrome. In the Tromsø Study [35], a population-based health survey, testosterone levels were inversely associated with anthropometric measurements, and the lowest levels of TT and FT were found in men with the most pronounced central obesity. TT was inversely associated with systolic blood pressure, and men with hypertension had lower levels of TT and FT. Furthermore, men with diabetes had lower testosterone levels compared with men without a history of diabetes, and an inverse association between testosterone levels and glycosylated hemoglobin was found. Thus, there are strong associations between low levels of testosterone and the different components of the metabolic syndrome. In addition, an independent association between low testosterone levels and the metabolic syndrome itself has recently been presented in cross-sectional and prospective population-based studies. Thus, testosterone may have a protective role in the development of metabolic syndrome and subsequent DM and CVD in aging men [35].

Premature ejaculation

PE is a timely topic. The epidemiology is under intense review. Two recent reviews have helped to synthesize the data [36,37].

Results from the Global Study of Sexual Attitudes and Behaviors (GSSAB) found PE to be the most common sexual dysfunction in six of seven worldwide geographic regions studied [17]. Only in the Middle East region was the prevalence of PE (12.4%) eclipsed by other sexual dysfunctions, including ED (14.1%) and lack of sexual interest (21.6%). The prevalence rates for the non-European West (27.4%), Central/South America (28.3%), East Asia (29.1%), and Southeast Asia (30.5%) regions were roughly equivalent and in agreement with the data from the National Health and Social Life Survey (NHSLS) [5]. The prevalence of PE in the Northern Europe (20.7%) and Southern Europe (21.5%) regions was slightly less. In 1999, Fugl-Meyer and colleagues [38] reported a prevalence of 4% (51 of 1281 subjects) in a large representative population study of Swedes aged 18 to 74 years. A remarkably low prevalence of other common forms of sexual dysfunction was also reported, with erectile difficulties reported only by 3% of men surveyed. These results suggest that Swedes have an unexplainably lower prevalence of PE and other sexual dysfunctions than can be found in the United States or other regions. Of course, this assumes that the study design allowed for an accurate representation of the entire Swedish population. Estimates of PE in the Unites States are that approximately 31% of the male population aged 18 to 59 years is afflicted with sexual dysfunction [5].

The definition of PE remains controversial. There currently exists a DSM-IV-TR definition of PE [39]. In the DSM-IV-TR, which is issued by the American Psychiatric Association, PE is defined as a "persistent or recurrent ejaculation with minimal sexual stimulation before, on, or shortly after penetration and before the person wishes it" [39]. "The clinician must take into account factors that affect duration of the excitement phase, such as age, novelty of the sexual partner or situation, and recent frequency of sexual activity" [39]. According to this definition, PE can only be diagnosed when "the disturbance causes marked distress or interpersonal difficulty" [39].

Historically, most clinicians have used 1 to 2 minutes as the cutoff for the diagnosis of PE. In a recent study, Patrick and colleagues [40] have attempted to offer time-related norms. In an attempt to define normal ejaculation time, a 4-week multicenter observational study of men (≥ 18 years old) and their female partners in monogamous relationships (≥ 6 months) was conducted using intravaginal ejaculatory latency time (IELT), as measured by a stopwatch held by the partner. The IELT was recorded for each sexual intercourse experience. The median IELT was 1.8 (range: 0–41) minutes for PE subjects and 7.3 (range: 0–53) minutes for non-PE subjects ($P < .0001$). More PE subjects versus non-PE subjects gave ratings of "very poor" or "poor" for control over ejaculation (72% versus 5%; $P < .0001$) and satisfaction with sexual intercourse (31% versus 1%; $P < .0001$). More subjects in the PE group versus the non-PE group gave ratings of "quite a bit" or "extremely" for personal distress (64% versus 4%; $P < .0001$) and interpersonal difficulty (31% versus 1%; $P < .0001$). Subject and partner assessments showed similar patterns and correlated moderately (IELT range: 0.36–0.57). These data would seem to support a 1- to 2-minute time frame, anteportal or using IELT, for PE. Of note, in this study, there was considerable overlap in IELT between the men with and without PE, suggesting that IELT alone may not be good discriminator between men with and without PE. IELT was a good discriminator for men who had IELTs of less than 1 minute. Many authorities believe that IELT alone is not sufficient to diagnose PE. Thus, PE should be a multidimensional diagnosis, including IELT, control, and distress. See the article by Waldinger elsewhere for further exploration of this topic.

In another article in this issue, Waldinger challenges the current definition of PE. A new proposal for the pending the DSM-V and ICD-11 definitions of PE has been put forward. According to this proposal, PE should be classified according to a "syndromal" approach incorporating well-controlled clinical and epidemiologic stopwatch studies [39–42].

Summary and recommendations

PE is a timely topic. A new definition has been proposed in lieu of the 1- to 2-minute time frame used historically. Many authorities rely on ejaculation time, patient control, and patient distress to define PE. Others incorporate questionnaires into the history. Most clinicians still use a 1- to 2-minute ejaculation time, combined with some element of distress, as the time frame for the diagnosis of PE.

Sexual medicine history and physical examination

The office evaluation consists of a series of direct questions about the nature of the sexual dysfunction complaint, as delineated in Box 1. The interview should take place in a quiet room, in a nonjudgmental fashion. These men are embarrassed and often need reassurance that this topic is acceptable to discuss. The questions should be asked in a gentile manner, avoiding any gestures or posturing that might be misconstrued.

In lieu of direct questions, many clinicians prefer to provide the patient with questionnaires that delve into the specific sexual complaint. The Sexual Health Inventory for Men (SHIM) is a simple five-question instrument that inquires about erectile function over the previous 6 months. The SHIM is an abridged and slightly modified version of the IIEF [43]. This simpler version allows the clinician to assess male ED with great security. This brief questionnaire is user-friendly and is most often completed by the patient in the examination room or waiting room before the interview. The SHIM is appended, and it is scored as follows:

> Score of 22 to 25: no ED
> Score of 17 to 21: mild ED
> Score of 12 to 16: mild to moderate ED
> Score of 8 to 11: moderate ED

A score of 0 to 7 represents severe ED, such as that seen after radical prostatectomy or pelvic surgery (in Dr. Seftel's personal experience, psychogenic ED should be considered). The SHIM gives a severity index, provides a common vocabulary, and has supplanted vascular testing in many cases. The SHIM, however, is not predictive of outcome.

The Androgen Deficiency in the Aging Male (ADAM) questionnaire, although not sensitive for hypogonadism, asks questions that are pertinent to the hypogonadal state [44].

The Centers for Epidemiologic Study-Depression (CES-D) is a useful screening tool for depression [45].

The American Urological Association (AUA) symptom index is familiar to most urologists. It queries the patient regarding the urologic voiding pattern [46].

Box 1. Initial evaluation of a man complaining of sexual dysfunction

Characterize the sexual dysfunction.
What type of sexual problem does the patient complain of?
Does he have ED?
If so, how long has he had the problem?
When was the last time he had intercourse?
When was the last time he had any sexual activity?
Does the erection problem bother him?
Does the erection problem bother his partner?
Did the problem arise suddenly (psychogenic), or has it arisen gradually?
Did the problem start when he started a new medication?
Does the problem occur with his partner only, or does it also occur without his partner,
   for example, with masturbation?
Does the problem occur because he has no partner or an uninterested partner?
Does he have a partner outside of his main relationship?
Can he get an erection? If so, is it firm enough for penetration?
Can he maintain the erection for intercourse?
Does he have a problem with sexual desire?
How long has he lost sexual desire?
Has he lost sexual desire with all partners?
Has he lost desire under all circumstances?
Has he lost desire because he cannot get or maintain an erection?
Has he lost desire because his partner has lost desire?
Does the patient complain of other associated symptoms, such as being tired, loss
   of stamina, loss of strength, loss of muscle mass, loss of muscle tone, recent weight gain,
   fatigue, or sleep issues?
Is the patient depressed?
Does he have a problem with ejaculation?
What type of ejaculation problem does the patient complain of?
When did the problem start?
Is the problem bothersome to the patient?
Is the problem bothersome to the partner?
Does the problem occur under all circumstances?

The Structured Interview on Erectile Dysfunction (SEIDY) is a useful 13-item structured interview, composed of three scales that identify and quantify organic, relational, and intrapsychic domains [47].

A brief side note is provided here. A study by Braun and colleagues [48] highlights another important epidemiologic association. Not only was there a significant prevalence of ED in this survey, but there was a strong association between ED and LUTSs. LUTSs are classic urinary symptoms associated with prostatic enlargement. The study by Braun and colleagues [48] noted that 72% of men with LUTSs had ED, whereas only 38% of those without LUTSs had ED. Recently, Vallancien and colleagues noted that ED and ejaculatory dysfunction (EjD) were common in men with LUTSs in a study of 1274 European men. Interestingly, the ED and EjD were quite bothersome, even in men with advanced age [49]. Thus, over the past several years, there was keen interest in understanding this relation. The vasoconstrictor RHo-kinase was thought to be a common mechanism for ED, EjD, and LUTSs [50]. This concept is still in its infancy.

The physical examination for a man with sexual dysfunction is relatively straightforward and is delineated as follows:

Height, weight, and waist size
Blood pressure
Auscultation of heart and lungs

Check pulses
Examination of breasts, thyroid, and lymph
nodes
Examination of abdomen
Examination of penis for plaques, lesions, and
urethral position
Examination of testis for size, lumps, masses,
and position
Examination of rectum for sphincter tone,
prostate size, masses, lesions, and bulboca-
vernosus reflex
Brief neurologic examination

Box 2 describes the laboratory work that is
suggested and that is optional for the patient.

Treatment of male sexual dysfunction

There are several articles in this issue that deal
specifically with the treatment of male ED.
Treatment includes the use of a phosphodiesterase

**Box 2. Laboratory work for a man
complaining of ED (if not performed
recently)**

Fasting lipid
Fasting glucose
TT and FT (morning testing preferred)
PSA: mandatory if considering
   testosterone supplementation;
   otherwise, it may be optional
Optional laboratory tests
Prolactin
Creatinine
Estradiol
Thyroid-stimulating hormone (TSH)
Follicle-stimulating hormone (FSH)
Luteinizing hormone (LH)
Dehydroepiandrosterone (DHEA)
25-hydroxyvitamin D level
SHBG
Albumin
Many clinicians use the following
   optional questionnaires to query the
   patient about his sexual complaints:
Sexual health inventory for men (IIEF-5,
   SHIM) [51]
CES-D [45]
AUA symptom index [46]
ADAM [52]
SEIDY [47]

---

type 5 inhibitor (PDE5i). These drugs include
sildenafil, vardenafil, and tadalafil. Alternative
options include the medicated system for erections
(MUSE), vacuum erection device (VED) therapy,
and operative insertion of a penile prosthesis. An
important adjunct to success of these therapies is
inclusion of the partner (male or female). Further,
brief psychotherapy is often a crucial adjunct to
successful treatment. Further, if the patient is
deemed to be depressed, referral to the primary
care clinician or psychotherapist is essential to
successful therapy. Box 3 delineates a simple treatment algorithm.

Erectile dysfunction

In the office, most men prefer any of the three
PDE5is [53]. Half-life, duration of activity, erection
hardness [54,55], intercourse satisfaction, number
of intercourse attempts, insurance coverage, and
side effect profile can assist the patient and the clinician in the decision-making process [56].

PDE5is cannot be offered to men taking
nitrates. PDE5is do not seem to be effective for
all men with ED, working in approximately 60%

**Box 3. Therapies for male sexual
dysfunction**

1. ED
   A. Treatment of male ED
      i. Start with oral PDE5i
      ii. Start with VED
      iii. Start with penile intracavernosal
         injections (ICITs)
      iv. Start with MUSE
      v. Consider a penile prosthesis
      vi. Consider combination of oral
         PDE5i with other therapies, such
         as testosterone replacement,
         VED, MUSE, or ICITs
2. Hypogonadism: consider testosterone
   replacement for hypogonadal men.
   Consider aiming for the levels noted
   previously in the text.
3. Referral for psychotherapy for
   depression.
4. Brief counseling for couple's issues.
5. Start oral selective serotonin reuptake
   inhibitor (SSRI) for PE, consider
   adjuvant psychotherapy.

to 70% of men. Further, many men do not remain on oral PDE5i therapy [57]. Thus, alternate first-line therapies include the VED, ICIT of vasoactive agents, and MUSE. These are all reasonable options and have time-honored success in specific patients [58–60]. Penile prosthesis insertion remains a viable second-line option in most cases [61]. Penile prostheses have been available for many years. They have undoubtedly withstood the test of time.

Several concerns have been raised regarding ED therapy, specifically the PDE5is. The two main concerns have centered around cardiovascular morbidity and mortality when using these drugs, whereas an additional concern has centered around nonarteritic anterior ischemic optic neuropathy (NAION). Regarding cardiovascular safety, several articles have been published that demonstrate long-term cardiovascular safety of the PDE5is. There were no cardiovascular signals in any of the populations studied, attesting to the cardiovascular safety of these medications [62,63].

Nonarteritic anterior ischemic optic neuropathy

NAION is the most common acute optic neuropathy among older adults in the United States [64–66]. An estimated 1500 to 6000 people develop NAION annually, of whom 1 in 4 go on to experience NAION in the fellow eye [67–69]. NAION manifests as acute painless monocular vision loss, optic disk edema, and a relative afferent pupillary defect. Presenting visual acuity is worse than 20/64 in approximately 50% of patients and may subsequently improve (in 30%–40% of patients), worsen (in 12%–22% of patients), or remain unchanged (in approximately 45% of patients) [70,71].

There have been several case reports suggesting a link between certain phosphodiesterase inhibitor ED medications (sildenafil and tadalafil) and NAION [72–76]. Visual side effects (eg, light sensitivity, color vision abnormalities) associated with these medications are well documented, but these effects, which have been traced to the fact that phosphodiesterase inhibitors seem to have an inhibitory influence, albeit weak, on enzymatic activity in the rod and cone cells, seem to be transient in nature [77,78]. The mechanism by which these medications might damage the optic nerve is not as well understood, however. It has been theorized that sildenafil, which works through the nitric oxide–cyclic guanosine monophosphate (GMP) pathway, may alter the perfusion of the optic nerve head by modifying nitric oxide levels. Given their similar properties, it can also be theorized that tadalafil might act similarly, although no explicit theories have been proposed.

A retrospective matched case-control study was conducted. Thirty-eight cases of NAION in male patients were identified from an academic ophthalmology practice in Birmingham, Alabama and matched (on age) to 38 controls without a history of NAION. Self-reported information regarding past and current use of sildenafil or tadalafil was obtained by means of a telephone questionnaire from interviewers who were not blinded to case status. Overall, male patients who had NAION were no more likely to report a history of sildenafil or tadalafil use compared with similarly aged controls (OR = 1.75, 95% confidence interval (CI): 0.48–6.30; OR = 1.82, 95% CI: 0.21–15.39). For those with a history of MI, however, a statistically significant association was observed (OR = 10.7, 95% CI: 1.3–95.8). A similar association was observed for those with a history of hypertension, although it lacked statistical significance (OR = 6.9, 95% CI: 0.8–63.6) [79].

In a review of its own database, Pfizer found the following. The incidence of NAION in men receiving sildenafil treatment for ED was estimated using pooled safety data from global clinical trials and European observational studies. Based on clinical trial data in more than 13,000 men and on more than 35,000 patient-years of observation in epidemiologic studies, an incidence of 2.8 cases of NAION per 100,000 patient-years of sildenafil exposure was estimated. This is similar to estimates reported in general US population samples (2.52 and 11.8 cases per 100,000 men aged ≥50 years). The data cited here do not suggest an increased incidence of NAION in men who took sildenafil for ED [80]. Thus, it seems unlikely that sildenafil caused NAION based on the data presented previously.

Summary

First-line treatment of ED can be safely provided by the 3 PDE5is. Reasonable first-line alternates include ICITs, VEPs, and, in certain instances, penile prostheses. Second-line therapies include combinations of these and addition of testosterone to the mix. Data do not suggest that PDE5is increase any aspect of cardiovascular morbidity or mortality, or increase the chances of NAION. PDE5is may not be given to men who are taking nitrates. Testosterone cannot be given to men with prostate or breast cancer. Counseling may be indicated for some men who are clearly psychogenic or depressed. Combined therapy, including the PDE5is plus counseling, may also be indicated for men using a PDE5i when the drug provides them with a good erection but they cannot seem to make use of the PDE5i with a partner.

Hypogonadism

Treatment of hypogonadism with testosterone in the United States is relegated to intramuscular injection of short-acting testosterone, testosterone patches, topical gels, or buccal preparations. All these treatment options are successful in restoring testosterone levels into the therapeutic range [81]. Patient preference, cost, ease of application or administration, and side effects are factors in the choice of therapy. The overriding concern in testosterone replacement has been the safety of testosterone with respect to the prostate [82].

Advocates of an increased risk for prostate cancer in hypogonadal men would recommend a prostate biopsy in hypogonadal men before initiation of testosterone supplementation therapy [83]. A standard monitoring regimen in men receiving testosterone supplementation is not universally accepted [84], however. Nonetheless, it is incumbent on the clinician to develop a standard monitoring regimen that provides adequate monitoring for optimal patient safety. PSA level, a complete blood cell count (CBC), and urinary symptoms are the three areas that have received the most attention for monitoring. Most data continue to support testosterone safety and a lack of development of prostate cancer in men who choose to use testosterone supplementation [85–87].

Recent studies have confirmed the long-held belief that adequate testosterone concentrations are important for sexual function and decreased testosterone concentrations are associated with decreased sexual health [88,89]. Testosterone replacement monotherapy has been shown to improve sexual desire and function in hypogonadal men [88,90], with effects persisting for up to 3 years [91].

To guide clinicians, recent data have emerged that provide goals for testosterone supplementation [88]. Researchers have explored the possibility that there might be a threshold average daily serum testosterone level for sexual response,

meaning a testosterone level at which the sexual response is no different from that of the group of subjects with the lowest serum testosterone level (0–300 ng/dL) as well as a level wherein there was a significant change compared with that of the group of subjects with the lowest serum testosterone level (Fig. 1).

This threshold level seemed to be approximately 400 ng/dL for nighttime erections, 500 ng/dL for sexual intercourse, and 600 ng/dL for sexual desire. In all three parameters, there was no significant difference in sexual function between the group of subjects with the lowest serum testosterone levels (0–300 ng/dL) and the group of subjects with the next highest serum testosterone levels (300–400 ng/dL for nighttime erections, 300–500 ng/dL for sexual intercourse, and 300–600 ng/dL for sexual desire; $P \geq .16$).

There were significant differences between the group of subjects with values greater than the threshold serum testosterone value and the group with the lowest serum testosterone levels (0–300 ng/dL; $P \leq .0028$), however. In addition, there were significant differences between the group of subjects with values greater than the threshold serum testosterone value and the group of subjects with serum testosterone levels between 300 ng/dL and the threshold for sexual desire and intercourse ($P \leq .0098$; see Fig. 1). These results indicate that the response functions for sexual desire and intercourse were relatively flat until the serum testosterone levels were restored to levels greater than the threshold value, whereas the response function for nighttime erections gave an indication of an increased response even with restoration of serum testosterone levels into the low-normal range (300–400 ng/dL).

Testosterone replacement therapy (TRT) given in combination with phosphodiesterase inhibitors is an evolving concept. TRT given in combination with phosphodiesterase inhibitors has been shown in early studies to improve sexual function in androgen-deficient men with suboptimal response to phosphodiesterase inhibitors alone, yielding greater potency, erectile function, orgasmic function, and overall satisfaction [92,93]. This effect may be related to the effects of TRT on endothelial function [94], as described in the preceding section on cardiovascular health. ED has been shown to be associated with biochemical markers of endothelial function and atherosclerosis [11]. In men with ED who take TRT with sildenafil, testosterone levels have been shown to correlate with penile arterial inflow [95]. Different degrees

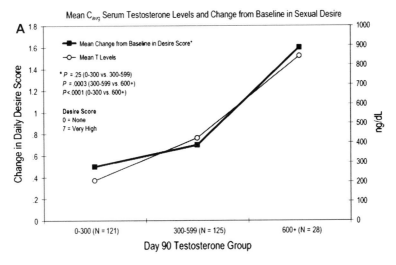

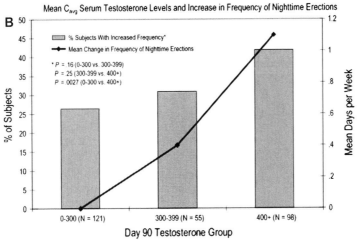

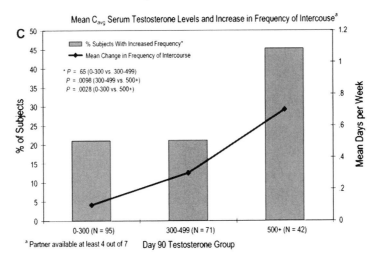

Fig. 1. (*A–C*) Mean change from baseline for daily sexual desire score and mean average concentration (C_{avg}; 0–24 hours) serum testosterone levels (ng/dL); percentage of subjects with increased frequency and mean change in frequency for nighttime erections and intercourse. (*From* Seftel AD, Mack RJ, Secrest AR, et al. Restorative increases in serum testosterone levels are significantly correlated to improvements in sexual functioning. J Androl 2004;25(6):970; with permission.)

of testosterone deficiency may determine a sequence of molecular penile events leading to a reduced capacity of penile smooth muscle relaxation and endothelial cells [96]. Therefore, improvement in hypogonadism might be expected to improve endothelial dysfunction and thereby improve erectile function.

Recent consensus panels have provided guidance regarding testosterone supplementation [33,97]:

1. Testosterone administration is absolutely contraindicated in men suspected of or having carcinoma of the prostate or breast.
2. Men with significant polycythemia, untreated sleep apnea, severe heart failure, severe symptoms of lower urinary tract obstruction as evidenced by high scores in the IPPS score, or clinical findings of bladder outflow obstruction (increased postmicturition residual volume, decreased peak urinary flow, or pathologic pressure flow studies) because of an enlarged clinically benign prostate should not be treated with testosterone. Moderate obstruction represents a partial contraindication. After successful treatment of the obstruction, the contraindication is lifted.
3. In the absence of definite contraindications, age, as such, is not a contraindication to initiate testosterone substitution.
4. Preparations of natural testosterone should be used for substitution therapy. Currently available intramuscular, subdermal, transdermal, oral, and buccal preparations of testosterone are safe and effective. The treating physician should have sufficient knowledge and adequate understanding of the pharmacokinetics and the advantages and drawbacks of each preparation. The selection of the preparation should be a joint decision of the patient and the physician.
5. Because the possible development of a contraindication during treatment (especially prostate carcinoma) requires rapid discontinuation of testosterone substitution, short-acting (transdermal, oral, or buccal) preparations are preferred over long-acting (intramuscular or subdermal) depot preparations in patients who have LOH.

Reassurance regarding testosterone supplementation in older men was recently documented by Marks and colleagues [98]. They determined the effects of TRT on prostate tissue of aging men with low serum testosterone levels. The trial was a randomized, double-blind, placebo-controlled trial of 44 men aged 44 to 78 years with screening serum testosterone levels lower than 300 ng/dL (<10.4 nmol/L) and related symptoms, which was conducted at a US community-based research center between February 2003 and November 2004. Participants were randomly assigned to receive testosterone enanthate at a dose of 150 mg or matching placebo intramuscularly every 2 weeks for 6 months. Of the 44 men randomized, 40 had prostate biopsies performed at baseline and at 6 months and qualified for per-protocol analysis (TRT, n = 21; placebo, n = 19). TRT increased serum testosterone levels to the midnormal range (median at baseline = 282 ng/dL [9.8 nmol/L]; median at 6 months = 640 ng/dL [22.2 nmol/L]), with no significant change in serum testosterone levels in matched placebo-treated men. Median prostate tissue levels of testosterone (0.91 ng/g) and dihydrotestosterone (6.79 ng/g) did not change significantly in the TRT group, however. No treatment-related change was observed in prostate histology, tissue biomarkers (androgen receptor, Ki-67, and CD34), gene expression (including AR, PSA, PAP2A, VEGF, NXK3, and CLU [Clusterin]), or cancer incidence or severity. Treatment-related changes in prostate volume, serum PSA, voiding symptoms, and urinary flow were minor. These preliminary data suggest that in aging men with LOH, 6 months of TRT normalizes serum androgen levels but seems to have little effect on prostate tissue androgen levels and cellular functions. Establishment of prostate safety for large populations of older men undergoing a longer duration of TRT requires further study [98].

Summary

Testosterone supplementation should be viewed with caution. The diagnosis of hypogonadism is controversial, and an undercurrent of concern remains, as evidenced by statements from the FDA. The diagnosis should be based on a low serum testosterone level, combined with some symptom complex suggestive and supportive of hypogonadism. Once the patient has agreed to start testosterone therapy, a planned program of monitoring should be started and adhered to. If testosterone supplementation is not deemed effective after a reasonable time, it would seem reasonable to reconsider the need for the testosterone therapy. The goal of testosterone supplementation should be to restore the testosterone to therapeutic levels. For guidance, data suggest that threshold levels seem to be approximately

400 ng/dL for nighttime erections, 500 ng/dL for sexual intercourse, and 600 ng/dL for sexual desire. Intramuscular testosterone injections usually are given at 2- to 3-week intervals at a rate of 100 to 200 mg per dose. Intramuscular testosterone has a slightly higher risk for polycythemia than do the patches or gels, because there may be a higher testosterone level achieved with intramuscularly administered testosterone than with patches or gels. Testosterone patches, testosterone gels, and buccal preparations are reasonable first-line choices for testosterone supplementation. Testosterone patches are applied daily. Approximately 5% to 10% of patients experience a rash at the site of application. A significant number of patients also need more than one patch to notice a perceivable therapeutic benefit. Because of twice-daily dosing, buccal preparations have fallen into disfavor. With respect to testosterone gels, Androgel and Testim have demonstrated long-term safety and efficacy records. Immediate side effects are limited to the site of application, in that 1% of patients experience a rash at the application site. If the patient does not perceive a subjective response to one packet of either of these products, he may move to two gel applications per day. Once there is a dose adjustment, monitoring should be vigorous to assess the change and assess any potential side effects [99,100]. An increase in the serum PSA beyond normally anticipated levels should signal the need to stop the testosterone supplementation and possibly perform a prostate biopsy. If using the gels, patients should be cautious about person-to person contact for a few hours after application, because the testosterone may be transferred to a partner or to a child. In younger men, the clinician should caution the patient that testosterone supplementation can lead to azoospermia. The azoospermia is usually reversible on cessation of the testosterone supplementation. If the CBC becomes an issue, it reasonable to stop the testosterone supplementation and readjust the dosing regimen. On occasion, phlebotomy may be necessary to control the CBC abnormalities. A low serum testosterone level might suggest the need to check a serum prolactin level. If the serum prolactin is elevated, one might consider pituitary MRI to look for a mass.

Premature ejaculation

There is no currently FDA-approved treatment for PE. Most clinicians commence therapy with an oral SSRI. These drugs can be used on an as-needed basis, taken a few hours before planned intercourse, or on a daily basis. Recent data suggest that men prefer the daily regimen [101]. In a small study of 88 men who had PE and were naive to treatment, with an average age of 37 ± 11 years (mean $\pm$ SD), 71 men (81%) preferred a drug for daily use, 14 men (16%) preferred a drug on demand, and 3 men preferred topical anesthetic cream. The most frequently reported argument for preferring daily drug treatment was that this strategy would have the least effect with regard to the spontaneity of having sex.

The choice of SSRI to use for PE treatment remains unclear. Dapoxetine has been proposed for FDA approval for PE. This drug did not receive an approvable letter from the FDA [102], however. Thus, the choice SSRI for use remains an off-label choice.

In a study of 154 men with PE, 127 (81%) of 157 subjects experienced a significant increase in their Arabic Index of Premature Ejaculation (AIPE) total score after sertraline treatment. Sixty-six (66%) of 100 patients available for follow-up experienced relapse of PE within 6 months after sertraline withdrawal. The active drug was generally well tolerated. Our relatively large study, using a validated questionnaire (AIPE), confirmed the useful effect of sertraline on PE [103].

It is important to note that the FDA has issued a "black-box" warning for SSRI drugs with respect to suicide. This warning can be viewed on-line [104].

This is the language that is used by the US Food and Drug Administration

Suicidality and antidepressant drugs

Compared with placebo, antidepressants increased the risk for suicidal thinking and behavior (suicidality) in children, adolescents, and young adults in short-term studies of major depressive disorder (MDD) and other psychiatric disorders. Anyone considering the use of any antidepressant in a child, adolescent, or young adult must balance this risk with the clinical need. Short-term studies did not show an increase in the risk for suicidality with antidepressants compared with placebo in adults older than 24 years; there was a reduction in risk with antidepressants compared with placebo in adults aged 65 years and older. Depression and certain other psychiatric disorders are themselves associated with increases in the risk for suicide. Patients of all ages who are started on antidepressant therapy should be monitored appropriately and observed closely for clinical worsening, suicidality, or unusual changes in behavior. Families and caregivers should be advised of the need for close observation and communication with the prescriber. Fluoxetine hydrochloride is approved for use in pediatric patients who have MDD and obsessive compulsive disorder (OCD). Sertraline hydrochloride is not approved for use in pediatric patients, except for patients who have OCD. Fluvoxamine is not approved for use in pediatric patients, except for patients who have OCD.

Topical anesthetic spray and cream therapy, such as the topical eutectic mixture for premature ejaculation (TEMPE), for PE is under study [105]. In a small study of men with PE, 35 (83%) of 42 patients considered the spray easy to use. Mild to moderate local numbness occurred in 3 (12%) of the TEMPE-treated patients but did not lead to discontinuation. Topical treatment with TEMPE produced a statistically and clinically significant increase in IELT compared with placebo and resulted in positive trends in ejaculatory control and quality of life. TEMPE was considered easy to use and was well tolerated. The data support the conduct of further large-scale studies to establish the utility of TEMPE as a first-line treatment for PE.

Lidocaine cream and a variety of other agents have been used for PE with limited success [106].

Summary

The prevalence of PE and the definition are evolving. To date, most authorities allow for an extravaginal or intravaginal latency of ejaculation of 1 to 2 minutes to define PE. Oral therapies remain off-label choices, and the recent black-box warning for SSRIs mandates a thoughtful approach to PE treatment. Data suggest that most men prefer a daily oral tablet and not an as-needed pill. Topical creams and aerosols remain in an investigational stage.

Clinical pearls

Most men with ED or hypogonadism present somewhere between the ages of 35 and 65 years. Although most men presenting with ED have organic disease, the possibility of psychogenic ED must be remembered. A significant minority of men with ED in this age group have psychogenic ED. Psychogenic ED can be successfully treated with short-term PDE5i therapy combined with counseling [107].

The contribution of the partner in the etiology of ED and the role of the partner in the ED treatment plan cannot be overemphasized. This point needs to be borne in mind when seeing a patient who has ED. Further, it is well established that inclusion of the partner in the ED evaluation and treatment process improves outcome. Inclusion of the partner is challenging but can be quite rewarding if successful [108].

Questionnaires for the diagnosis of PE and other ejaculatory disorders exist but have not found their way into the mainstream of evaluation and treatment of PE or other ejaculatory disorders [109–111].

Young men in unconsummated marriages who have "ED" can be managed with PDE5is [112].

Adolescents presenting with ED are a new and challenging group to evaluate and treat. Usually, these young men, aged 13 to 18 years, present for an ED evaluation accompanied by a concerned parent. The utmost of care and compassion must be used in these cases, because these young men may have sexual concerns beyond ED that are specific to their age group.

Psychotherapy has been mentioned as adjuvant therapy for men with sexual dysfunction. Psychotherapy is helpful for men with ED, for men with PE, and possibly for men with hypogonadism who have a mild degree of depression [107,113].

With respect to depression, various degrees of depression are associated with male sexual dysfunction. ED, PE, and hypogonadism are all associated with some degree of depression [9,99,114]. Please refer to the articles by Segraves, Neiderberger and colleagues in this issue that deal with several of these issues. Suffice it to say that it is prudent to screen for depression when men present for a sexual medicine evaluation.

Overall summary

Male sexual health, now an office evaluation, requires a thorough understanding of the implications of ED, hypogonadism, and PE. It is hoped that the data presented here can guide the clinician and allow for successful evaluation and management of the patient.

References

[1] Krane RJ, Goldstein I. Saenz de Tejada I. Impotence. N Engl J Med 1989;321:1648–59.

[2] Rosen RC, Leiblum SR. Erectile disorders: an overview of historical trends and clinical perspectives. In: Rosen RC, Leiblum SR, editors. Erectile disorders: assessment and treatment. New York: Guilford; 1992. p. 3–26.

[3] NIH Consensus Conference. Impotence. NIH Consensus Development Panel on Impotence. JAMA 1993;270(1):83–90.

[4] Feldman HA, Goldstein I, Hatzichristou DG, et al. Impotence and its medical and psychosocial correlates: results of the Massachusetts Male Aging Study. J Urol 1994;151(1):54–61.

[5] Laumann E, Paik A, Rosen RC. Sexual dysfunction in the United States: prevalence and predictors. JAMA 1999;281(6):537–44.

[6] Masumori N, Tsukamoto T, Kumamoto Y, et al. Decline of sexual function with age in Japanese men compared with American men—results of two community-based studies. Urology 1999;54: 335–44.

[7] Marumo K, Nakashima J, Murai M. Age-related prevalence of erectile dysfunction in Japan: assessment by the International Index of Erectile Function. Int J Urol 2001;8(2):53–9.

[8] Saigal CS, Wessels H, Pace J, et al. Predictors and prevalence of erectile dysfunction in a racially diverse population. Arch Intern Med 2006;166: 207–12.

[9] Seftel AD, Sun P. Swindle R. The prevalence of hypertension, hyperlipidemia, diabetes mellitus and depression in men with erectile dysfunction. J Urol 2004;171(6 Pt 1):2341–5.

[10] Esposito K, Giugliano F, Di Palo C, et al. Effect of lifestyle changes on erectile dysfunction in obese men: a randomized controlled trial. JAMA 2004; 291(24):2978–84.

[11] Eaton CB, Liu YL, Mittleman MA, et al. A retrospective study of the relationship between biomarkers of atherosclerosis and erectile dysfunction in 988 men. Int J Impot Res 2007;19(2):218–25.

[12] Min JK, Williams KA, Okwuosa TM, et al. Prediction of coronary heart disease by erectile dysfunction in men referred for nuclear stress testing. Arch Intern Med 2006;166:201–6.

[13] Grover SA, Lowensteyn I, Kaouache M, et al. The prevalence of erectile dysfunction in the primary care setting. Arch Intern Med 2006;166:213–9.

[14] Thompson IM, Tangen CM, Goodman PJ, et al. Erectile dysfunction and subsequent cardiovascular disease. JAMA 2005;294(23):2996–3002.

[15] Montorsi P, Ravagnani PM, Galli S, et al. Association between erectile dysfunction and coronary artery disease. Role of coronary clinical presentation and extent of coronary vessels involvement: the COBRA trial. Eur Heart J 2006;27(22):2632–9.

[16] Kostis JB, Jackson G, Rosen R, et al. Sexual dysfunction and cardiac risk (the Second Princeton Consensus Conference). Am J Cardiol 2005;96(2): 313–21.

[17] Laumann EO, Nicolosi A, Glasser DB, et al. Sexual problems among women and men aged 40–80 y: prevalence and correlates identified in the global study of sexual attitudes and behaviors. Int J Impot Res 2005;17:39–57.

[18] de Boer BJ, Bots ML, Lycklama a Nijeholt AA, et al. The prevalence of bother, acceptance, and need for help in men with erectile dysfunction. J Sex Med 2005;2:445–50.

[19] Korenman SG. New insights into erectile dysfunction: a practical approach. Am J Med 1998;105: 135–44.

[20] Fugl-Meyer AR, Lodnert G, Branholm IB, et al. On life satisfaction in male erectile dysfunction. Int J Impot Res 1997;9:141–8.

[21] Rosen RC. Quality of life assessment in sexual dysfunction trials. Int J Impot Res 1998;10:S21–3.

[22] Gades NM, Nehra A, Jacobson DJ, et al. Association between smoking and erectile dysfunction: a population-based study. Am J Epidemiol 2005; 161(4):346–51.

[23] Bacon CG, Mittleman MA, Kawachi I, et al. A prospective study of risk factors for erectile dysfunction. J Urol 2006;176(1):217–21.

[24] Hatzichristou D, Rosen RC, Broderick G, et al. Clinical evaluation and management strategy for sexual dysfunction in men and women. J Sex Med 2004;1(1):49–57.

[25] Mulligan T, Frick MF, Zuraw QC, et al. Prevalence of hypogonadism in males aged at least 45 years: the HIM study. Int J Clin Pract 2006;60(7):762–9.

[26] Seftel AD. Male hypogonadism. Part I: epidemiology of hypogonadism. Int J Impot Res 2006;18(2): 115–20.

[27] Rhoden EL, Morgentaler A. Risks of testosterone-replacement therapy and recommendations for monitoring. N Engl J Med 2004;350:482–92.

[28] Harman SM, Metter EJ, Tobin JD, et al. Longitudinal effects of aging on serum total and free testosterone levels in healthy men. Baltimore Longitudinal Study of Aging. J Clin Endocrinol Metab 2001;86:724–31.

[29] Morley JE, Kaiser FE, Perry HM III, et al. Longitudinal changes in testosterone, luteinizing hormone, and follicle-stimulating hormone in healthy older men. Metabolism 1997;46:410–3.

[30] Snyder PJ. Effects of age on testicular function and consequences of testosterone treatment. J Clin Endocrinol Metab 2001;86:2369–72.

[31] Vermeulen A. Androgen replacement therapy in the aging male: a critical evaluation. J Clin Endocrinol Metab 2001;86:2380–90.

[32] Bremner WJ, Vitiello MV, Prinz PN. Loss of circadian rhythmicity in blood testosterone levels with aging in normal men. J Clin Endocrinol Metab 1983;56:1278–81.

[33] Bhasin S, Cunningham GR, Hayes F, et al. Testosterone therapy in adult men with androgen deficiency syndromes: an Endocrine Society clinical

practice guideline. J Clin Endocrinol Metab 2006; 91:1995–2010.

[34] Shames D, Gassman A, Handelsman H. Commentary: guideline for male testosterone therapy: a regulatory perspective. J Clin Endocrinol Metab 2007; 92(2):414–5.

[35] Svartberg J. Epidemiology: testosterone and the metabolic syndrome. Int J Impot Res 2007;19(2): 124–8.

[36] Carson C, Gunn K. Premature ejaculation: definition and prevalence. Int J Impot Res 2006;18(Suppl 1):S5–13.

[37] Segraves RT. Rapid ejaculation: a review of nosology, prevalence and treatment. Int J Impot Res 2006;18(Suppl 1):S24–32.

[38] Fugl-Meyer AR, Sjogren K, Fugl-Meyer KS. Sexual disabilities, problems, and satisfaction in 18–74 year old Swedes. Scand J Sexol 1999;3: 79–105.

[39] American Psychiatric Association. Diagnostic and statistical manual of mental disorders. 4th edition. Text revision (DSM-IV-TR). Washington, DC: American Psychiatric Association; 2000.

[40] Patrick DL, Althof SE, Pryor JL, et al. Premature ejaculation: an observational study of men and their partners. J Sex Med 2005;2(3):358–67.

[41] Waldinger MD, Schweitzer DH. Changing paradigms from an historical DSM-III and DSM-IV view towards an evidence based definition of premature ejaculation. Part II: proposals for DSM-V and ICD-11. J Sex Med 2006;3:693–705.

[42] Waldinger MD. Emerging drugs for premature ejaculation. Expert Opin Emerg Drugs 2006; 11(1):99–109.

[43] Rosen RC, Cappelleri JC, Smith MD, et al. Development and evaluation of an abridged, 5-item version of the International Index of Erectile Function (IIEF-5) as a diagnostic tool for erectile dysfunction. Int J Impot Res 1999;11(6):319–26.

[44] Morley JE, Charlton E, Patrick P, et al. Androgen deficiency in aging males (ADAM): validation of a screening questionnaire for androgen deficiency in aging males. Metabolism 2000;49(9):1239–42.

[45] Weissman MM, Sholomskas D, Pottenger M, et al. Assessing depressive symptoms in five psychiatric populations: a validation study. Am J Epidemiol 1977;106(3):203–14.

[46] Nitti VW, Kim Y, Combs AJ. Correlation of the AUA symptom index with urodynamics in patients with suspected benign prostatic hyperplasia. Neurourol Urodyn 1994;13(5):521–7 [discussion 527–9].

[47] Corona G, Mannucci E, Petrone L, et al. Psychobiological correlates of free-floating anxiety symptoms in male patients with sexual dysfunctions. J Androl 2006;27(1):86–93.

[48] Braun M, Wassmer G, Klotz T, et al. Epidemiology of erectile dysfunction: results of the 'Cologne Male Survey'. Int J Impot Res 2000;12:305.

[49] van Moorselaar RJ, Hartung R, Emberton M, et al. ALF-ONE Study Group. Alfuzosin 10 mg once daily improves sexual function in men with lower urinary tract symptoms and concomitant sexual dysfunction. BJU Int 2005;95(4):603–8.

[50] Rees RW, Foxwell NA, Ralph DJ, et al. Y-27632, a Rho-kinase inhibitor, inhibits proliferation and adrenergic contraction of prostatic smooth muscle cells. J Urol 2003;170(6 Pt 1):2517–22.

[51] Cappelleri JC, Rosen RC. The Sexual Health Inventory for Men (SHIM): a 5-year review of research and clinical experience. Int J Impot Res 2005;17(4):307–19.

[52] Morley JE, Charlton E, Patrick P, et al. Validation of a screening questionnaire for androgen deficiency in aging males. Metab Clin Exp 2000;49(9): 1239–42.

[53] Martin-Morales A, Haro JM, Beardsworth A, et al. EDOS Group. Therapeutic effectiveness and patient satisfaction after 6 months of treatment with tadalafil, sildenafil, and vardenafil: results from the Erectile Dysfunction Observational Study (EDOS). Eur Urol 2007;51(2):541–50.

[54] Lowy M, Collins S, Bloch M, et al. Quality of erection questionnaire correlates: change in erection quality with erectile function, hardness, and psychosocial measures in men treated with sildenafil for erectile dysfunction. J Sex Med 2007;4(1):83–92.

[55] Padma-Nathan H. Sildenafil citrate (Viagra) treatment for erectile dysfunction: an updated profile of response and effectiveness. Int J Impot Res 2006; 18(5):423–31.

[56] Eardley I, Montorsi F, Jackson G, et al. Factors associated with preference for sildenafil citrate and tadalafil for treating erectile dysfunction in men naive to phosphodiesterase 5 inhibitor therapy: post hoc analysis of data from a multicentre, randomized, open-label, crossover study. BJU Int 2007; 100(1):122–9.

[57] Seftel AD. Challenges in oral therapy for erectile dysfunction. J Androl 2002;23(6):729–36.

[58] Levine SB, Althof SE, Turner LA, et al. Side effects of self-administration of intracavernous papaverine and phentolamine for the treatment of impotence. J Urol 1989;141(1):54–7.

[59] Turner LA, Althof SE, Levine SB, et al. External vacuum devices in the treatment of erectile dysfunction: a one-year study of sexual and psychosocial impact. J Sex Marital Ther 1991;17(2):81–93.

[60] Padma-Nathan H, Hellstrom WJ, Kaiser FE, et al. Treatment of men with erectile dysfunction with transurethral alprostadil. Medicated Urethral System for Erection (MUSE) Study Group. N Engl J Med 1997;336(1):1–7.

[61] Sadeghi-Nejad H. Penile prosthesis surgery: a review of prosthetic devices and associated complications. J Sex Med 2007;4(2):296–309.

[62] Jackson G, Montorsi P, Cheitlin MD. Cardiovascular safety of sildenafil citrate (Viagra): an

updated perspective. Urology 2006;68(Suppl 3): 47–60.

[63] Kloner RA, Jackson G, Hutter AM, et al. Cardiovascular safety update of tadalafil: retrospective analysis of data from placebo-controlled and open-label clinical trials of tadalafil with as needed, three times-per-week or once-a-day dosing. Am J Cardiol 2006;97(12):1778–84.

[64] Hayreh SS. Anterior ischemic optic neuropathy. New York: Springer Verlag; 1975.

[65] Hayreh SS. Anterior ischemic optic neuropathy. Arch Neurol 1981;38:675–8.

[66] Hayreh SS. Anterior ischemic optic neuropathy: differentiation of arteritic from non-arteritic type and its management. Eye 1990;4:25–41.

[67] Johnson LN, Arnold AC. Incidence of non-arteritic anterior ischemic optic neuropathy: population based study in the state of Missouri and Los Angeles County, California. J Neuroophthalmol 1994;14:38–44.

[68] Ischemic Optic Neuropathy Decompression Trial (IONDT) Research Group. Manual of operations. Baltimore: University of Maryland at Baltimore, 1992;1:1–2.

[69] Hattenhauser MG, Leavitt JA, Hodge DO, et al. Incidence of nonarteritic anterior ischemic optic neuropathy. Am J Ophthalmol 1997;123:103–7.

[70] Buono LM, Foroozan R, Sergott RC, et al. Nonarteritic anterior ischemic optic neuropathy. Curr Opin Ophthalmol 2002;13:357–61.

[71] Rucker JC, Biousse V, Newman NJ. Ischemic optic neuropathies. Curr Opin Neurol 2004;17:27–35.

[72] Cunningham AV, Smith KH. Anterior ischemic optic neuropathy associated with Viagra. J Neuroophthalmol 2001;21:22–5.

[73] Egan RA, Pomeranz HD. Sildenafil (Viagra) associated anterior ischemic optic neuropathy. Arch Ophthalmol 2000;118:291–2.

[74] Pomeranz HD, Smith KH, Hart WM, et al. Sildenafil-associated nonarteritic anterior ischemic optic neuropathy. Ophthalmology 2002;109:584–7.

[75] Pomeranz HD, Bhavsar AR. Nonarteritic ischemic optic neuropathy developing soon after use of sildenafil (Viagra): a report of seven new cases. J Neuroophthalmol 2005;25:9–13.

[76] Escaravage GK, Wright JD, Givre SJ. Tadalafil associated with anterior ischemic optic neuropathy. Arch Ophthalmol 2005;123:399–400.

[77] Laties AM, Zrenner E. Viagra (sildenafil citrate) and ophthalmology. Prog Retin Eye Res 2002;21: 485–506.

[78] Marmor MF, Kessler R. Sildenafil (Viagra) and ophthalmology. Surv Ophthalmol 1999;44:153–62.

[79] McGwin G, Vaphiades MS, Hall TA, et al. Non-arteritic anterior ischaemic optic neuropathy and the treatment of erectile dysfunction. Br J Ophthalmol 2006;90(2):154–7.

[80] Gorkin L, Hvidsten K, Sobel RE, et al. Sildenafil citrate use and the incidence of nonarteritic anterior ischemic optic neuropathy. Int J Clin Pract 2006; 60(4):500–3.

[81] Miner MM, Sadovsky R. Evolving issues in male hypogonadism: evaluation, management, and related comorbidities. Cleve Clin J Med 2007; 74(Suppl 3):S38–46.

[82] Miner MM, Seftel AD. Testosterone and ageing: what have we learned since the Institute of Medicine report and what lies ahead? Int J Clin Pract 2007;61(4):622–32.

[83] Morgentaler A, Rhoden EL. Prevalence of prostate cancer among hypogonadal men with prostate-specific antigen levels of 4.0 ng/mL or less. Urology 2006;68(6):1263–7.

[84] Morales A. Monitoring androgen replacement therapy: testosterone and prostate safety. J Endocrinol Invest 2005;28(Suppl 3):122–7.

[85] Wiren S, Stocks T, Rinaldi S, et al. Androgens and prostate cancer risk: a prospective study. Prostate 2007;67(11):1230–7.

[86] Travis RC, Key TJ, Allen NE, et al. Serum androgens and prostate cancer among 643 cases and 643 controls in the European Prospective Investigation into Cancer and Nutrition. Int J Cancer 2007; 121(6):1331–8.

[87] Gann PH, Hennekens CH, Ma J, et al. Prospective study of sex hormone levels and risk of prostate cancer. J Natl Cancer Inst 1996;88(16):1118–26.

[88] Seftel AD, Mack RJ, Secrest AR, et al. Restorative increases in serum testosterone levels are significantly correlated to improvements in sexual functioning. J Androl 2004;25:963–72.

[89] Barqawi A, O'Donnell C, Kumar R, et al. Correlation between LUTS (AUA-SS) and erectile dysfunction (SHIM) in an age-matched racially diverse population: data from the Prostate Cancer Awareness Week (PCAW). Int J Impot Res 2005; 17:370–4.

[90] Gray PB, Singh AB, Woodhouse LJ, et al. Dose-dependent effects of testosterone on sexual function, mood, and visuospatial cognition in older men. J Clin Endocrinol Metab 2005;90:3838–46.

[91] Wang C, Cunningham G, Dobs A, et al. Long-term testosterone gel (AndroGel) treatment maintains beneficial effects on sexual function and mood, lean and fat mass, and bone mineral density in hypogonadal men. J Clin Endocrinol Metab 2004; 89:2085–98.

[92] Rosenthal BD, May NR, Metro MJ, et al. Adjunctive use of AndroGel (testosterone gel) with sildenafil to treat erectile dysfunction in men with acquired androgen deficiency syndrome after failure using sildenafil alone. Urology 2006;67: 571–4.

[93] Shabsigh R, Kaufman JM, Steidle C, et al. Randomized study of testosterone gel as adjunctive therapy to sildenafil in hypogonadal men with erectile dysfunction who do not respond to sildenafil alone. J Urol 2004;172:658–63.

[94] Bocchio M, Desideri G, Scarpelli P, et al. Endothelial cell activation in men with erectile dysfunction without cardiovascular risk factors and overt vascular damage. J Urol 2004;171:1601–4.

[95] Aversa A, Isodori AM, Spera G, et al. Androgens improve cavernous vasodilation and response to sildenafil in patients with erectile dysfunction. Clin Endocrinol (Oxf) 2003;58:632–8.

[96] Aversa A, Isidori AM, Greco EA, et al. Hormonal supplementation and erectile dysfunction. Eur Urol 2004;45:535–8.

[97] Nieschlag E, Swerdloff R, Behre HM, et al. Investigation, treatment, and monitoring of late-onset hypogonadism in males: ISA, ISSAM, and EAU recommendations. J Androl 2006;27(2):135–7.

[98] Marks LS, Mazer NA, Mostaghel E, et al. Effect of testosterone replacement therapy on prostate tissue in men with late-onset hypogonadism: a randomized controlled trial. JAMA 2006;296(19):2351–61.

[99] Seftel A. Male hypogonadism. Part II: etiology, pathophysiology, and diagnosis. Int J Impot Res 2006;18(3):223–8.

[100] Seftel A. Testosterone replacement therapy for male hypogonadism: part III. Pharmacologic and clinical profiles, monitoring, safety issues, and potential future agents. Int J Impot Res 2007;19(1): 2–24.

[101] Waldinger MD, Zwinderman AH, Olivier B, et al. The majority of men with lifelong premature ejaculation prefer daily drug treatment: an observation study in a consecutive group of Dutch men. J Sex Med 2007;4(4i):1028–37.

[102] Pryor JL, Althof SE, Steidle C, et al. Dapoxetine Study Group. Efficacy and tolerability of dapoxetine in treatment of premature ejaculation: an integrated analysis of two double-blind, randomised controlled trials. Lancet 2006;368(9539):929–37.

[103] Arafa M, Shamloul R. Efficacy of sertraline hydrochloride in treatment of premature ejaculation: a placebo-controlled study using a validated questionnaire. Int J Impot Res 2006;18(6):534–8.

[104] Available at: http://www.fda.gov/cder/drug/antide pressants/antidepressants_label_change_2007.pdf. Accessed October 18, 2007.

[105] Dinsmore WW, Hackett G, Goldmeier D, et al. Topical eutectic mixture for premature ejaculation (TEMPE): a novel aerosol-delivery form of lidocaine-prilocaine for treating premature ejaculation. BJU Int 2007;99(2):369–75.

[106] Morales A, Barada J, Wyllie MG. A review of the current status of topical treatments for premature ejaculation. BJU Int 2007;100(3):493–501.

[107] Banner LL, Anderson RU. Integrated sildenafil and cognitive-behavior sex therapy for psychogenic erectile dysfunction: a pilot study. J Sex Med 2007; 4(4 Pt 2):1117–25.

[108] Althof SE. When an erection alone is not enough: biopsychosocial obstacles to lovemaking. Int J Impot Res 2002;14(Suppl 1):S99–104.

[109] Althof S, Rosen R, Symonds T, et al. Development and validation of a new questionnaire to assess sexual satisfaction, control, and distress associated with premature ejaculation. J Sex Med 2006;3(3): 465–75.

[110] Symonds T, Perelman M, Althof S, et al. Further evidence of the reliability and validity of the premature ejaculation diagnostic tool. Int J Impot Res 2007;19(5):521–5.

[111] Rosen RC, Catania JA, Althof SE, et al. Development and validation of four-item version of Male Sexual Health Questionnaire to assess ejaculatory dysfunction. Urology 2007;69(5):805–9.

[112] Ghanem H, Zaazaa A, Kamel I, et al. Short-term use of sildenafil in the treatment of unconsummated marriages. Int J Impot Res 2006;18(1):52–4.

[113] Althof SE, Weider M. Psychotherapy for erectile dysfunction: more relevant than ever. Endocrine 2004;23(2–3):131–4.

[114] Sato Y, Tanda H, Kato S, et al. Prevalence of major depressive disorder in self-referred patients in a late onset hypogonadism clinic. Int J Impot Res 2007; 19(4):407–10.

ELSEVIER
SAUNDERS

Urol Clin N Am 34 (2007) 483–496

UROLOGIC
CLINICS
of North America

Centrally Acting Mechanisms for the Treatment of Male Sexual Dysfunction

Martin M. Miner, MD[a],*, Allen D. Seftel, MD[b]

[a]Division of Biology and Medicine, Department of Family Medicine, Warren Alpert Medical School of Brown University, Providence, RI, USA
[b]Department of Urology, University Hospitals School of Medicine, Case Western Reserve University, Cleveland, OH, USA

The development of pharmacologic therapy for erectile dysfunction (ED) has been possible because of incremental growth in our understanding of the physiology of normal erections and the complex pathophysiology of ED. Although the oral phosphodiesterase type 5 (PDE5) inhibitors have provided safe, effective treatment of ED for some men, a large proportion of men who have ED do not respond to PDE5 inhibitors or become less responsive or less satisfied as the duration of therapy increases. Also, men who are receiving organic nitrates and nitrates, such as amyl nitrate, cannot take PDE5 inhibitors because of nitrate interactions. The current options for treatment beyond PDE5 inhibitors are invasive, unappealing to some patients, and sometimes ineffective. Search for other options by which ED can be treated has branched out and now encompasses centrally acting mechanisms that control erectile function. Drugs available in Europe include apomorphine. This article focuses on the mechanism of centrally acting agents and reviews clinical data on potential new centrally acting drugs for men who have ED. For the purposes of this discussion, the definition of ED is that issued at the National Institutes of Health Consensus Development Conference on Impotence in 1992: "the

inability to achieve and/or maintain an erection sufficient for satisfactory sexual performance [1]."

Erectile dysfunction: epidemiology and current treatments

Epidemiology

As many as 20 million Americans may have ED [2]. In the National Health and Social Life Survey, a demographically representative, probability sample study that included 1410 men aged 18 to 59 years, nearly one third (31%) reported some form of sexual dysfunction. The three most common sexual disorders reported in this male cohort were hypogonadism (5% of the total), ED (5%), and premature ejaculation (21%) [3]. The Massachusetts Male Aging Study (MMAS) was a random sample observation study conducted over a 2-year period in and around Boston among community-dwelling men aged 40 to 70 years. Investigators found that of the variables examined, age was the one associated most strongly with ED. Overall, the prevalence of ED in the MMAS cohort was 52%. The prevalence of complete (total) ED increased from 5.1% among 40-year-old subjects to 15% among those aged 70 years. The prevalence of moderate ED increased from 17% to 34% in the same age groups, and the prevalence of mild ED was 17% in all age groups. Only one third of 70-year-old subjects reported experiencing no ED [4]. The robust association between age and increasing risk for ED has been confirmed by several other studies [2].

Several groups of investigators have attempted to determine whether age per se increases the risk

This work was supported by a grant from Palatin Technologies, Inc. and King Pharmaceuticals, Inc.

* Corresponding author. Department of Family Medicine, Brown University School of Medicine, Swansea Family Practice, 479 Swansea Mall Drive, Swansea, MA 02777.

E-mail address: martin_miner@brown.edu (M.M. Miner).

for ED or whether other factors also come into play. In the MMAS, the risk for ED was correlated significantly with higher incidence among men who had diabetes, heart disease, and hypertension and the use of the associated medications, as well as with measures of anger and depression, even after controlling for age. ED risk correlated inversely with high-density lipoprotein cholesterol level and serum dehydroepiandrosterone. Among men who had heart disease and hypertension, cigarette smoking increased the risk for complete ED [4].

The strong association between ED and age is not explained fully. The fundamental structure and function of the penis may change with age in ways that diminish erectile function or the common concomitant illnesses that increase in incidence with advancing age may be at fault. It is likely that age and comorbid illnesses contribute to ED. In a study conducted among 225 men at a general medical clinic, ED was reported by 26% of men younger than 65 years, by 27% of those aged 65 to 75 years, and by 50% of those aged 75 years and older. Logistic regression revealed that overall sexual dysfunction was related significantly to subjective poor health, diabetes, and incontinence while controlling for age. These investigators concluded that sexual dysfunction is more common in older men, but often is related more strongly to comorbid illness than to aging [5].

ED also is associated strongly with lower urinary tract symptoms (LUTS), which can be associated with prostatic enlargement. In a study conducted in Cologne, Germany that involved nearly 4500 survey respondents, 72% of men who had LUTS also reported ED [6]. Conversely, LUTS occurred in only 38% of men who did not have ED. The nature of the relationship between ED and LUTS remains unclear. In the Multinational Study of the Aging Male, LUTS was an independent predictor of sexual dysfunction other than age, and 49% of 12,815 men experienced ED, and 46% of 11,114 men experienced ejaculatory dysfunction [7].

Current treatments

The American Urological Association (AUA) guidelines for the management of ED stipulate that in a patient who has ED, any organic comorbidities and psychosexual dysfunctions should be identified and treated [8]. In particular, ED and cardiovascular disease (CVD) may share some etiologic factors, and many men have ED

and CVD. The Princeton Consensus Panel developed guidelines for the management of ED in patients who have CVD, noting that most patients who have ED are at low risk for a cardiovascular event during sex. Examples include men who have controlled hypertension or uncomplicated past myocardial infarction, who can be treated safely for ED. Men of indeterminate or high risk for CVD should be assessed or treated as necessary before ED treatment is initiated [9]. Accumulating evidence shows that changes in lifestyle, especially weight loss and increased physical activity, can improve erectile function [10]. The Princeton Consensus Panel places a special emphasis on these recommendations in men seeking help for ED [9].

Nonsurgical treatments for ED that are currently available in the United States and that were reviewed by the AUA panel include the PDE5 inhibitors sildenafil, tadalafil, and vardenafil; alprostadil intraurethral suppositories; intracavernous alprostadil, papaverine, or phentolamine injection or combination injections; vacuum constriction; trazodone; and yohimbine and other herbal therapies. The AUA identified the PDE5 inhibitors as first-line therapy for ED and noted that evidence supporting the efficacy of one over another is lacking [8].

Alprostadil suppositories are recommend by the AUA for men who are not candidates for PDE5 inhibitors or who have used PDE5 inhibitors without success [8]. The AUA notes that intracavernous injection therapy with alprostadil, papaverine, or phentolamine is the single most effective nonsurgical treatment for ED. Vacuum constriction devices are sometimes effective and generally low-cost alternatives to drugs and injections for the management of ED.

The AUA panel recommended against the use of trazodone, testosterone, yohimbine, and other herbal remedies for the treatment of ED, citing the lack of evidence of efficacy [8]. The AUA document discussed the uses of noninflatable (malleable) and inflatable penile prostheses. It recommended against penile venous reconstructive surgery and noted that arterial reconstructive surgery was an option only in men who had ED of recent onset with a focal arterial occlusion and no evidence of systemic vascular disease.

Benefits and limitations of current treatments

The three available PDE5 inhibitors are potent and reversible inhibitors of PDE5. All are metabolized by the liver. Although none exhibits superiority over the others, the agents differ in the pharmacokinetic and adverse event profiles. Sildenafil and vardenafil each have a T_{max} of 1 hour and a half-life of approximately 4 hours. The T_{max} of tadalafil is approximately 2 hours, and its half-life is approximately 18 hours [8]. Sildenafil, vardenafil, and tadalafil are significantly more effective than placebo in producing erections that are strong enough and of sufficient duration to permit successful intercourse. The overall efficacy rate of PDE5 inhibitors is estimated at 60% to 75%. Efficacy rates are lower in patients who have severe neurologic damage, diabetes, or severe vascular disease [11]. In patients who have diabetes, those with better glycemic control and fewer diabetic complications are more likely to have a good response to PDE5 inhibitors than are patients with poor glycemic control and many complications [11].

High-fat meals and alcohol reduce the absorption of sildenafil and vardenafil. Tadalafil has no interactions with food and can be taken without regard to meals, the fat content of meals, or alcohol consumption. The beneficial effects of tadalafil on erectile function may persist for as long as 36 hours. Most men notice an improvement in ED with the first or second dose of a PDE5 inhibitor, whereas others experience no response until taking six or eight doses [12].

PDE5 inhibitor therapy for ED is simple and convenient for most men. When PDE5 inhibitors are effective, the benefits of treatment may persist for months to years [13]. Nonetheless, 30% to 35% of men who receive a prescription for a PDE5 inhibitor fail to respond to an adequate trial of the drug [13]. Overall, at least 50% of men taking sildenafil, vardenafil, or tadalafil discontinue treatment [2]. For the first 3 to 4 months of treatment, prescription renewal rates for PDE5 inhibitors are in the range of 60%. Within 6 to 12 months of treatment, however, renewal rates decrease to approximately 30%. Treatment failure is one of several reasons why patients may discontinue the use of PDE5 inhibitors [13].

Treatment failure with PDE5 inhibitors has several important implications. Patients may perceive failure as a sign that they will never again have satisfactory sexual function. Others may no longer trust the physician who prescribed the medication. As a result, their intimate relationships may suffer [11].

Some patients seem to develop resistance to the effects of a PDE5 inhibitor over time, possibly by a tachyphylactic mechanism [14]. In one study,

17% of sildenafil users discontinued its use because it became ineffective after 2 years of use [15,16]. Tachyphylaxis has not been confirmed clinically with PDE5 inhibitor users [16]; however, data suggest that sildenafil dosages must be increased to up to 200 mg when the initial dose (50 mg; 25 mg for the elderly or patients who have renal or hepatic impairment) is no longer effective. Typically, vardenafil and tadalafil are started at 10 mg and increased, if necessary, to 20 mg. Yet, this approach may work for fewer than 25% of patients in whom the initial dose is no longer effective. Further, the higher dose often is accompanied by an increased incidence of side effects. Among men taking more than 100 mg of sildenafil, for example, at least 30% discontinue treatment because of adverse effects [12,16]. When treatment with one PDE5 inhibitor fails, the chance that another PDE5 inhibitor will provide successful treatment is estimated at less than 5% [14]. Worsening comorbid illnesses also have been advanced as a cause of diminished efficacy of PDE5 inhibitors over time. Atherosclerosis and diabetes, for example, may cause further declines in erectile function over time that override the effects of PDE5 inhibitors [16].

The adverse events associated with the PDE5 inhibitors are a consequence of the vasodilatory properties of these agents, including headache, flushing, and nasal congestion. Other adverse effects include dyspepsia and abnormal color vision. Nonarteritic anterior ischemic optic neuropathy (NAION) is the most common acute optic neuropathy and is one of the most common causes of sudden blindness in older adults. Possible risk factors for NAION include some that also are associated with ED: diabetes, hypertension, arteriosclerosis, and hypercholesterolemia. The US Food and Drug Administration (FDA) has received reports of NAION developing in at least 43 cases of ischemic optic neuropathy in patients taking PDE5 inhibitors. Most of these events occurred in men who had risk factors for NAION; however, in some, a temporal relationship may have existed between the onset of vision loss and the use of a PDE5 inhibitor. The FDA asked the manufacturers of all three PDE5 inhibitors for new labeling to acknowledge the possible risk.

A major impediment to the use of PDE5 inhibitors is the contraindication for their use in patients who take any of the many available formulations of nitrates. PDE5 inhibitors may enhance the vasodilatory properties of nitrates and induce severe hypotension. For patients taking sildenafil or vardenafil, at least 24 hours must pass after the most recent dose before a nitrate can be administered, even with close patient observation and monitoring; for tadalafil, 48 hours must pass after the last dose [8]. The lack of population estimates of the number of men who have ED and who are taking nitrates makes it difficult to quantify how many men who have ED may be impacted by this drug interaction. One prospective study at a clinic dedicated to giving sexual advice to men who have cardiac disease and ED found that 88 of 425 (21%) men were taking long-acting oral nitrates as well as carrying sublingual nitrates [17].

The treatment options for patients, beyond PDE inhibitor therapy, are limited. The use of an alprostadil intraurethral suppository is one option. A synthetic vasodilator, alprostadil should be used the first time under medical supervision to ensure prompt treatment of hypotension or syncope in response to the first dose, an event that occurs in about 3% of treated patients. Alprostadil suppositories have been used in conjunction with penile constriction devices and PDE5 inhibitors, with some reports suggesting better efficacy than that obtained with alprostadil alone [8].

Intracavernous injections also are an option, but one that many men find unacceptable. Although intracavernous injections often are effective, they are more likely than other ED treatments to cause priapism. Injections cannot be given more than once every 24 hours. Typically, the first dose is administered under the supervision of a physician to monitor for side effects and to assess the risk for priapism. The consequences of priapism can be severe, and AUA recommends that physicians who prescribe these medications prepare a formal plan for intervening early and effectively when a patient develops this complication [8].

Vacuum constriction devices represent another treatment option. Most of the devices in this category are reasonably priced. Vacuum constriction devices can generate high negative pressures on the penis, however, causing serious injury. The AUA recommends that vacuum limiters be incorporated into all vacuum constriction devices to prevent this complication. Patient acceptability for this method is low [8].

The antidepressant trazodone has been studied as a treatment for ED but is not recommended. Although it showed better efficacy than placebo in some studies, these improvements were not statistically significant in a recent meta-analysis [18]. Little data exist to support the role of testosterone in treating ED, although it may improve the efficacy of the PDE5 inhibitors in hypogonadal men who undergo repletion. Yohimbine has little evidence in favor of its role as a possible treatment for ED, and it may cause blood pressure and heart rate elevations and tremor, among other adverse effects.

Several surgical therapies are available, including penile implants. Possible complications include autoinflation and pump displacement. Infection is the most serious complication of surgical implants. The risk for infection persists while the implant is in place.

Treatment gaps

Treatment options for patients in whom PDE5 inhibitors have not produced satisfactory improvements in erectile function or in whom PDE5 inhibitor efficacy has diminished with use are limited, and no pharmacologic options beyond those discussed above exist in the United States. If an adequate trial of one PDE5 inhibitor has not produced improvements in erectile function, it is unlikely that another drug from the same class will be effective. If the patient cannot tolerate the side effects of a particular PDE5 inhibitor, he is likely to experience the same problems with other agents in this class. Men who are obese may have improvements in ED or become more responsive to PDE5 inhibitors if they make recommended lifestyle changes with respect to weight loss, physical activity, and smoking cessation [19]. These changes typically are recommended to the patient at the time he reports ED; however, men often are noncompliant.

Patients who have ED that is the result of a radical prostatectomy or other abdominal surgery or diabetes are most likely to be unresponsive to PDE5 inhibitors. The response rate in these patients is in the 40% to 65% range.

After exhausting the PDE5 inhibitor possibilities, effective treatment choices are restricted to alprostadil suppositories, intracavernous injections, and implantation of a prosthetic device. Few patients are candidates for arterial reconstructive surgery. Many, if not most, of these choices are unpalatable to men and their partners. They attempt to treat the mechanical aspects of erectile function but could have damaging effects on the emotional and psychosocial facets of intimate relationships. The need for effective pharmacologic therapies other than PDE5 inhibitors seems clear.

Central targets: mechanistic considerations and historical perspectives

Cavernosal smooth muscle relaxation is the last in a series of complex, interrelated events that lead to a full erection. Peripheral autonomic and somatic pathways contribute to the balance between contractile and relaxing elements that result in an erection or flaccidity. Central stimuli initiate the normal erectile process, however [20]. Recent advances in our understanding of erectile physiology underscore the importance of the supraspinal pathways and centers that also contribute to erectile function. Animal studies suggest that the medial preoptic area (MPOA), the hippocampus, and the paraventricular nucleus of the hypothalamus (PVN) are involved in various facets of sexual activity, including erection. Neurons within the MPOA, for example, are known to concentrate androgens. They also maintain connections to the limbic areas and lower autonomic brainstem [20].

Data collected in rat studies showed that stimulation of the PVN, MPOA, or hippocampus causes erections, whereas damage at these sites severely impaired sexual function. In humans, damage caused to these areas by stroke or Parkinson's disease also can lead to erectile dysfunction [21]. Based on these and other findings, investigators have accumulated considerable data about how neurotransmitters, impulse propagation, and transduction of neural signals act to induce relaxation of cavernosal smooth muscle relaxation [22]. Research into how components of the central nervous system (CNS) are involved in the genesis of erections is beginning to shed light on potential targets for pharmaceutical agents that might enhance erectile function.

Dopamine

The dopaminergic system acts at the supraspinal and spinal levels to trigger erections. Dopaminergic neurons connect the MPOA and PVN to the lumbosacral portion of the spinal cord. Several types of dopamine receptors (eg, D_1, D_2, and so forth) are key components of the autonomic and somatic erection arc. In the MPOA, D_1 receptors seem to be involved primarily in erectile responses. In the PVN, D_2 receptors take on this function [22]. In rats and probably also in humans, stimulation of the D_2 receptor has an erectogenic effect [23]. Stimulation of D_2 receptors also causes stretching and yawning reflexes that are associated with the erectile response [22]. In rat and other animal models, administration of low-dose dopamine D_2 receptor agonists promotes erection [23]. The erectogenic effects of D_2 stimulation in the PVN are impeded by oxytocin antagonists, as well as by depletion of central oxytocin content, suggesting that oxytocin pathways mediate D_2 receptor function.

The D_1/D_2 receptor agonist apomorphine causes penile erections in animal models (rats) and humans, a process in which nitric oxide (NO) also is involved. Subcutaneous apomorphine administration increases PVN levels of NO and NO synthase (NOS). Inhibition of NOS blocks the apomorphine-induced increase in NO and NOS. Confirmation that apomorphine works in the CNS was obtained from data showing that two centrally acting dopamine antagonists, haloperidol and clozapine, block the erectogenic effects of apomorphine. In contrast, the peripherally acting dopamine antagonist domperidone has no effect on erections triggered by apomorphine.

Melanocortin system

The melanocortins are widely distributed and involved in various activities, including steroidogenesis, exocrine secretion, analgesia, inflammation, neuromuscular regeneration, and gastrointestinal (GI) and sexual function, among others. The precursor of all melanocortins is proopiomelanocortin (POMC), a polyhormone that may generate as many as eight peptides, depending on the cleavage sites. POMC precursor and mRNA is localized in the pituitary gland as well as the hypothalamus, (arcuate nucleus), brainstem (commissural nucleus), melanocytes, immune system, lung, and GI tract [24,25]. The term "melanocortin system" refers collectively to the melanocortin peptides, corticotropin, melanocortin receptors (MCRs), melanocortin antagonists, and several ancillary proteins. The melanocortin peptides include α-, β-, and γ-melanocyte stimulating hormone (MSH). The melanocortins are highly tissue-specific and share the amino acid sequence, His-Phe-Arg-Trp, which seems to be the minimum required sequence for binding to receptors, stimulating activation, and producing biologic effects [24].

Some 40 years ago it was discovered that intraventricular injection of corticotropin and α-MSH triggered erections, grooming behavior, stretching, and yawning in several animal species [26,27]. A role for the melanocortins in human erectile function was discovered accidentally among men enrolled in a clinical dermatology study. They received a compound called melano-tan- II (MT-II), which was designed to trigger tanning and, thus, protect the skin from the effects of UV radiation. Study subjects reported having unexpected erections [28].

Five MCRs have been characterized, and all are coupled to G-protein. The melanocortin receptors increase target cell cyclic AMP levels when activated [24]. Each receptor type has a different affinity for the various melanocortin peptides. All MCRs are activated by corticotropin, and MC-2 is the only receptor not activated by α-MSH [25]. MC3R and MC4R receptors are located in the hypothalamus and PVN in areas that play a pivotal role in erectile function. After exposure to a dose of a melanocortin that causes an erection, the PVN and supraoptic nuclei of the hypothalamus in rats express early gene products indicative of stimulation [29]. MC4Rs also are found in other areas of the brain. MC4R mRNA has been detected throughout the entire spinal cord of the rat and is the only receptor subtype for which mRNA is detectable. The MC4R concentration is particularly dense in the thoracic spinal cord, the outer part of the dorsal horn, the dorsal root ganglia, and the ventral horn. MC4R also has been localized to the penis and major pelvic ganglion, part of the autonomic relay pathway to the penis. Evidence of MC4R mRNA also is present in free nerve endings and mechanoreceptors in the rat penis [25,30]; however, several lines of evidence mitigate against a role for penile melanocortin receptors in erectile function. Injection of MT-II directly into cavernosal tissue has no effect on erections in rats, but is effective in causing erections when injected IV or ICV [29]. It is possible that the MC4Rs found in penile tissue have an effect on afferent nerve activity by way of sensory fibers [25].

Injections of corticotropin and α-MSH into the PVN cause yawning and erections [22]. Evidence supporting the role of MC3R and MC4R in erectile function includes the observation that antagonists of these receptors block erections induced by MT-II. MC4R-knockout mice demonstrate less mounting and more latency in intromission [30]. In addition, mRNA from MC4R occurs in the penises of human males and rats and has been located in the spinal cord and pelvic ganglia of rats. Selective MC4R agonists greatly increase erectile activity in rats, an action that is impeded by MC4R antagonists [22].

Evidence exists that erections stimulated by MC4R are mediated by way of the oxytocinergic system [31]. When oxytocin antagonists are administered in conjunction with MC4R agonists, erectile activity is diminished [22]. Melanocortin activity also seems to be testosterone dependent. Corticotropin does not cause erectile activity in animals that have been castrated; erectile function in response to corticotropin is restored, however, when testosterone is replaced [26].

Other neurotransmitters also seem to act in conjunction with the melanocortin system to control erectile function. For example, administration of an NOS inhibitor blocks erections in response to corticotropin. It has been postulated that NO activation is the common denominator in erection-controlling pathways involving melanocortins, oxytocin, and dopamine [25]. Calcium channel blockers also block erections caused by corticotropin. Other inhibitors of corticotropin-induced erections include compounds that open potassium channels and muscarinic receptor antagonists.

Serotonin

Evidence that serotonin or 5-hydroxytryptamine (5-HT) is involved in erectile activity includes the observation that 5-HT–containing neurons are located in the supraspinal areas and are involved in sexual activity. Some sacral preganglionic neurons and motoneurons have synapses with 5-HT–containing neurons. Many subtypes of the 5-HT receptor exist, and stimulation of different receptor subtypes can inhibit or promote erectile function. This may depend, in some part, on where in the spinal cord the different 5-HT subtype receptors are located. For example, stimulation of the 5-HT_{1A} receptor blocks erectile function, whereas stimulation of the 5-HT_{1C} and 5-HT_{2C} receptors enhance erectile function. NO and oxytocin also contribute to stimulation induced by 5-HT_{1C} activation. Trazodone, an inhibitor of 5-HT uptake, has been investigated as a potential therapy for ED. One of its metabolites is a 5-HT_{2C} agonist. Some preclinical data suggest that this trazodone metabolite may be a candidate for clinical investigation [22].

Noradrenaline

According to data obtained in animal models, noradrenergic transmission modulates sexual activity on the α_1- and α_2-adrenergic receptors. Noradrenergic activation of the α_1-adrenergic receptors promotes mating behavior, whereas stimulation of the α_2-adrenergic receptors curtails sexual behavior. Clonidine, a known α_2-adrenergic receptor agonist, inhibits sexual activity when introduced directly into the MPOA. This inhibitory action is blocked by the use of an α_2-adrenergic antagonist. Yohimbine is an antagonist of α_2-adrenergic activity, from which it may gain its putative benefits as a treatment of ED.

Excitatory amino acids

Excitatory amino acids, such as N-methyl-D-aspartate (NMDA), work in the PVN to enhance erectile function. Because NO levels increase in the PVN after NMDA administration, it is likely that the actions of NMDA are facilitated by an NOS signaling pathway. This is supported by the fact that the effects of NDMA can be blocked by administration of an oxytocin antagonist or NOS inhibitor [22].

Nitric oxide

NO has a dual role in erectile function. Functioning as an intercellular modulator, NO is a cornerstone of peripheral erectile physiology. Functioning as an intracellular modulator, it also acts as a CNS transmitter. Several lines of evidence point to its role in central mechanisms. When introduced into the PVN and MPOA, inhibitors of NOS prevent erections that are triggered by dopamine agonists, corticotropin, NMDA, and 5-HT$_{2C}$ agonists. This suggests the wide-ranging role played by NO in the centrally acting system. Levels of NO increase in the PVN and the MPOA during certain types of sexual activity in rats. Neurons containing NOS populate much of the spinal cord. NO has been implicated in many pathways that influence erectile activity, including preganglionic sympathetic and parasympathetic pathways and somatosensory and visceral sensory arcs.

Despite the major role played by NO in erectile function in the periphery and CNS, potential therapeutic NO agents have not been identified.

Growth hormone–releasing peptide

In animal studies, analogs of several growth hormone–releasing peptides stimulate penile erection when introduced directly into the PVN. The character of the erections is similar to those caused by dopamine receptor antagonists and oxytocin, and growth hormone–releasing peptides are believed to function by way of the oxytocinergic system and involve NO production by NOS in the relevant neurons within the PVN [22].

Opioid peptides

Morphine and other opioids have a notoriously deleterious effect on erectile function in humans and rats. Furthermore, opioids also antagonize the yawning- and erection-promoting effects of oxytocin and dopamine in animal models. Yawning and erectile function was restored when animals were pretreated with the opioid antagonist naloxone [32]. Morphine also reduces NO concentrations in the PVN.

Centrally acting drugs for erectile dysfunction: clinical experience

Apomorphine

Receptor activation in the hypothalamus is believed to be the mechanism by which the postsynaptic dopamine receptor agonist apomorphine causes erections in rats and men with and without ED. Apomorphine stimulates D$_1$ and D$_2$ dopamine receptors, but its erection-stimulating effect seems to occur by way of D$_2$ receptor stimulation [23,27].

In 1984, the findings of a placebo-controlled trial demonstrated that apomorphine caused erections in healthy men in doses of 0.25 to 0.75 mg [33]. Apomorphine also potentiates erections caused by visual stimuli in men [34]. Based on evidence that began to accumulate in the 1980s showing that subcutaneously administered apomorphine induced and enhanced erections, apomorphine was investigated as a potential treatment for ED. Orally administered apomorphine is not effective [22]. Injected formulations of the drug were determined to be effective but caused numerous side effects, including emesis, yawning, drowsiness, nausea, lacrimation, facial flushing, and dizziness. When 2- or 3-mg doses of apomorphine are absorbed through the oral mucosa, however, it remains effective and causes fewer side effects, because the drug avoids first-pass metabolism when entering the bloodstream this way [22,35].

Early confirmation of the clinical efficacy of apomorphine came from a 10- to 12-week double-blind, randomized, cross-over efficacy study of sublingual apomorphine, 2 mg, in 252 men who had ED [36]. Compared with men taking placebo, 10% more men in the apomorphine group experienced erections firm enough for intercourse (SEP-2); this difference was statistically significant ($P < .001$). The proportion of successful intercourse attempts (SEP-3) also was higher in the apomorphine group than in the placebo group. The 3-mg dose of sublingual apomorphine was tested in a similar study [37]. Erections firm enough for intercourse were experienced by 47% of the apomorphine group and 32% of the placebo group, a significant difference at the $P < .001$ level. Successful intercourse rates were 48% and 34% in the apomorphine and placebo groups, respectively.

Apomorphine dose-response effects have been observed in a double-blind, dose-escalation study that enrolled 507 patients [35]. Participants were randomized to receive placebo or increasing doses of apomorphine during the 8-week study period. Those randomized to apomorphine were given apomorphine, 2 mg or 3 mg, for separate 2-week periods. The 3-mg dose was superior. Among men using the 3-mg dose, 40.9% achieved successful intercourse on at least 50% of their attempts; among those taking the 2-mg dose, only 32.9% were able to complete intercourse on at least half of the attempts. No additional improvements in erectile function were noted when the apomorphine dose was increased to 4 mg. The frequency of adverse effects increased markedly, however. The incidence of nausea, for example, increased from approximately 3% to 14% with the 3- and 4-mg doses, respectively [37].

Apomorphine is notable for the speed with which it becomes effective. In one study, one third of men achieved an erection within 10 minutes of administration, and an additional 37% of men responded in the second 10 minutes [38]. Overall, 71% of participants in this trial had functional erections within 20 minutes. Repeat administration does not lead to tolerance. Unlike the PDE5 inhibitors, apomorphine causes no interactions with nitrates, food, or alcohol [22].

Several groups of investigators have compared the efficacy of sildenafil and apomorphine. The results have varied, with a benefit usually seen for sildenafil [22]. In an unblinded cross-over study, the rate of successful sexual encounters was 73.1% to 62.7% in favor of sildenafil over apomorphine [39]. A second study, which included men who had iatrogenic ED, had more divergent results, with a 63.7% versus 32.1% advantage for sildenafil compared to apomorphine [40]. These investigators noted that in the subgroup of subjects who had abnormal findings on the penile Doppler examination, thereby suggesting vasculogenic ED, the success rate of apomorphine was only 14% compared to 76% for sildenafil.

Further, 80% of men assigned to receive apomorphine exercised their option of increasing their dosages from 2 mg to 3 mg. In contrast, more than half of men assigned to sildenafil maintained the 50-mg starting dose. These findings were notable for the fact that 20% of participants were not satisfied with the study drugs.

An open-label cross-over study of sildenafil and apomorphine was conducted by Eardley and colleagues [41] and included 139 men who had never been treated for ED. Each of the two treatment periods was 8 weeks in length, and a 2-week washout period separated the two. The primary end point was the erectile function (EF) domain of the International Index of Erectile Function (IIEF). Participants were allowed to titrate the dosage of each of the study drugs. The rate of successful intercourse was 75% postsildenafil and 35% postapomorphine. The EF domain score was 25.2 for sildenafil and 15.9 for apomorphine. While taking sildenafil, 52% of subjects increased their dosage to 100 mg. While on apomorphine, 89% increased the dosage of that drug to 3 mg. Overall, 96% of subjects preferred sildenafil to apomorphine.

Another cross-over study that enrolled treatment-naive patients had similar results [42]. Compared with apomorphine, statistically significant improvements in rigidity, capacity to get and maintain an erection, and sexual confidence were found in men taking sildenafil. Satisfaction with sildenafil treatment was 90% compared with only 46% for apomorphine. Overall, 95% of subjects stated a preference for sildenafil over apomorphine at the end of the study. Sixty five adverse events were reported from 45 patients while taking sildenafil, and 35 adverse events occurred among 27 patients while taking apomorphine. The leading adverse events associated with sildenafil were headache, flushing, dyspepsia, and rhinitis. The most common ones associated with apomorphine were headache and nausea.

A study by Gontero and colleagues [43] investigated the efficacy of sublingual apomorphine in 130 men who had diabetes and ED. Participants were randomized to receive placebo or four 3-mg tablets of apomorphine. Responses on the EF domain of the IIEF and the single-item global efficacy question were used to assess efficacy. The results showed no difference between the efficacy of apomorphine and placebo. Overall, 22% of men who received apomorphine did experience a clinically significant erection. Younger men and men with lower hemoglobin A1c levels were more likely than older ones and men with higher hemoglobin A1c levels to have erections with treatment. The investigators concluded that apomorphine has "a limited use" in men who have diabetes and ED.

Crossover, double-blind, phase III clinical trials of apomorphine have included more than 854 men, aged 18 to 70 years, who took 8263 tablets of sublingual apomorphine in 2-and 4-mg doses [44,45]. Outcome measures included intercourse and erection rates. In this cohort, 74.1% of patients had moderate or severe grades of ED, 31% had hypertension, 16% had CAD, 16% had dyslipidemia, 16% had diabetes, and 16% had benign prostatic hypertrophy. Erections suitable for intercourse were obtained in 54.4% of attempts with the 4-mg apomorphine dose compared with 33.8% with placebo, a difference that was significant ($P < .001$). More than 50% of intercourse attempts were successful with the 4-mg dose, which was twice the baseline rate ($P < .001$). The 2-mg dose also was associated with significant improvements in the prevalence of successful intercourse attempts (41.5%). Nausea was the most common adverse reaction, occurring in more than 20% of patients at the 4-mg dose, compared with 2.1% at the 2-mg dose. Other side effects noted in studies of apomorphine include dizziness, headache, and yawning [22].

Patients who seem to benefit from apomorphine are those who are younger and have mild/moderate ED. Because of its associated adverse effects, apomorphine is not widely accepted among patients. An intranasal formulation is being developed as a possible means of diminishing adverse effects and prolonging its half-life [22].

Bremelanotide (formerly PT-141)

Following up on the finding that patients who received MT-II in a dermatologic clinical trial often experienced unexpected erections, investigators enrolled 10 subjects aged 37 to 67 years who had organic ED in a double-blind, placebo-controlled, cross-over study to assess the safety, erectogenic properties, and affect on libido of MT-II [46]. Organic risk factors for ED that were present in the 10 subjects included hypercholesterolemia, obesity, hypertension, peripheral neuropathic injury, diabetes, cigarette smoking, and heart disease, among others. Placebo and MT-II (0.25 mg/kg) were injected subcutaneously twice daily. MT-II was injected 19 times into the 10 subjects, and placebo was administered 21 times. Erections occurred in response to 12 of 19 MT-II

injections (63%) but with only 1 of 21 placebo injections ($P = .001$). On a scale of 1 to 10, erections had a mean rigidity score of 6.9. Mean duration of the induced erections was 64.1 minutes (range, 2 minutes to 4 hours of intermittent erectile activity). Tip rigidity greater than 80% was maintained for a mean of 45.3 minutes compared to 1.9 minutes for placebo. Sexual desire levels were elevated after 13 of 19 MT-II doses (68%) compared with 4 of 21 placebo injections (19%; $P = .0034$). Nausea, stretching, and yawning were more common among men taking MT-II than placebo, and 4 of 19 injections of MT-II were associated with severe nausea.

A similar placebo-controlled, cross-over study was conducted among men with ED that was judged to be psychogenic based on the observation of at least one nocturnal erection lasting at least 10 minutes and with 70% tip rigidity during pretrial monitoring [47]. Ten men, with an average age of 47.4 years, were enrolled and given two subcutaneous abdominal injections each of MT-II and placebo. MT-II doses ranged from 0.025 to 0.157 mg/kg. Eight of the 10 participants reported erections after MT-II injections; no erections were reported after placebo injections. The time to onset of erection among the 8 men who responded to MT-II ranged from 15 to 270 minutes (mean, 127.5 minutes), and the average erection duration was 144 minutes. All but one of the responders experienced an erection after both MT-II injections. Fifteen of the 20 total MT-II injections caused sustained tip rigidity. Severe side effects were not reported, but nausea, yawning, and decreased appetite occurred more often after MT-II administration. No participants reported vomiting.

Bremelanotide, an active metabolite of MT-II, was shown to be an agonist at the MC3R and MC4R receptors, and a formulation was developed for intranasal administration [48]. Early tests were conducted in healthy men and in sildenafil-responsive men who had ED. Erectile response was assessed in healthy men and in sildenafil-responsive patients who had ED with the help of visual stimulation. In both groups of patients, bremelanotide caused a statistically significant erectile response compared to placebo at doses exceeding 7 mg. Erections typically occurred about 30 minutes after dosing. Bremelanotide was well-tolerated; flushing and nausea were the most common adverse events.

Rosen and colleagues [49] evaluated the erectogenic potential of subcutaneously administered bremelanotide in healthy men who did not have ED (phase I study) and in men who had moderate-to-severe ED in whom sildenafil had provided less than adequate treatment, or a functional erection no more than 50% of the time while taking 100 mg of sildenafil (phase IIa study). The mean erection rate with sildenafil in this group was 25%. In the phase I study, 36 healthy subjects received doses ranging from 0.3 to 10 mg subcutaneously in the lower right abdominal quadrant, and 12 subjects received placebo. Doses higher than 1.0 mg caused a statistically significant erectile response without visual sexual stimulation (VSS). In the phase IIa study, patients who had ED received placebo (n = 25) or bremelanotide, 4 mg (n = 24) or 6 mg (n = 21), in a cross-over design. Men who had ED were provided with VSS during the assessments. Dosing site was the same as in the healthy men. Among men who had ED, the mean duration of maintaining at least 60% base rigidity was 28 minutes and 41 minutes for patients on the 4- and 6-mg doses, respectively (Fig. 1). Among men who had ED taking placebo, this degree of rigidity had a mean duration of 6 minutes. Base rigidity of at least 80% lasted for a mean of 14 and 17 minutes for men taking the 4- and 6-mg doses, respectively, and 3 minutes for men on placebo. Ten of the study subjects were categorized as having severe ED (IIEF EF domain score, 6–10). The 6-mg dose of bremelanotide was associated with at least 60% base rigidity that lasted for 36 minutes and at least 80% base rigidity that lasted for 15 minutes (Fig. 2). The corresponding times for placebo were 8 minutes and 2 minutes, respectively. The erectile response induced by bremelanotide was statistically significant compared with placebo at both doses. Bremelanotide was safe and well-tolerated in both groups of participants.

Bremelanotide also has been investigated as an intranasal formulation in healthy men (phase I study) and in men who have sildenafil-responsive ED (phase IIa study) [48]. In the phase I study, patients were randomized to receive placebo (n = 8) or single-dose administration of bremelanotide, 4 mg (n = 6), 7 mg (n = 6), 10 mg (n = 6), or 20 mg (n = 6). In the phase IIa study, patients were randomized to receive placebo (n = 24) or single-dose administration of bremelanotide, 7 mg (n = 24) or 20 mg (n = 24). Among the healthy men in the phase I study, mean C_{max} and AUC_{0-t} for bremelanotide increased in a dose-dependent manner. The median T_{max} was 0.50 hour, and the mean $t_{1/2}$ ranged from 1.85 to 2.09 hours. Compared with placebo in the healthy men and those who had ED, erectile responses associated with bremelanotide were statistically significant at the 10- and 20-mg dose in the phase I study and at the 20-mg dose in the phase IIa study (Figs. 3 and 4). Erection onset occurred in approximately 30 minutes. Bremelanotide was safely administered and well tolerated in both groups of patients. The most common adverse events were flushing and nausea (17% for each).

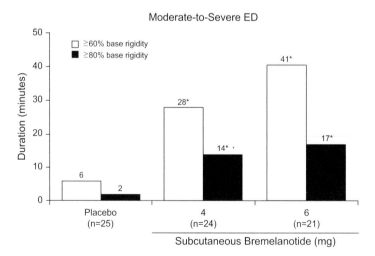

Fig. 1. Duration of at least 60% and at least 80% base rigidity in patients who had moderate-to-severe ED and received single doses of subcutaneous bremelanotide. RigiScan monitoring session was 2.5 hours duration with VSS. *$P < .001$ versus placebo.

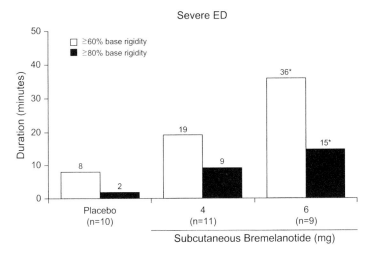

Fig. 2. Duration of at least 60% and at least 80% base rigidity in patients who had severe ED and received single doses of subcutaneous bremelanotide. RigiScan monitoring session was 2.5 hours duration with VSS. *$P < .01$ versus placebo.

The safety and efficacy of coadministration of subtherapeutic doses of bremelanotide plus sildenafil was assessed in 19 men who had ED [50]. Participants were randomized to receive sildenafil, 25 mg, plus intranasal bremelanotide, 7.5 mg; sildenafil, 25 mg, plus placebo spray; and placebo plus intranasal placebo spray in a triple crossover protocol. All subjects had ED that was responsive to sildenafil with a mean efficacy of 75%; on average, three of every four doses of sildenafil produced an erection sufficient for intercourse. Patients had a baseline IIEF EF domain

score of 21.2, which was not representative of baseline ED severity in this patient population. Comorbid conditions among the participants included smoking (50%), hyperlipidemia (50%), hypertension (20%), obesity (10%), and diabetes mellitus (10%). Erectile responses generated by coadministration of sildenafil plus bremelanotide were significantly greater than the responses generated by sildenafil alone. Patients receiving bremelanotide plus sildenafil had a significantly longer duration of base rigidity of at least 60% compared with sildenafil alone and placebo (113

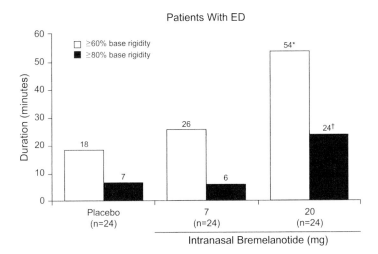

Fig. 3. Duration of at least 60% and at least 80% base rigidity in patients who had ED and received single doses of intranasal bremelanotide. Two 30-minute RigiScan monitoring sessions with VSS. *$P < .001$ versus placebo. †$P < .01$ versus placebo.

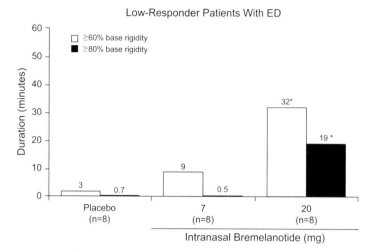

Fig. 4. Duration of at least 60% and at least 80% base rigidity in low-responder patients who had ED and received single doses of intranasal bremelanotide. Low-responder patients were defined by the inability to achieve at least 20% base rigidity for at least 3 consecutive minutes during 30 minute of VSS after administration of placebo. Two 30-minute RigiScan monitoring sessions with VSS. *P < .05 versus placebo.

versus 70 [P < .01] and 37 [P < .001] minutes). Results from the self-assessment of erection quality instrument (scale 1–10 with 1 = lowest and 10 = highest quality erection) after each VSS session indicated that erection quality was significantly greater in patients receiving bremelanotide plus sildenafil compared with sildenafil alone or placebo (8.2 versus 6.8 [P < .05] and 5.7 [P < .001], respectively). Coadministration of the two agents did not increase the frequency or severity of adverse events that have been observed with monotherapy. No new adverse events occurred.

Summary

ED is a highly prevalent condition associated with numerous risk factors, including age, diabetes, CVD, and LUTS, among others. The range of medical and surgical options for men is limited in the United States primarily to oral PDE5 inhibitors and several more invasive medical and surgical remedies, such as alprostadil suppositories and penile implants. The response to PDE5 inhibitors varies, depending on the drug, the etiology of ED, and the duration of the condition. Response rates are lower in men who have diabetes or a history of pelvic surgery. Only about half of men who receive a prescription for sildenafil continue the treatment long-term. PDE5 inhibitors are contraindicated in men who take nitrates, and possible adverse effects include

flushing, headache, and visual disturbances. As our understanding of normal erectile physiology and ED pathophysiology has grown, it is clear that one or more centrally acting agents may have a role to play in the treatment of ED. Evidence suggests that bremelanotide, with or without sildenafil cotherapy, may be a viable treatment option for men who have ED.

References

[1] Impotence. NIH Consensus Statement. 1992;10:1.
[2] Seftel AD, Mohammed MA, Althof SE. Erectile dysfunction: etiology, evaluation, and treatment options. Med Clin North Am 2004;88:387–416.
[3] Laumann EO, Paik A, Rosen RC. Sexual dysfunction in the United States: prevalence and predictors. JAMA 1999;281(6):537–44.
[4] Feldman HA, Goldstein I, Hatzichristou DG, et al. Impotence and its medical and psychological correlates: results of the Massachusetts Male Aging Study. J Urol 1994;151(1):54–61.
[5] Mulligan T, Retchin SM, Chinchilli VM, et al. The role of aging and chronic disease in sexual dysfunction. J Am Geriatr Soc 1988;36(6):520–4.
[6] Braun M, Wassmer G, Klotz T, et al. Epidemiology of erectile dysfunction: results of the Cologne Male Survey. Int J Impot Res 2000;12:305–11.
[7] Rosen R, Altwein J, Boyle P, et al. Lower urinary tract symptoms and male sexual dysfunction. The Multinational Study of the Aging Male (MSAM-7). Eur Urol 2003;44(6):637–49.

[8] Montague DK, Jarow JP, Broderick GA, et al. The management of erectile dysfunction: an AUA update. J Urol 2005;174:230–9.

[9] Kostis JB, Jackson G, Rosen R, et al. Sexual dysfunction and cardiac risk (the Second Princeton Consensus Conference). Am J Cardiol 2005;96(2): 313–21.

[10] Esposito K, Giugliano F, Di Palo C, et al. Effect of lifestyle changes on erectile dysfunction in obese men. A randomized controlled trial. JAMA 2004; 291(24):2978–84.

[11] Hatzimouratidis K, Hatzichristou D. Phosphodiesterase type 5 inhibitors: the day after. Eur Urol 2007;51:75–89.

[12] McMahon CG. High dose sildenafil citrate as a salvage therapy for severe erectile dysfunction. Int J Impot Res 2002;14(6):533–8.

[13] Masson P, Lambert SM, Brown M, et al. PDE-5 inhibitors: current status and future trends. Urol Clin North Am 2005;32:511–25.

[14] Lau DHW, Kommu K, Mumtaz FH, et al. The management of phosphodiesterase-5 (PDE-5) inhibitor failure. Curr Vasc Pharmacol 2006;4:89–93.

[15] El-Galley R, Rutland H, Talic R, et al. Long-term efficacy of sildenafil and tachyphylaxis effect. J Urol 2001;166(3):927–31.

[16] McMahon CN, Smith CJ, Shabsigh R. Treating erectile dysfunction when PDE5 inhibitors fail. BMJ 2006;332:589–92.

[17] Jackson G, Martin E, McGing E, et al. Successful withdrawal of oral long-acting nitrates to facilitate phosphodiesterase type 5 inhibitor use in stable coronary disease patients with erectile dysfunction. J Sex Med 2005;2(4):513–6.

[18] Fink HA, MacDonald R, Rutks IR, et al. Trazodone for erectile dysfunction: a systematic review and meta-analysis. Br J Urol 2003;92(4):441–6.

[19] Kloner RA. Erectile dysfunction and cardiovascular risk factors. Urol Clin North Am 2005;32:397–402.

[20] Stief CG. Is there a common pathophysiology of erectile dysfunction and how does this relate to new pharmacotherapies? Int J Impot Res 2002; 14(suppl 1):S11–6.

[21] Dean RC, Lue TF. Physiology of penile erection and pathophysiology of erectile dysfunction. Urol Clin North Am 2005;32:379–95.

[22] Kendirci M, Walls MM, Hellstrom WHG. Central nervous system agents in the treatment of erectile dysfunction. Urol Clin North Am 2005;32:487–501.

[23] Andersson KE, Hedlund P. New directions for erectile dysfunction therapies. Int J Impot Res 2002; 14(suppl 1):S82–92.

[24] Getting SJ. Targeting melanocortin receptors as potential novel therapeutics. Pharmacol Ther 2006; 111:1–15.

[25] Giuliano F. Control of penile erection by the melanocortinergic system: experimental evidences and therapeutic perspectives. J Androl 2004;25(5): 683–91.

[26] Bertolini A, Gessa GL. Behavioral effects of ACTH and MSH peptides. J Endocrinol Invest 1981;4(2): 241–51.

[27] Andersson KE, Wagner G. Physiology of penile erection. Physiol Rev 1995;75:191–236.

[28] Gura T. Having it all. Science 2003;299(5608):850.

[29] Shadiack A, Sharma SD, Earle DC, et al. Melanocortins in the treatment of male and female sexual dysfunction. Curr Top Med Chem 2007;7:1137–44.

[30] Van der Ploeg LH, Martin WJ, Howard AD, et al. A role for the melanocortin 4 receptor in sexual function. Proc Natl Acad Sci U S A 2002;99(17):11381–6.

[31] Martin WJ, McGowan E, Cashen DE, et al. Activation of melanocortin MC(4) receptors increases erectile activity in rats ex copula. Eur J Pharmacol 2002; 454(1):71–9.

[32] Melis MR, Stancampiano R, Gessa GL, et al. Prevention by morphine of apomorphine- and oxytocin-induced penile erection and yawning: site of action in the brain. Neuropsychopharmacology 1992;6(1):17–21.

[33] Lal S, Ackman D, Thavundayil JX, et al. Effect of apomorphine, a dopamine receptor agonist, on penile tumescence in normal subjects. Prog Neuropsychopharmacol Biol Psychiatry 1984;8(4-6):695–9.

[34] Danjou P, Alexandre L, Warot D, et al. Assessment of erectogenic properties of apomorphine and yohimbine in man. Br J Clin Pharmacol 1988; 26(6):733–9.

[35] Heaton JP. Recovery of erectile function by the oral administration of apomorphine. Urology 1995;45: 200–6.

[36] Mirone VG, Stief CG. Efficacy of apomorphine SL in erectile dysfunction. BJU Int 2001;88(Suppl 3): 25–9.

[37] Dula E, Bukofzer S, Perdok R, et al. Apomorphine SL Study Group. Double-blind, crossover comparison of 3 mg apomorphine SL with placebo and with 4 mg apomorphine SL in male erectile dysfunction. Eur Urol 2001;39:558–64.

[38] Dula E, Keating W, Siami PF, et al. Efficacy and safety of fixed-dose and dose-optimization regimens of sublingual apomorphine versus placebo in men with erectile dysfunction. The Apomorphine Study Group. Urology 2000;56(1):130–5.

[39] Perimenis P, Markou S, Gyftopoulos K, et al. Efficacy of apomorphine and sildenafil in men with non-arteriogenic erectile dysfunction. A comparative crossover study. Andrologia 2004;36(3):106–10.

[40] Perimenis P, Gyftopoulos K, Giannitsas K, et al. A comparative, crossover study of the efficacy and safety of sildenafil and apomorphine in men with evidence of arteriogenic erectile dysfunction. Int J Impot Res 2004;16(1):2–7.

[41] Eardley I, Wright P, MacDonagh R, et al. An open-label, randomized, flexible-dose, crossover study to assess the comparative efficacy and safety of sildenafil citrate and apomorphine in men with erectile dysfunction. BJU Int 2004;93:1271–5.

[42] Porst H, Bebre HM, Jungwirth A, et al. Comparative trial of treatment satisfaction, efficacy, and tolerability of sildenafil versus apomorphine in erectile dysfunction. An open, randomized crossover study with flexible dosing. Eur J Med Res 2007;12:61–7.

[43] Gontero P, D'Antonio R, Pretti G, et al. Clinical efficacy of apomorphine SL in erectile dysfunction of diabetic men. Int J Impot Res 2005;17:80–5.

[44] Heaton JPW. Key issues from the clinical trials of apomorphine SL. World J Urol 2001;19(1):25–31.

[45] Briganti A, Chun FK, Salonia A, et al. A comparative review of apomorphine formulations for erectile dysfunction. Recommendations for use in the elderly. Drugs Aging 2006;23(4):309–19.

[46] Wessells H, Gralnek D, Dorr R Hruby VJ, et al. Effect of an alpha-melanocyte stimulating hormone analog on penile erection and sexual desire in men with organic erectile dysfunction. Urology 2000;56: 641–6.

[47] Wessells H, Fuciarelli K, Hansen J, et al. Synthetic melanotropic peptide initiates erections in men with psychogenic erectile dysfunction: double-blind, placebo-controlled crossover study. J Urol 1998;16: 389–93.

[48] Diamond LE, Earle DC, Rosen RC, et al. Double-blind, placebo-controlled evaluation of the safety, pharmacokinetic properties and pharmacodynamic effects of intranasal PT-141, a melanocortin receptor agonist, in healthy males and patients with mild-to-moderate erectile dysfunction. Int J Impot Res 2004;16(1):51–9.

[49] Rosen RC, Diamond LE, Earle DC, et al. Valuation of the safety, pharmacokinetics and pharmacodynamic effects of subcutaneously administered PT-141, a melanocortin receptor agonist, in healthy male subjects and in patients with an inadequate response to Viagra. Int J Impot Res 2004;16: 135–42.

[50] Diamond LE, Earle DC, Garcia WD, et al. Co-administration of low doses of intranasal PT-141, a melanocortin receptor agonist, and sildenafil to men with erectile dysfunction results in an enhanced erectile response. Urology 2005;65:755–9.

ELSEVIER
SAUNDERS

Urol Clin N Am 34 (2007) 497–506

UROLOGIC
CLINICS
of North America

Female Sexual Disorders: Assessment, Diagnosis, and Treatment

Sheryl A. Kingsberg, PhD*, Jeffrey W. Janata, PhD

*Departments of Reproductive Biology and Psychiatry, University Hospitals Case Medical Center,
Case Western Reserve University School of Medicine, Cleveland, OH, USA*

"Some men spend a lifetime in an attempt to comprehend the complexities of women. Others pre-occupy themselves with somewhat simpler tasks, such as understanding the theory of relativity!"

Albert Einstein

"The great question that has never been answered and which I have not yet been able to answer, …is 'What does a woman want?'"

(Sigmund Freud)

Despite the increased popular attention that sexual dysfunction has received in the recent past, more often than not physicians and their patients remain avoidant of the topic in clinical visits, although there is evidence that healthy sexual functioning is an important contributor to women's sense of well-being and quality of life [1] and that sexual dysfunction in women is strikingly prevalent [2–5]. Women are hesitant to initiate discussions with their clinicians about sexual concerns, apparently fearful that time constraints, lack of effective treatments, or physician embarrassment stand as obstacles to a successful resolution to the distress that women and their partners are experiencing [6].

The patient hesitancy in this dynamic suggests that clinicians can best serve their patients by routinely initiating discussions about sexual function during clinical visits. When physicians appreciate the distress patients might be experiencing with sexual problems and when assessment of sexual function becomes a priority, even time-constrained visits can include a few moments to inquire about sexual concerns. Although many women experience sexual difficulties, sexual dysfunctions diagnostically include a sexual problem and that the woman or her partner experience distress as a function of that sexual problem. In this article, we provide an overview of the female sexual dysfunctions and address screening and treatment options.

Historical perspective

Female sexuality, as a research area and experientially, has historically been given short shrift. This is in large part due to our long-held western cultural beliefs regarding female sexuality as essentially inconsequential or inappropriate unless it is tied to the notion of pleasing one's husband. When it was determined during the Victorian era that female orgasm was not necessary for conception, female sexuality was further demonized.

Kinsey's research in the 1950s on the sexual practices of American men and women helped to dispel the myth that women are not interested in sex, but it has taken our culture a long time to catch up and accept the notion that women have a right to their sexuality [7]. The struggle for sexual equality continues today, as may be evident by the fact that research on female sexuality lags behind research on male sexuality and the difficulty our culture has in accepting that female sexual problems are as disruptive to a woman's quality of life as male sexual problems are to men.

There are a number of reasons why research has focused more on male sexual problems than female sexual problems. First is the difficulty in

* Corresponding author.
E-mail address: sherly.kingsberg@uhhs.com (S.A. Kingsberg).

0094-0143/07/$ - see front matter © 2007 Elsevier Inc. All rights reserved.
doi:10.1016/j.ucl.2007.08.016

measuring appropriate endpoints in clinical trials. For example, until recently there have been few valid outcome measures for assessing female sexual desire. In contrast, assessment of male arousal is relatively uncomplicated. Second, current models for conceptualizing the female sexual response reveal how complicated and multifactorial it is. The traditional linear models of Masters and Johnson [8], Kaplan [9], and Leif [10] suggested that the sexual response is invariant and is the same for males and females in that desire always precedes arousal (Fig. 1).

More recently, Basson [11] has developed a new, nonlinear model of female sexual response that integrates emotional intimacy, sexual stimuli, and relationship satisfaction Fig. 2. This model recognizes that female sexual functioning is more complex and is not as linear as male sexual functioning and that many women initially begin a sexual encounter from a point of sexual neutrality. The decision to be sexual may come from a conscious wish for emotional closeness or as a result of seduction or suggestion from a partner. Women have numerous reasons for engaging in sexual activity other than sexual drive.

Sexual neutrality or being receptive to rather than initiating sexual activity is considered a normal variation of female sexual functioning. In addition, it is frequently the case that subjective and physiologic sexual arousal precedes desire.

Sexual dysfunction: an overview of classification

According to the DSM IV TR [12], which is based on the linear model of sexual response posed by Masters and Johnson, there are six sexual disorders that encompass dysfunctions across the sexual response cycle (Table 1).

Human Sexual Response: Classic Models

- Excitement → Divided ↗ Desire
  ↘ Arousal
- Plateau
- Orgasm
- Resolution

Linear progression

Fig. 1. Human sexual response: classic models.

Female Sexual Response Cycle

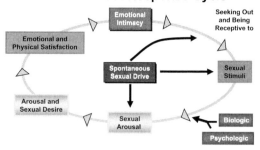

Fig. 2. Female sexual response cycle.

Hypoactive sexual desire disorder

Hypoactive sexual desire disorder (HSDD) is defined in the DSM IV TR as persistent or recurrent deficient or absent sexual fantasies/thoughts or desire for or receptivity to sexual activity. The judgment of "deficiency" is subjective and made by a clinician only after taking into account factors that affect sexual functioning such as age, physical condition, and the context of a person's life. As with all sexual disorders, prevalence is difficult to determine. Although

Table 1
DSM IV TR classifications of female sexual dysfunctions

Disorder	Description
Sexual desire disorders	
Hypoactive sexual desire disorder	Absence or deficiency of sexual fantasies and/or desire
Sexual aversion disorder	Aversion to and avoidance of genital sexual contact with a partner
Sexual arousal disorders	
Female sexual arousal disorder	Inability to attain or maintain adequate lubrication-swelling response of sexual excitement
Orgasmic disorders	
Female orgasmic disorder	Delay in or absence of orgasm after a normal sexual excitement phase
Pain disorders	
Dyspareunia	Genital pain associated with sexual intercourse
Vaginismus	Involuntary contraction of the perineal muscles preventing vaginal penetration

there have been a number of population surveys within the United States and worldwide, the prevalence estimates vary. Hayes and colleagues [13] and Segraves and Woodard [14] point to differences between studies in definition of hypoactive desire, methods of data collection, age group studied, and other defined criteria as the reason for such discrepancies. Segraves and Woodard [14] suggest that if the population of women who have HSDD were restricted to those reporting frequent problems with desire, the prevalence of HSDD would vary between 5.4% and 13.6%.

In clinical practice, women often present with the complaint of loss of desire but with little awareness of how, when, or why the problem occurred. One of the reasons that desire disorders remain elusive is that desire is a relatively complex concept that requires delineating the components for the patient and the clinician. Levine [15] suggests that desire is comprised of three distinct but interrelated components.

The first component is *drive*, which is the biologic component based on nueroendocrine mechanisms and evidenced by spontaneous sexual interest. That is, a person's body signals through sexual thoughts, fantasies, dreams, or sensations, such as genital tingling, that it wants to be sexual. Patients know this as feeling "horny." Drive is relative. Each individual has a certain drive level that normally declines with age in men and women.

The second component is *cognitive*. This component reflects a person's expectations, beliefs, and values about sex. For example, a 60-year-old happily married woman whose kids have finally left home and who adores her husband and believes that sex is healthy and fun will likely have more desire than a 60-year-old widow who believes that grandmothers aren't supposed to be sexual and doesn't believe in premarital sex.

The third component of desire is the emotional or interpersonal component of desire, which is subsumed under the category of *motivation* and characterized by the willingness of a person to engage in sexual activity. This is often the most important and is affected by the quality of a relationship, psychologic functioning, worries about health, and children.

This distinction between drive and desire is essential for any physician assessing or treating sexual problems because treatment is vastly different based on which component or components of desire have been impaired. For example, a woman might have a very strong sexual drive, but if she is not motivated to be sexual (eg, if she is angry with her partner, dealing with a stressful work problem, or suffering from depression), she will not act on the drive. On the other hand, if a woman has lost some of her drive but remains motivated to be close and intimate with her partner, then despite having little physical cues or interest, she still enjoys the sexual experience.

Hypoactive sexual desire disorder is the sexual dysfunction that is often assumed to correspond to menopause. This assumption has been challenged by recent longitudinal studies that suggest that age has a stronger impact on sexual desire than does menopause alone [16]. Nevertheless, menopause, particularly surgical menopause, may negatively effect sexual desire in some women primarily due to the significant and often sudden (with surgical or chemical menopause) decline in testosterone levels.

Testosterone is necessary for a normal sex drive in men and women, playing a role in motivation, desire, and sexual sensation. Women achieve peak androgen production in their mid-20s. Beginning in their early 30s, they gradually lose testosterone in an age-related fashion. By the time most women reach their 50s, their testosterone levels are half of what they were in their 20s [17].

Treatments include individual or couples psychotherapy/sex therapy, hormone therapy (exogenous testosterone replacement for postmenopausal women or tibolone, a synthetic selective estrogen and androgen modulator) and centrally acting pharmacologic agents that may have prosexual effects by inhibiting serotonergic activity, facilitating dopaminergic activity, or binding to melanocyte receptors [11]. There are no FDA-approved pharmacologic treatments for the treatment of any female sexual disorder, but a number of treatments are in clinical trials, and Procter & Gamble's testosterone patch (Intrinsa) has been approved and in use in Europe.

Sexual aversion disorder

DSM-IV-TR criteria for sexual aversion include persistent or recurrent aversive response to any genital contact with a sexual partner and emphasize the role of avoidance. As with all sexual disorders, personal or relationship distress is a required criterion. The Sexual Function Health Council of the American Foundation for Urologic Disease convened the Consensus Development Panel on Female Sexual Dysfunction

[18], and, in response to these criteria, the panel added a distinction between psychogenic- and organically based disorders. Although the incidence and prevalence of sexual aversion disorder are not known, the disorder is considered widespread [19].

Sexual aversion disorder is sometimes conceptualized as sexual phobia, yet aversion implies the element of abhorrence and disgust, whereas phobia does not. In our experience, sexual aversion routinely is characterized by women as including elements of revulsion and disgust in ways that phobias rarely are. The DSM IV-TR criteria, however, do not require the physiologic responses that we often associate with aversion. Although sexual aversion typically encompasses these responses (eg, nausea, revulsion, shortness of breath), aversion can also be expressed as persistent avoidance of partnered sexual behavior and a situationally specific panic response. For an individual, whatever painful or traumatic event gave rise to the association of sexual behavior with aversion, the disorder can be conceptualized as maintained by ongoing avoidance of sexual behavior.

Sexual aversions can be general or specific and may develop in response to any sexual stimulus, overt or covert, such that a patient may present with a circumscribed aversion to a highly specific sexual thought or behavior or may exhibit more global revulsion to sexual behavior.

Assessment emphasizes careful sexual history that concentrates on the distinction between events that may have initiated aversion and current behavior that may continue to reinforce the aversive response. Behavioral treatment follows from the conceptualization. Because avoidance of sexual behavior is reinforcing aversion, a graduated exposure paradigm is used in which patients pair relaxation exercises with a graded and patient-controlled reintroduction of sexual behavior. This strategy is often facilitated by the use of a selective serotonin reuptake inhibitor.

Female sexual arousal disorder

Female sexual arousal disorder is the inability to complete sexual activity with adequate lubrication. Absent or impaired genital responsiveness to sexual stimulation is the essential DSM-IV-TR diagnostic criterion. To qualify for the diagnosis, these symptoms must cause personal or relationship distress. Women who have sexual arousal disorder often report having almost no subjective experience of arousal, and the disorder is frequently associated with pain and avoidance of sexual contact. Subjective experience of arousal is not a component of the diagnosis, which has become a source of controversy in the field because it seems that physiologic response and subjective arousal are not highly correlated in women [20].

Female arousal disorder is better understood by using the subtypes of combined arousal disorder (no subjective or physiologic arousal), missed arousal disorder (physiologic arousal but no subjective arousal), and genital arousal disorder (subjective arousal but no physiologic arousal) [18,21]. Clinically, it can be difficult to distinguish between arousal and orgasmic disorder, and either or both can be diagnosable in an individual. A careful sexual history is required for adequate diagnostic clarity.

Treatment of female sexual arousal disorder generally follows the work of Masters and Johnson [22], who emphasized the importance of learning to attend adequately to sexual sensations (sensate focus) using masturbation training while working to improve communication with one's partner. Success rates using these strategies are good, although there has been little evidence-based research after the initial reports by Masters and Johnson.

More recently, physiologic strategies have been introduced, propelled by the success of pharmacologic treatments for male erectile dysfunction. The phosphodiesterase inhibitors have dominated pharmacologic trials as researchers have sought to address the vasocongestion problems that define female sexual arousal disorder. Although vaginal engorgement in the presence of sexual stimuli was demonstrated, subjective experience of arousal was not reliably achieved, and, ultimately, clinical trials of Sildenafil were abandoned [23]. Estrogen therapy, systemic or local, is often an effective treatment for arousal disorder that is acquired after menopause and can improve vaginal blood flow and lubrication. Over-the-counter lubricants may be recommended when lubrication has been diminished. Other topical pharmacologic treatments that are being studied have included the use of L-arginine, Zestra, alprostadil, and androgens.

Female orgasmic disorder

Female orgasmic disorder as defined in the DSM IV TR is the persistent or recurrent delay in or absence of orgasm after a normal excitement phase. It is difficult to determine the incidence of orgasmic difficulties due to the lack of well controlled studies and the variability of definitions and criteria used for orgasmic disorder. Results from the National Health and Social Life Survey (2) indicated that 24% of the 1749 United States women (ages 18–59) had experience a lack of orgasm in the past year.

Despite its importance in our lives, orgasm is simply a transient peak sensation of intense pleasure [24] and might best be viewed as a reflex. Similar to reflex centers serving other functions, the orgasmic reflex center is subject to multiple inhibitory and facilitory influences from direct sensory input and higher neural centers.

It may be helpful to view orgasmic attainment in women as a normal distribution. This distribution reflects women who have no physical problems that might interfere with achieving orgasm. On the left are women who have never experienced orgasm. On the other end of the curve are women who can experience orgasm under almost any circumstance, including fantasy without any physical stimulation. The rest of the population falls somewhere in between.

A large percentage of women are situationally orgasmic. That is, they can achieve orgasm readily and reliably with some forms of stimulation but not others. For example, often women are reliably orgasmic with manual stimulation or cunnilingus but not with intercourse. Intercourse is not a reliable way for many women to achieve an orgasm.

The cause of orgasmic difficulties is likely multifactorial and different for each woman. Many women develop performance anxiety around having an orgasm with a partner. If they start to worry that they are taking too long or will embarrass themselves by making sounds or faces when they do orgasm, anxiety and distraction creep in, and desire and arousal are lost. A number of psychosocial factors, including age, social class, personality, and relationship status, have been most commonly considered to be related to orgasmic ability. In addition, religiosity has been found to be negatively correlated with orgasmic ability due to excessive guilt about participating in sexual activity [24].

Treatment of female orgasmic disorder

Success rates for treatment are high. First-line treatment includes basic education and permission given by a physician. The most effective treatment is a cognitive-behavioral approach in which a woman learns to be comfortable with her body and her own sexuality by altering negative attitudes and decreasing anxiety. The behavioral treatments include directed masturbation, sensate focus exercises, and systematic desensitization [24], all of which women can do in the privacy of their own homes with the goal of helping them discover what stimulation is pleasing and effective. Debunking myths about masturbation as bad is also a common theme in treatment. Masturbation is an extremely effective way for the woman who has never achieved orgasm to experience her first climax. In private and without the pressure of performing for or pleasing a partner, the woman is free to explore her own body and responsivity.

Dyspareunia

Coital pain is the defining symptom of two sexual disorders: dyspareunia and vaginismus. Dyspareunia is defined as persistent, recurrent urogenital pain occurring before, during, or after sexual intercourse that is not caused exclusively by lack of lubrication or by vaginismus. Dyspareunia can be difficult to distinguish from vaginismus because vaginismus can be secondary to a history of dyspareunia and because vaginismus often coexists with dyspareunia. Adequate diagnosis includes establishing whether the dyspareunia is acquired or lifelong and whether it is generalized or situational.

Although dyspareunia has long been considered to be psychogenic, biologic factors often contribute to the presentation. Recent perspectives have characterized vaginismus and dyspareunia as pain disorders that interfere with sexuality rather than as sexual disorders characterized by pain [25]. Conceptualized as such, dyspareunia is seen as a specific pain disorder, with interdependent psychologic and biologic contributions and context-dependent etiologies. Identification of the initiating and maintaining factors is central to the diagnostic process. The differential diagnoses include vaginismus, atrophy, inadequate lubrication, and vulvodynia. Urethral disorders, cystitis, and interstitial cystitis can also present with painful intercourse. Less common etiologies are adhesions, infections, endometriosis, and pelvic congestion.

Dyspareunia may be described by patients as involving pain on entry or deep pain. Painful entry is most typical of vulvodynia, inadequate

lubrication, and vaginismus. A physical examination often reproduces the pain when the vagina is
touched with a cotton swab or insertion of a finger.
Palpation of the walls of the vagina, uterus, and
urethral structures can help identify physiologic
contributions.

Any understanding of the organic etiology
must be integrated with an appreciation of the
ongoing behavioral contributions. Initiating factors, such as trauma or unpleasant experiences
with intercourse, can be identified by taking
a careful sexual history. Maintaining factors,
such as avoidance of intercourse (which can
contribute to anticipatory anxiety), fear, phobic
response to coital intimacy, and negative sexual
expectation contribute to an appreciation of the
factors and negative expectations and attitudes
that perpetuate the pain cycle. Loss of libido and
arousal disorders associated with dyspareunia
may contribute to the worsening of coital pain
over time; these are further magnified by the
distress experienced by the patient and her partner. The psychobiology of sexual pain should be
addressed with a comprehensive, integrated, and
patient-centered perspective.

Vaginismus

Vaginismus is defined as involuntary, recurrent, and persistent spasm of the outer third of the
vaginal musculature that interferes with vaginal
penetration. There has been much criticism of this
definition and whether the musculature actually
spasm. In July 2003, at the 2nd International
Consultation on Erectile and Sexual Dysfunction,
a committee of experts in female sexual function
proposed an alternate definition: "The persistent
or recurrent difficulties of the woman to allow
vaginal entry of a penis, a finger, and/or any
object, despite the woman's expressed wish to do
so. There is often (phobic) avoidance and antic-
ipation/fear of pain. Structural or physical abnormalities must be ruled out/addressed" [26]. This
committee also reported prevalence rates, based
on few studies, to range from 1% to 6%. Although it is categorized under pain disorders, it
is not technically a pain disorder because women
may not feel pain.Vaginismus essentially occurs
as a result of the anticipation of pain. Women
can enjoy sexual activity and be orgasmic despite
having vaginismus, although penetration is not
possible.

For some women, vaginismus is limited to
sexual activity; these women have little difficulty

with pelvic examinations. Similarly, some women
have no difficulty with intercourse but have
vaginismus related to fear of pelvic examinations.
Many women have vaginismus that is generalized
to both circumstances.

Regardless of etiology, the treatment of choice
is a combination of cognitive and behavioral
psychotherapy approaches. The goal is to de-
sensitize a woman to her panic and to help her
achieve a sense of control over a sexual encounter
or a pelvic examination and an understanding that
she is in no danger of experiencing pain so that
she feels safe and calm. Her body can then learn to
relax; the vaginal muscle contractions will no
longer be a necessary automatic defense, and she
will be able to feel in more control of her muscles.
One of the most commonly used treatment
techniques is systematic desensitization. In this
case, women are first taught deep muscle relaxation and then taught to very gradually insert
objects (usually dilators) of increasing diameter
into the vagina.

Initial assessment of sexual problems

The following section describes what to include
in a brief and a detailed sexual history. There are
a number of communication strategies that enhance the efficiency and effectiveness of the
assessment.

Make the environment conducive

The establishing of rapport and putting patients at ease helps to make the environment
conducive for a discussion of sexual problems. If
a physician is comfortable with sexual terminology, patients are more likely to feel comfortable
reporting their sexual concerns. Physicians may
benefit by practicing the use of explicit sexual
terminology to reduce embarrassment, hesitation
in delivery, or other signs of discomfort. A
balance can be found between terminology that
is so formal as to be distancing and so informal as
to be offensive or inappropriate.

When to take a sexual history/assessment

Taking even a brief sexual history during a new
patient visit is effective and indicates to the patient
that the discussion of sexual concerns is appropriate and is a routine component of an office
visit. Many health-related conditions, life-events,
or developmental milestones put patients at
higher risk for sexual problems and provide the

opportunity to inquire about associated changes in sexual function. Urologic surgeries or problems, such as menopause and depression, are risks for the development of sexual problems, and physicians can normalize the frequency with which women find that medical issues give rise to sexual issues.

How to take a sexual history and assess current sexual function

The brief assessment (2–3 minutes)

A sexual history can be a part of the review of systems and should take place in a private setting Sin which confidentiality is assured. The patient should be clothed to eliminate the anxiety and sense of vulnerability that are commonly experienced when sitting in an examination gown [6,27].

We encourage all practitioners to address sexual function in their patients. Even time-constrained visits can include basic assessment of sexual function, which can be limited to a few specific questions. Opening the discussion by mentioning the importance of assessing sexual function as part of your usual history and physical with all patients may help put patients at ease [28,29]. The questions listed in Fig. 3 [29] can suffice for the initial assessment.

It is important that physicians not assume the gender of sexual partners or that the woman's sexual behavior is limited to an identified partner or spouse. For example, if a physician assumes that a 68-year-old widow may only seek out sexual relationships with men, she may be reluctant to discuss any other behavior to the contrary. The implication that the physician does not hold preconceived notions may give patients the courage to discuss a sexual concern at a later time.

It can be helpful to link a woman's current reproductive stage or presenting issue to her sexual function. For example, "Following surgery, many women experience discomfort with sexual intercourse or decreased sexual desire. Have you noticed any such problems yourself?" [6].

When a sexual problem is identified during initial screening, it should be determined whether (1) the concern can be addressed during the current appointment, (2) a follow-up visit is needed to allow more time to address the concern adequately, or (3) the sexual problem is beyond physician's scope of training and the patient should be referred to a specialist. It is helpful to legitimize the sexual problem and to attend to patient discomfort by deferring sensitive questions to a subsequent visit or by supplying alternative terminology for patients who seem too embarrassed to provide explicit sexual details [28].

Elements of a complete sexual history

Because sexual functioning is multifactorial, a thorough sexual history should cover medical, reproductive, surgical, psychiatric, social, and sexual information (Box 1) [30–33]. Although in the past most sexual dysfunctions were thought to be primarily psychologic in nature, biologic factors contribute to the onset or maintenance of sexual problems and must be considered.

Current use of medicines, including prescription, over-the-counter, and alternative medicines, should be identified as a function of the potential

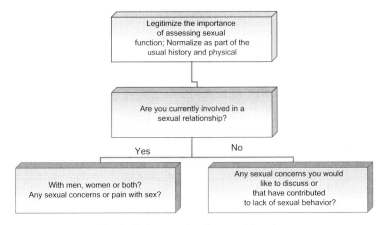

Fig. 3. Basic screening for sexual function.

Box 1. Relevant medical information
for a thorough sexual assessment

Past medical history.
Current health status.
Reproductive history and current status,
   including age at menarche, menstrual
   history, pregnancies, pregnancy
   losses, consequences of deliveries (eg,
   episiotomies), infertility, birth control/
   contraception, sexually transmitted
   illnesses, urogynecologic pain,
   surgeries, and the urologic system.
Endocrine system (eg, diabetes can
   impair arousal and orgasm, androgen
   insufficiency has been linked to
   hypoactive desire, and estrogen
   deficiency has been linked to vaginal
   atrophy and arousal problems).
Thyroid conditions can impair sexual
   desire. Neurologic diseases (eg,
   multiple sclerosis and spinal cord
   injuries) can impair arousal and
   orgasm. Cardiovascular disease has
   been linked to arousal disorder [33].
Psychiatric illnesses (eg, depression) can
   impair sexual desire.

Box 2. Some medications known
to have sexual side-effects

Psychotropic medications
Antidepressants and mood stabilizers
Selective serotonin reuptake inhibitors
   (SSRIs), Serotonin- norepinephrine
   reuptake inhibitors (SNRAs), Tricyclic
   antidepressants, Monoamine oxidase
   inhibitors (MAOi's)
Antipsychotics
Benzodiazepines
Antiepileptics
Antihypertensives
Beta-blockers
Alpha-blockers
Diuretics
Cardiovascular agents
Lipid-lowering agents
Digoxin
Histamine H2-receptor blockers
Hormones
Oral contraceptives, estrogens,
   progestins, antiandrogens, GnRH
   agonists
Narcotics
Amphetamines
Anticonvulsants
Steroids

sexual side effects that many have. Box 2 lists some commonly prescribed medications associated with sexual side effects [32,34–36].

A patient's history may not be sufficient to assess her sexual function, and a physical examination or laboratory testing may help in determining the physiologic factors involved in a sexual complaint [34,35]. Table 2 [35] lists the elements to be included specifically in a urogynecologic physical examination and related conditions that may cause sexual problems. The examination should include evaluation of blood pressure, heart rate, peripheral pulses, edema, and a neurologic screen to assess sensation [31]. Suggested laboratory tests include a hormonal profile, fasting glucose, thyroid function, liver function, cholesterol, and lipids [31]. Androgen levels should be measured when they are at their highest (on days 8 through 10 of the menstrual cycle).

Elements of a complete sexual assessment

Box 3 lists questions that help identify the essential components of a sexual complaint [30,36].

These questions help elicit the patient's perceptions of theproblem, determine its timeline, and reveal current health problems that might affect sexual function. These questions also help identify which components of the sexual response (desire, arousal, orgasm) are compromised. This information can help determine etiology and provide the basis for treatment considerations (eg, education, psychotherapy, medication).

Scales, questionnaires, and checklists

Waiting room questionnaires allow for a quick initial screening of sexual function, and responses can be discussed during the consultation. Moreover, patients learn early in the office visit that sexual health is of importance to the physician and appropriate to discuss. For example, The Brief Sexual Symptom Checklist [31], a short screening tool, can be incorporated into a patient intake form.

Table 2
Elements of a urogynecologic examination and conditions that may impair sexual function

Examination	Condition to consider
Inspection of external genitalia	
Muscle tone, skin color/texture, skin turgor and thickness, pubic hair amount, vaginal pH	Vaginismus, vulvar atrophy, vulvar dystrophy
Cotton swab test of vulva, vestibule, hymenal ring, Bartholin's and Skene's glands (pain mapping)	Vulvar vestibulitis
Expose clitoris	Adhesions
Examine posterior forchette and hymenal ring	Episiotomy scars, strictures
Monomanual examination	
Palpate rectovaginal surface, levator muscles, bladder/urethra	Rectal disease, vaginismus, levator ani myalgia, interstitial cystitis, urinary tract infection
Evaluate vaginal depth	Postoperative or postradiation changes, stricture
Bimanual examination	
Palpate uterus and adnexa and perform rectovaginal examination	Fibroids, endometriosis, masses, cysts
Speculum examination and Papanicolaou smear	Atrophy, human papilloma virus infection, cancer, cystocele, rectocele, uterine prolapse

Adapted from Phillips NA. The clinical evaluation of dyspareunia. Int J Impot Res 1998;10(Suppl 2):S117–20; with permission.

Box 3. Essential questions to include in a sexual assessment

How does the patient describe the problem?

How long has the problem been present?

Was the onset sudden or gradual?

Is the problem specific to a situation/partner, or is it generalized?

Were there likely precipitating events (biologic or situational)?

Are there problems in the woman's primary sexual relationship (or any relationship in which the sexual problem is occurring)?

Are there current life stressors that might be contributing to sexual problems?

Is there guilt, depression, or anger that is not being directly acknowledged?

Are there physical problems such as pain?

Are there problems in desire, arousal, or orgasm?

Is there a history of physical, emotional, or sexual abuse?

Does the partner have any sexual problems?

Meston [37] has developed a slide kit that describes the most commonly used and well validated sexual function assessment tools. This kit is available at http://www.femalesexualdysfunctiononline.org, in the section labeled "Clinician Resources." The website is sponsored by Baylor College of Medicine. The site includes the validity and reliability of the assessment tools, their recommended uses, and information about how to obtain the tools.

Referrals

The decision to refer a patient who has sexual dysfunction depends on the physician's comfort and level of expertise and the complexity of the dysfunction. Some sexual problems are best treated by specialists (eg, a sex therapist or a marital therapist) alone or in the context of a multidisciplinary approach. Referrals are more likely to be accepted by patients when the physician normalizes the nature of the patient's problem and the process of referral to a specialist [6].

References

[1] Kingsberg SA. Loss of sexual desire and menopause: prevalence, causes and impact on quality of life. The Female Patient 2005;30(4):57–63.
[2] Laumann EO, Paik A, Rosen RC. Sexual dysfunction in the United States: prevalence and predictors. JAMA 1999;281(6):537–44.

[3] Bancroft J, Loftus J, Long JS. Distress about sex: a national survey of women in heterosexual relationships. Arch Sex Behav 2003;32(3):193–208.

[4] Simons J, Carey M. Prevalence of sexual dysfunctions: results from a decade of research. Arch Sex Behav 2001;30(2):177–219.

[5] Rosen RC. Prevalence and risk factors of sexual dysfunction in men and women. Curr Psychiatry Rep 2000;3:189–95.

[6] Kingsberg SA. Taking a sexual history. Obstet Gynecol Clin North Am 2006;33(4):535–47.

[7] Kinsey AC. Sexual behavior in the human female. Philadelphia: W.B. Saunders Company; 1953.

[8] Masters WH, Johnson VE. Human sexual response. Boston: Little Brown; 1966.

[9] Kaplan HS. Hypoactive sexual desire. J Sex Marital Ther 1977;3:3–9.

[10] Leif HI. Inhibited sexual desire. Med Aspects Hum Sex 1977;7:94–5.

[11] Basson R. Female sexual response: the role of drugs in the management of sexual dysfunction. Obstet Gynecol 2001;98:350–3.

[12] American Psychiatric Association. Diagnostic and statistical manual of mental disorders. 4th edition, text revision (DSM-IV-TR). Washington, DC: American Psychiatric Association; 2000.

[13] Hayes RD, Bennett CM, Fairley CK, et al. What can prevalence studies tell us about female sexual difficulty and dysfunction? J Sex Med 2006;3: 589–95.

[14] Segraves R, Woodard T. Female hypoactive sexual desire disorder: history and current status. J Sex Med 2006;3:408–18.

[15] Levine SB. Sexual life. New York: Plennum Press; 1992.

[16] Hayes R, Dennerstein L. The impact of aging on sexual function and sexual dysfunction in women: a review of population based studies. J Sex Med 2005;2(3):317–30.

[17] Zumoff B, Strain GW, Miller LK, et al. Twenty-four-hour mean plasma testosterone concentration declines with age in normal premenopausal women. J Clin Endocrinol Metab 1995;80: 1429–30.

[18] Basson R, Berman J, Burnett A, et al. Report of the international consensus development conference on female sexual dysfunction: definitions and classifications. J Urol 2000;163(3):888–93.

[19] Crenshaw TL. The sexual aversion syndrome. J Sex Marital Ther 1985;11:285–92.

[20] Laan E, Everaerd W. Determinants of female sexual arousal: psychophysiological theory and data. Annu Rev Sex Res 1995;6:32–76.

[21] Basson R, Leiblum S, Brotto L, et al. Definitions of women's sexual dysfunction reconsidered: advocating expansion and revision. J Psychosom Obstet Gynecol 2003;24:221–9.

[22] Masters W, Johnson V. Human sexual inadequacy. Boston: Little Brown; 1970.

[23] Laan E, Everaerd W, Both S. Female sexual arousal disorder. In: Balon R, Segraves RT, editors. Handbook of sexual dysfunction. New York: Marcel Dekker, Inc.; 2005. p. 123–54.

[24] Meston CM, Levin RJ. Female orgasmic dysfunction. In: Balon R, Segraves RT, editors. Handbook of sexual dysfunction. New York: Marcel Dekker, Inc.; 2005. p. 193–214.

[25] Binik YM, Reissing E, Pukall C, et al. The female sexual pain disorders: genital pain or sexual dysfunction? Arch Sex Behav 2002;31(5):425–9.

[26] Lue TF, Basson R, Rosen R, et al, editors. Sexual medicine: sexual dysfunctions in men and women. 2nd international consultation on sexual dysfunctions. Paris: Health Publications; 2004. p. 932.

[27] Tomlinson J. ABC of sexual health: taking a sexual history. BMJ 1998;317:1573–6.

[28] Basson R. Sexuality and sexual disorder. Update in Women's Health Care 2003;11:91–4.

[29] Kingsberg SA. Just ask! Talking to patients about sexual function. Sexuality, Reproduction & Menopause 2004;2(4):1–5.

[30] Basson R. Taking the sexual history, part 1: eliciting the sexual concerns of your patient in primary care. Medical Aspects of Human Sexuality 2000;1(1): 13–8.

[31] Hatzichristou D, Rosen RC, Broderick G, et al. Clinical evaluation and management strategy for sexual dysfunction in men and women. J Sex Med 2004;1(1):49–57.

[32] Clayton A. Sexual function and dysfunction in women. Psychiatr Clin North Am 2003;26:673–82.

[33] Berman JB, Berman L, Goldstein I. Female sexual dysfunction: incidence, pathophysiology, evaluation and treatment options. Urology 1999;54:381–91.

[34] Pauls RN, Kleeman SD, Karram MM. Female sexual dysfunction: principles of diagnosis and therapy. Obstet Gynecol Surv 2005;60(3):196–205.

[35] Phillips NA. The clinical evaluation of dyspareunia. Int J Impot Res 1998;10(Suppl 2):S117–20.

[36] Plaut SM, Graziottin A, Heaton JPW. FastFacts: sexual dysfunction. Oxford (UK): Health Press; 2004.

[37] Meston C. Validated instruments for assessing female sexual function (slide kit). Available at: http://www.femalesexualfunctiononline.org. Accessed August 13, 2007.

ELSEVIER
SAUNDERS

Urol Clin N Am 34 (2007) 507–515

UROLOGIC
CLINICS
of North America

Phosphodiesterase Type 5 Inhibitors: State of the Therapeutic Class

Culley C. Carson III, MD

Division of Urology, Department of Surgery, University of North Carolina, Chapel Hill, NC, USA

The introduction of oral agents for the treatment of erectile dysfunction (ED) has revolutionized the treatment of men with erection problems of all severities and etiologies. Sildenafil, available on the world market since 1998, was joined in 2003 by tadalafil and vardenafil as effective safe and reliable oral agents for the treatment of ED. Although these agents have the same mechanism of action, there are differences between the three agents. Sildenafil has the longest patient experience and the most robust data confirming its activity, safety, and tolerability [1]. It has recently been released for use in pulmonary hypertension in addition to ED. Vardenafil, the most biochemically potent of the molecules, has also been demonstrated to be effective in men with severe ED. Tadalafil is unique in its longer half-life and is safe and effective for all severities and etiologies of ED. Tadalafil is also unique in its inhibition of phosphodiesterase type 11 (PDE11), a characteristic of unknown but probably negligible importance [1]. Newer data have also suggested that these agents may be helpful in the treatment of lower urinary tract symptoms (LUTSs), and sildenafil is approved for use in pulmonary hypertension [2].

ED is defined as the recurrent inability to obtain and maintain an erection for sexual function [3]. ED affects more than 150 million men across the world. Although effective treatment is available, most men with ED receive no treatment. ED has a major impact on the quality of life for patients and partners and is often a harbinger of other diseases, including such

cardiovascular conditions as type 2 diabetes mellitus (DM) and hypertension (Table 1) [3].

Among the earliest recognized PDE inhibitors were caffeine and theophylline [4]. The PDE3 inhibitors milrinone and amrinone were investigated in the 1980s as positive inotropic agents for patients who have heart failure. Although PDE5 inhibiting agents have only been available clinically since 1998, the basic science of these drugs began more than a half century ago with the discovery of the enzyme (PDE) that blocked the activity of the second messenger cyclic adenosine $3',5'$-monophosphate (cAMP) in animal models [5]. PDEs are enzymes that regulate physiologic functions in a many tissues and organ systems and can be divided into 100 families. PDE5 is widely distributed, with localization primarily in the pulmonary and visceral smooth muscle, kidney, platelets, and cerebellum. Intracellular levels of cyclic nucleotides, including cAMP and cyclic guanosine $3',5'$-monophosphate (cGMP), determine the activity of these agonist agents. cGMP is the second messenger for the smooth muscle relaxation activity of nitric oxide (NO) in the corpora cavernosa. The connection of NO with smooth muscle relaxation starts with synthesis of NO by nitric oxide synthase (NOS) from L-arginine and oxygen with sexual stimulation. NO originates from nonadrenergic noncholinergic (NANC) nitrergic neurons and endothelial cells. NO is a highly unstable, transient, gaseous mediator produced by endothelial-cell NOS (eNOS) and neural NOS (nNOS). NO crosses the cell membrane and binds with sGC in the smooth muscle cell cytoplasm. Binding of NO and sGC activates this enzyme, with increased formation of cGMP. cGMP initiates the events of penile vasodilation

E-mail address: carson@med.unc.edu

508
CARSON

Table 1
PDE5 inhibitors: selectivity for PDE5 versus other PDE isoenzymes[a]

PDE isoenzyme	Sildenafil	Tadalafil	Vardenafil
PDE1	80	>4000	690
PDE2	>19,000	>4000	62,000
PDE3	4628	>4000	40,000
PDE4	2057	>4000	47,000
PDE6 (rod)	11	188	35
(cone)	10	153	6
PDE7	6100	>14,000	>300,000
PDE8	8500	>14,000	>300,000
PDE9	750	>14,000	5800
PDE10	2800	>14,000	30,000
PDE11[b]	780	6	1620

[a] Selectivity ratio for PDE5 = 1 for all inhibitors; higher ratios indicate lower selectivity.
[b] Physiologic role and clinical relevance are not yet known.
From Francis SH, Corbin JD. Molecular mechanisms and pharmacokinetics of phosphodiesterase-5 antagonists. Curr Urol Rep 2003;4:459; with permission.

and increased penile blood flow, with ultimate storage of blood by direct compression of emissary veins. Erection resolves with the breakdown of cGMP by the PDE5 enzymes. Because PDE5 is the principle PDE in the corpus cavernosum [6], selective inhibition of the PDE5 isoenzyme increases intracellular cGMP concentrations in smooth muscle cells and facilitates NO-medicated relaxation, and thus erection.

The first PDE used clinically for the treatment of ED was papaverine, a nonselective inhibitor of PDE5. Papaverine is administered by means of injection into the corpora cavernosa of the penis alone or in combination with other vasoactive agents. Sildenafil, the first oral PDE5 inhibitor,

was approved for use in men with ED in 1998 [1]. The addition of vardenafil and tadalafil to the market has increased the number of approved PDE5 inhibitors to three agents used throughout the world. Each of these agents has a similar mechanism of action but has pharmacologic and clinical differences. The molecular structures of sildenafil, vardenafil, tadalafil, and cGMP are shown in Fig. 1. Although the structure of tadalafil is different from that of sildenafil and vardenafil, all three PDE5 inhibitors have heterocyclic nitrogen-containing double-ring systems [7]. The structure of the central ring is similar to that of cGMP and competes with PDE5 at the same catalytic site. The principal difference between sildenafil and vardenafil is in the core rings. N-1 of the purine ring in cGMP binds to Gln-817 of the catalytic site [7]. Differences in the core ring of the vardenafil molecule permit stronger binding with one or more of the binding sites. Tadalafil is a β-carboline–based PDE5 inhibitor with modifications of a nitrogen-containing hydantoin ring of sildenafil to form a piperazinedione ring in tadalafil [7].

All three approved agents in this class have similar pharmacokinetic and pharmacodynamic profiles, and each is effective for patients who have ED of all ages, severities, and etiologies. Although there are clear pharmacokinetic and pharmacodynamic differences between these three agents, clinical differences are somewhat more difficult to identify [1]. Indeed, the data of preference trials, head-to-head clinical trials, and selection trials are few. The differences in pharmacokinetics, although having distinct advantages in marketing each drug, may be difficult for clinicians and patients to identify. With the lack of data and well-done clinical trials, it is difficult

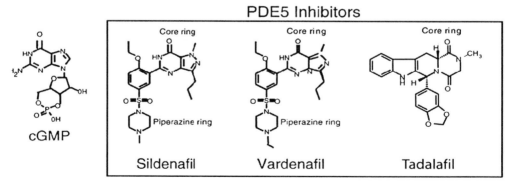

Fig. 1. PDE5 inhibitors: molecular structure.

for the clinician to differentiate between the three agents and to select a PDE5 inhibitor for a specific patient who has ED or a specific agent to switch to if an initial PDE5 agent is unsuccessful or poorly tolerated. This discussion summarizes some of the current data on PDE5 inhibitors and their efficacy, safety, and use in other conditions.

Pharmacokinetics

Specificity

One classification of differences between the three PDE5 inhibitors is that of specificity for PDE inhibition. Because the PDE enzyme is a participant in erectile function, inhibition is a method of facilitating erectile function. cGMP facilitates the relaxation of smooth muscle cells in the corpus cavernosum through the NO pathway. Sildenafil and vardenafil have excellent selectivity for PDE5 versus all PDEs except PDE6, which has some degree of inhibition from both agents, most significantly for sildenafil [8]. This selectivity for PDE6 produces a dose-related impairment of blue-green color discrimination and leads to the blue vision that some patients report. This inhibition is not related to the blindness reported with some PDE5 agents. Tadalafil, a weak inhibitor of PDE6, has a less than 0.1% occurrence of color vision abnormalities [9]. Tadalafil, however, has a higher selectivity for PDE11 than does sildenafil or vardenafil. Although the clinical effect of inhibition of PDE11 is unclear, PDE11 is known to exist in cardiac myosites, the pituitary gland, and the testis [10]. Studies have demonstrated no effect on spermatogenesis or testicular function; however, more robust long-term studies are needed to identify any other effects, if any, of PDE11 inhibition [11]. To date, however, there is no signal that this inhibition is dangerous to patients.

Absorption

Because of differences in gastrointestinal absorption with fatty meals and time of absorption, the three drugs have differences in ultimate plasma peak concentration (T_{max}) based on food intake [12]. Sildenafil, when taken with a high-fat meal has a reduction in maximum concentration (C_{max}) of approximately 29%, with delays of T_{max} that can be as long as 1 hour [13]. This interaction may result in delayed onset or reduced efficacy because of a decrease in serum T_{max}.

This reduction may result in treatment failure in some patients. Thus, patients taking sildenafil should be instructed take sildenafil 1 to 2 hours after eating or with a reduced-fat meal.

Vardenafil, although having less effect with a high-fat meal, has some reduction in C_{max} and T_{max} after eating. A high-fat meal with vardenafil may reduce C_{max} by 18% and delay T_{max} by 1 hour. With a moderate-fat meal, however, there seems to be no clinically significant effect on gastrointestinal absorption [14]. Indeed, clinical phase III trials did not reduce food intake other than high-fat meals, and there seemed to be no change in clinical efficacy with moderate- or low-fat food intake associated with vardenafil dosing [15].

Tadalafil, because of its longer half-life and absorption, is unaffected by high-fat food and can be taken with food. Although there is some measurable decline in C_{max} because of its long half-life, this change is not clinically significant [12].

Duration of action

The three available PDE5 inhibitors have some significant differences in serum half-life. Sildenafil and vardenafil have similar half-lives of 4 hours, whereas tadalafil's half-life measures approximately 17.5 hours for healthy men and 21.5 hours for elderly male patients. Although this change in half-life results in a longer clinical activity period, complete data on the advantages and risks for longer half-life are limited. Long-term and short-term studies of tadalafil, however, do not suggest any untoward concern of increased morbidity with tadalafil's longer half-life. The clinician must be aware, however, that emergent treatment with nitrate medications after ingestion of tadalafil should be delayed for 48 hours compared with 24 hours for sildenafil and vardenafil [13].

Onset of action

Multiple studies have been performed to evaluate the onset of activity of the three PDE5 inhibitors. Because of the artificial nature of these studies, clinical relevance continues to be controversial. Onset of action studies are designed to use stopwatch evaluations by patients or partners after ingestion of the PDE5 agent. Significance in onset of action is measured as first measurement of a statistically significant difference in erectile function compared with placebo. Although this statistically significant difference may occur as early as 11 minutes with sildenafil and 14 minutes with vardenafil and tadalafil, success at this early time point occurs for fewer than 40% of patients treated [16,17]. In patients who have significant risk factors and comorbidities for ED, counseling them to begin sexual activity at 15 minutes or earlier leads to treatment failure; it may also create performance anxiety, and patients may inappropriately lose confidence in the treatment.

Adverse events

The adverse events (AEs) of the three PDE5 inhibitors are quite similar (Table 2). Most AEs are a result of the vasoactive nature of these agents, producing vasodilation in vascular beds other than the corpora cavernosa. Additionally, a small number of patients report visual color changes with sildenafil, fewer still report visual color changes with vardenafil, and there are rare reports of visual color changes with tadalafil. Additional AEs include gastroesophageal reflux disease (GERD)–like symptoms and sinus congestion. All agents are contraindicated with nitrate medications as a result of the risk for additive vasodilation and significant, and occasionally catastrophic, hypotension. All three agents have similar AE profiles. Indeed, long-term studies with sildenafil, vardenafil, and tadalafil have found similar AEs. Because tadalafil and vardenafil have not been available for as long as sildenafil, longer term marketing studies may change these safety profiles; however, after large numbers of

prescriptions, no signal to concern seems to be emerging. AEs seem to decline over time in studies published with vardenafil and sildenafil [18,19].

Safety

Extensive treatment of patients who have vascular risk factors using all three PDE5 inhibitors has demonstrated safety with patients who have cardiac disease. Indeed, sildenafil was originally designed as a cardioprotective agent, and clinical and laboratory studies have confirmed this safety [20–22]. The Princeton Consensus Guideline Conference II carefully reviewed the risks, AEs, and safety of PDE5 inhibitors in men with cardiac disease [23]. This expert conference with meta-analysis of available phase III studies demonstrated no increased risk for cardiac events in patients taking PDE5 inhibitors compared with placebo-treated patients or patients in the general age-adjusted population with similar age and risk factor profiles. Indeed, in several of the studies reviewed, patients taking regular PDE5 inhibitors were demonstrated to have fewer cardiac events than those not taking PDE5 inhibitors.

In laboratory exercise stress tests and monitored electrocardiographic studies, significant risks have not been demonstrated with sildenafil, vardenafil, and tadalafil. Such evaluations have indeed demonstrated an improved treadmill time and increased time to cardiac ischemia and symptoms in patients who have stable coronary artery disease and are taking PDE5 inhibitors, however [13].

Based on these and other studies performed in patients taking PDE5 inhibitors, it is apparent that these drugs are safe in patients with various etiologies, including cardiac patients not taking nitrate medications. Although there is a slight trend of increased QTc noticed with vardenafil, this increase remains within a safe range; only those patients who have congenital QTc abnormalities should be treated with care when prescribing vardenafil for ED [24].

Clinical data

The US Food and Drug Administration approved sildenafil in March 1998 after extensive clinical trials. Vardenafil was approved in August 2003, whereas tadalafil was approved in November 2003. Because sildenafil has a 6-year history of safety and efficacy, it has more extensive clinical and laboratory data to demonstrate its use in

Table 2
Adverse events: PDE5 inhibitors

Adverse event	Reported by more than 2% of patients (%)		
	Sildenafil (flexible dose)	Tadalafil (20 mg)	Vardenafil (flexible dose)
Headache	16	15	15
Flushing	10	3	11
Nasopharyngitis/ rhinitis/nasal congestion	4	3	9
Dyspepsia	7	8	4
Abnormal vision	3		
Sinusitis			3
Flu syndrome			3
Diarrhea	3		
Myalgia		3	

varied etiologies, populations, and severities of ED. In clinical reviews published over the past 5 years, however, it is apparent that tadalafil and vardenafil have similar efficacy and similar safety profiles to sildenafil [1,8,25]. The drug side effects are similar, with some unique differences, but all three agents share a common contraindication for use with nitrate medications [1,26–28]. All three PDE5 inhibitors have vasodilatory action that can potentiate the hypotensive effects of nitrate medications and are absolutely contraindicated in patients using organic nitrates or other NO donors, including recreational NO use. Although hypotension is not inevitable, the blood pressure changes can be dangerous, especially in older patients who have cardiovascular disease [1].

Early data for sildenafil include a 12-week, randomized, placebo-controlled study at a dose of 50 mg that demonstrated a 65% rate of successful intercourse attempts compared with 20% in a placebo group [29]. A 12-week study of vardenafil using middle and high doses of 10 and 20 mg reported similar outcomes, with 65% of patients recording successful intercourse compared with 32% receiving placebo [30]. A similarly designed study using tadalafil at 10 and 20 mg demonstrated successful intercourse in 61% of patients receiving 10 mg and in 68% to 75% of those receiving 20 mg; only 32% of those receiving placebo were successful [16]. Although each of these studies included different populations of patients, had somewhat different inclusion and exclusion criteria, and PDE5 inhibitors excluded sildenafil failures in the latter two, it is clear that all three agents have efficacy in the treatment of ED with all severities and etiologies of ED. In reviewing these studies, however, it is clear that 25% to 35% of patients in these clinical study protocols had inadequate responses to PDE5 inhibitors.

The cytochrome P 450 (CYP) pathway is the principle metabolic system for sildenafil, tadalafil, and vardenafil. Vardenafil is metabolized to a desmethyl-piperazine derivative that accounts for approximately 7% of overall vardenafil pharmacologic activity [31]. Similarly, sildenafil has a desmethyl metabolite that accounts for approximately 20% of its overall pharmacologic activity [32]. Tadalafil is metabolized to a catechol derivative that is extensively methylated and glucuronidated, but metabolites contribute only minimally to tadalafil's pharmacologic activity [33]. Potent inhibitors of CYP3A4, including HIV protease inhibitors like indinavir and ritonavir, azole antifungals, and macrolide antibiotics like erythromycin, can increase system levels of PDE5 inhibitors 2- to 16-fold. CYP3A4 stimulators, including rifampin, can reduce available serum PDE5 inhibitor levels. Grapefruit juice can inhibit CYP metabolism in the gastrointestinal tract and can increase the bioavailability of PDE5 inhibitors. A randomized crossover trial evaluated the effects of taking a sildenafil as a single 50-mg dose 1 hour before, or at the same time as, grapefruit juice (250 mL) in 24 healthy male volunteers. Compared with water, grapefruit juice increased the serum concentration of sildenafil and its metabolites by 24% and prolonged time to T_{max} by 15 minutes [34]. Combination with alcohol, especially red wine, does not seem to hamper absorption or efficacy or to increase AEs [35].

Long-term efficacy

With the increasing experience of PDE5 inhibitor treatment for ED, efficacy over time is becoming better documented. Long-term studies, including 5- and 6-year data from sildenafil and long-term data from the other two PDE5 inhibitors, have demonstrated no clinical evidence for tachyphylaxis with any of these agents. Indeed, the long-standing efficacy of sildenafil, which is the oldest PDE5 inhibitor on the market, strongly suggests that this class of agents continues to be effective with long-term use. Because these agents are used only on an as-needed basis, few patients have taken daily doses for long periods. The few long-term daily dosing studies, however, have not demonstrated conclusively any evidence for tolerability or tachyphylaxis [36,37].

Difficult-to-treat patients

All three PDE5 inhibitors have been demonstrated to be effective in patients who have severe ED. Indeed, after radiation therapy or radical surgery, patients who have prostate cancer and patients who have severe vascular disease, diabetes, or depression are all treated satisfactorily with these agents. Although the efficacy declines in these patients who have severe ED, these agents are safe and effective; however, consideration in these patients should be given to increasing dosage levels to the maximum acceptable dose [1,38,39].

Men with DM are at elevated risk for ED and are difficult to treat. Sildenafil, tadalafil, and vardenafil have all been demonstrated as effective therapies for men with diabetic ED [1]. In the study of men with ED and DM reported by Saenz de Tejada and colleagues [40], tadalafil at a dose of 10 mg or 20 mg significantly improved the International Index of Erectile Function (IIEF) erectile function domain score by 6.4 and 7.3, respectively, compared with 0.1 for placebo ($P<.001$). The erectile function domain scores were similar to those reported in a retrospective analysis of 12 randomized controlled trials (RCTs) involving 637 men with ED and DM [41]. Similarly, 452 men with diabetic ED treated with vardenafil for 12 weeks had significant increases in the erectile function domain score of 5.9 for vardenafil at a dose of 10 mg and 7.8 for vardenafil at a dose of 20 mg compared with 1.4 for placebo ($P<.0001$) [42]. The Sildenafil Diabetes Study Group [43] reported that 56% of men with diabetic ED who received sildenafil (25–100 mg) treatment for 12 weeks reported improved erections in contrast to 10% of patients receiving placebo ($P<.001$). In this study, 61% of men randomized to sildenafil reported at least one successful attempt at sexual intercourse compared with 22% of controls ($P<.001$).

Because intact innervation to the penis is necessary for physiologic erectile responses, substantial proportions of patients who have prostate cancer experience ED after nerve-sparing radical retropubic prostatectomy (NS-RRP) or radiation therapy [44]. Patients who have prostate cancer and are treated with each of the PDE5 inhibitors have significant improvement in erectile function. In an open-label sildenafil study involving 84 men (mean age = 62 years) with ED 2.1 years after prostatectomy, 53% of patients receiving treatment at doses of 50 to 100 mg reported improved erections and 40% reported an enhanced ability to achieve and maintain erections [44]. Erectile function was directly related to the degree of nerve sparing, with bilateral NS-RRP patients tending to respond better than those receiving unilateral or non–nerve-sparing procedures [44]. Lower pathologic stage and older patient age were also predictive of improved outcomes.

A double-blind RCT involving 303 men with ED seen 12 to 48 months after bilateral NS-RRP showed that treatment with tadalafil at a dose of 20 mg for 12 weeks significantly enhanced EF [45]. Among all patients receiving tadalafil, 62% reported improved erections at the completion of study compared with 23% of controls ($P<.001$). Approximately 41% of intercourse attempts were successfully completed among patients receiving tadalafil compared with 19% among controls ($P<.001$) [45]. Treatment benefits were

significant and more pronounced in the approximately two thirds of patients who have postoperative penile tumescence. A total of 71% of patients who have postoperative tumescence receiving tadalafil at a dose of 20 mg reported improved erections at end point compared with 24% of controls ($P<.001$). In these same groups, approximately 69% of intercourse attempts resulted in successful penetration at end point and 52% of attempts resulted in successful intercourse ($P<001$ for each comparison versus placebo) [45].

Mean Erectile Dysfunction Inventory of Treatment Satisfaction (EDITS) scores ranged from 58 in all patients receiving tadalafil to 64 in those with postoperative tumescence, in which a score of 50 or greater indicates treatment satisfaction; corresponding values in placebo controls were 34 and 37, respectively ($P<.001$ for each comparison). Using a single EDITS question rather than the entire instrument, Hong and colleagues [46] documented a sildenafil treatment satisfaction rate of only 26% between 0 and 6 months after NS-RRP, which rose to a maximum of 60% between the 18th and 24th postoperative months.

Therapy with vardenafil at a dose of 10 and 20 mg for 12 weeks also significantly enhanced EF in 440 men with ED associated with bilateral or unilateral NS-RRP [47]. Using the global assessment question (GAQ), approximately 65% of patients who completed vardenafil treatment at a dose of 20 mg reported improved erections, in contrast to 13% of placebo controls ($P<.001$). At study completion, successful vaginal penetration (SEP 2) was reported in 48% of attempts with vardenafil at a dose of 20 mg compared with 22% of attempts with placebo ($P<.001$) and successful intercourse (SEP 3) was reported in 34% of attempts with vardenafil at a dose of 20 mg compared with 10% of attempts with placebo ($P<.001$).

Phosphodiesterase type 5 failure

Because as many as 30% to 40% of patients do not respond to PDE5 inhibitors alone, strategies must be considered to enhance responses [1]. Most importantly, patients must be counseled in the proper administration of PDE5 inhibitors. For vardenafil and sildenafil, patients should be counseled to avoid high-fat meals, and for all three agents, patients who have significant comorbidities should be advised to delay sexual stimulation for 1 hour after administration. Similarly, patients should be counseled that sexual stimulation is necessary. Studies with sildenafil have demonstrated an improvement in response after patients have taken sildenafil six or more times. Because many patients have had prolonged ED, they should be counseled that multiple doses may be necessary before an optimum response is achieved [48]. If a particular PDE5 inhibitor continues to be ineffective, change to another PDE5 inhibitor may improve response. Indeed, in a study of sildenafil failure, more than 60% of patients responded to vardenafil.

Patients who continue to be poorly responsive to PDE5 inhibitors should be further evaluated for hypogonadism. Indeed, sildenafil has been demonstrated to function poorly in the presence of low testosterone levels. Normalizing testosterone with testosterone gel therapy and maximizing the sildenafil dose to 100 mg should increase responses substantially. Indeed, Shabsigh and colleagues [49] showed an improvement in the EF domain scores of IIEF in patients treated with testosterone and sildenafil of 4.4 points compared with sildenafil and placebo of 2.1 points, which is a statistically significant difference. Additionally, these patients treated with a combination had an improvement in ejaculatory function.

Future directions

PDE5 inhibitors were introduced in an effort to improve EF. Their efficacy and safety have been well recorded in millions of patients worldwide. These agents, however, should not be confined only to the treatment of ED. The recent approval of sildenafil for use in pulmonary hypertension has led to the safe, effective, and low-morbidity treatment of patients who have a severe chronic condition, with improvement in their lifestyle and functional status. Sildenafil and tadalafil have also been demonstrated to improve LUTSs caused by benign prostatic hyperplasia (BPH). In two clinical studies, sildenafil has demonstrated effectiveness in improving International Prostate Symptom Scores (IPSSs) and bothersomeness, even though taken only on demand [50,51]. McVary and colleagues [52] reported a 12-week study of tadalafil given daily to men with LUTSs. These patients demonstrated statistically and clinically significant improvement in IPSSs after 12 weeks of treatment but had no statistically significant change in maximum flow rate (Q_{max}). Additional data have demonstrated the importance of chronic dosing of

PDE5 inhibitors in patients after radical prostatectomy. Prophylaxis using sildenafil was demonstrated to improve EF after radical prostatectomy by sevenfold in a study performed by Padma-Nathan and colleagues [53]. A similar pilot study at the author's institution has confirmed the effectiveness of tadalafil taken three times weekly beginning 1 day after radical prostatectomy, with improved erectile function at 6 months [54]. PDE5 inhibitors, especially sildenafil, have shown promise in treating pulmonary hypertension, Reynolds disease, and altitude sickness [2,55–57]. Finally, early data support the improvement of endothelial cell–mediated flow in peripheral arteries, suggesting a possible use for these agents as treatment for conditions known to limit endothelial function [58]. A recent in vitro study has shown ureteral smooth muscle relaxation, suggesting a role for PDE5 inhibitors in facilitating the passage of ureteral stones [59].

Newer PDE5 inhibitors

Two new agents are undergoing phase II and III trials for ED. Udenafil is a rapid-onset agent with a long-acting profile of up to 24 hours [60]. Selectivity is similar to that of sildenafil, with no PDE11 inhibition and minimal myalgia. Having completed phase III trials, udenafil is approved for clinical use in Korea. Avanafil, a fast-acting PDE5 inhibitor, has completed phase II trials, demonstrating a pharmacologic profile similar to sildenafil in efficacy and AEs. Phase III trials are being recruited [61].

Summary

With three effective and safe PDE5 inhibitors, the clinician now has multiple choices in the treatment of patients who have ED of all severities and etiologies. Based on pharmacokinetics, pharmacodynamics, efficacy, and safety, each of these agents can be used. Because no well-controlled head-to-head selection or patient preference studies are available, each clinician must choose an agent based on the profile of the patient, his tolerance, risk factors, and side effects. For patients concerned with timing of sexual activity, tadalafil has the longest duration of action, with a mean half-life of 17.5 hours. In patients concerned with early onset of action, counseling about morbidity and efficacy should be undertaken. Because all three agents have similar onset of action, choices are difficult to make based on early onset. Patients in whom activity is limited because of cardiac disease should be evaluated before prescribing PDE5 inhibitors, and no PDE5 inhibitor should be prescribed in patients taking nitrate medications.

References

[1] Carson CC, Lue TF. Phosphodiesterase type 5 inhibitors for erectile dysfunction. BJU Int 2005; 96(3):257–80.

[2] Bella AJ, Deyoung LX, Al-Numi M, et al. Daily administration of phosphodiesterase type 5 inhibitors for urological and nonurological indications. Eur Urol 2007;52(4):990–1005.

[3] Lue TF. Erectile dysfunction. N Engl J Med 2000; 342(24):1802–13.

[4] Butcher RW, Sutherland EW. Adenosine 3′,5′-phosphate in biological materials. I. Purification and properties of cyclic 3′,5′-nucleotide phosphodiesterase and use of this enzyme to characterize adenosine 3′,5′-phosphate in human urine. J Biol Chem 1962; 237:1244–50.

[5] Sutherland EW, Rall TW. Fractionation and characterization of a cyclic adenine ribonucleotide formed by tissue particles. J Biol Chem 1958;232(2):1077–91.

[6] Corbin JD. Mechanisms of action of PDE5 inhibition in erectile dysfunction. Int J Impot Res 2004; 16(Suppl 1):S4–7.

[7] Francis SH, Turko IV, Corbin JD. Cyclic nucleotide phosphodiesterases: relating structure and function. Prog Nucleic Acid Res Mol Biol 2001;65:1–52.

[8] Seftel AD. Phosphodiesterase type 5 inhibitor differentiation based on selectivity, pharmacokinetic, and efficacy profiles. Clin Cardiol 2004;27(4 Suppl 1):I14–9.

[9] Carson CC, Rajfer J, Eardley I, et al. The efficacy and safety of tadalafil: an update. BJU Int 2004; 93(9):1276–81.

[10] Gresser U, Gleiter CH. Erectile dysfunction: comparison of efficacy and side effects of the PDE-5 inhibitors sildenafil, vardenafil and tadalafil—review of the literature. Eur J Med Res 2002;7(10):435–46.

[11] Hellstrom WJ, Overstreet JW, Yu A, et al. Tadalafil has no detrimental effect on human spermatogenesis or reproductive hormones. J Urol 2003;170(3):887–91.

[12] Corbin JD, Francis SH. Pharmacology of phosphodiesterase-5 inhibitors. Int J Clin Pract 2002;56(6): 453–9.

[13] Padma-Nathan H, Giuliano F. Oral drug therapy for erectile dysfunction. Urol Clin North Am 2001; 28(2):321–34.

[14] Rajagopalan P, Mazzu A, Xia C, et al. Effect of high-fat breakfast and moderate-fat evening meal on the pharmacokinetics of vardenafil, an oral phosphodiesterase-5 inhibitor for the treatment of erectile dysfunction. J Clin Pharmacol 2003;43(3):260–7.

[15] Corbin JD, Beasley A, Blount MA, et al. Vardenafil: structural basis for higher potency over sildenafil in inhibiting cGMP-specific phosphodiesterase-5 (PDE5). Neurochem Int 2004;45(6):859–63.

[16] Brock GB, McMahon CG, Chen KK, et al. Efficacy and safety of tadalafil for the treatment of erectile dysfunction: results of integrated analyses. J Urol 2002;168(4 Pt 1):1332–6.

[17] Porst H, Padma-Nathan H, Giuliano F, et al. Efficacy of tadalafil for the treatment of erectile dysfunction at 24 and 36 hours after dosing: a randomized controlled trial. Urology 2003;62(1):121–5 [discussion: 125–6].

[18] Carson CC SR, Orazem J. Sildenafil citrate treatment for erectile dysfunction: rate of adverse events decreases with time. J Urol 2002;167:167–79.

[19] Stief C, Porst H, Saenz De Tejada I, et al. Sustained efficacy and tolerability with vardenafil over 2 years of treatment in men with erectile dysfunction. Int J Clin Pract 2004;58(3):230–9.

[20] Pfizer. Sildenafil citrate (Viagra) US prescribing information. Available at: http://www.pfizer.com/download/uspi_viagra.pdf. Accessed July 6, 2007.

[21] ICOS L. Tadalafil (Cialis) US prescribing information. Available at: http://www.lilly.com/us/cialis-pi.pdf. Accessed July 6, 2007.

[22] GSK. Vardenafil hydrochloride (Levitra) US prescribing information. Available at: http://www.univgraph.com/bayer/inserts/levitra.pdf. Accessed July 6, 2007.

[23] Kostis JB, Jackson G, Rosen R, et al. Sexual dysfunction and cardiac risk (the Second Princeton Consensus Conference). Am J Cardiol 2005;96(2): 313–21.

[24] Carson CC 3rd. Cardiac safety in clinical trials of phosphodiesterase 5 inhibitors. Am J Cardiol 2005; 96(12B):37M–41M.

[25] Sussman DO. Pharmacokinetics, pharmacodynamics, and efficacy of phosphodiesterase type 5 inhibitors. J Am Osteopath Assoc 2004;104(3 Suppl 4): S11–5.

[26] Ishikura F, Beppu S, Hamada T, et al. Effects of sildenafil citrate (Viagra) combined with nitrate on the heart. Circulation 2000;102(20):2516–21.

[27] Webb DJ, Muirhead GJ, Wulff M, et al. Sildenafil citrate potentiates the hypotensive effects of nitric oxide donor drugs in male patients with stable angina. J Am Coll Cardiol 2000;36(1):25–31.

[28] Kloner RA, Hutter AM, Emmick JT, et al. Time course of the interaction between tadalafil and nitrates. J Am Coll Cardiol 2003;42(10):1855–60.

[29] Padma-Nathan H, Steers WD, Wicker PA. Efficacy and safety of oral sildenafil in the treatment of erectile dysfunction: a double-blind, placebo-controlled study of 329 patients. Sildenafil Study Group. Int J Clin Pract 1998;52(6):375–9.

[30] Hellstrom WJ, Gittelman M, Karlin G, et al. Vardenafil for treatment of men with erectile dysfunction: efficacy and safety in a randomized, double-blind, placebo-controlled trial. J Androl 2002;23(6): 763–71.

[31] Bayer. Vardenafil hydrochloride (Levitra) US prescribing information. Available at: http://www.univgraph.com/bayer/inserts/levitra.pdf. Accessed September 24, 2004.

[32] Pfizer. Sildenafil citrate (Viagra). US prescribing information. Available at: http://www.pfizer.com/download/uspi_viagra.pdf. Accessed July 6, 2007.

[33] Lilly, ICOS, LLC. Cialis (tadalafil). US prescribing information. Available at: http://pi_lilly.com/us/cialis-pi.pdf. Accessed July 6, 2007.

[34] Jetter A, Kinzig-Schippers M, Walchner-Bonjean M, et al. Effects of grapefruit juice on the pharmacokinetics of sildenafil. Clin Pharmacol Ther 2002; 71(1):21–9.

[35] Leslie SJ, Atkins G, Oliver JJ, et al. No adverse hemodynamic interaction between sildenafil and red wine. Clin Pharmacol Ther 2004;76(4):365–70.

[36] Carson CC. Long-term use of sildenafil. Expert Opin Pharmacother 2003;4(3):397–405.

[37] Hellstrom WJ, Gittelman M, Karlin G, et al. Sustained efficacy and tolerability of vardenafil, a highly potent selective phosphodiesterase type 5 inhibitor, in men with erectile dysfunction: results of a randomized, double-blind, 26-week placebo-controlled pivotal trial. Urology 2003;61(4 Suppl 1):8–14.

[38] Carson CC 3rd. Efficacy and safety of tadalafil in men with severe erectile dysfunction in tertiary care academic centers. Curr Urol Rep 2005;6(6):437–8.

[39] Carson C, Shabsigh R, Segal S, et al. Efficacy, safety, and treatment satisfaction of tadalafil versus placebo in patients with erectile dysfunction evaluated at tertiary-care academic centers. Urology 2005;65(2): 353–9.

[40] Saenz de Tejada I, Anglin G, Knight JR, et al. Effects of tadalafil on erectile dysfunction in men with diabetes. Diabetes Care 2002;25(12):2159–64.

[41] Fonseca V, Seftel A, Denne J, et al. Impact of diabetes mellitus on the severity of erectile dysfunction and response to treatment: analysis of data from tadalafil clinical trials. Diabetologia 2004;47(11):1914–23.

[42] Goldstein I, Young JM, Fischer J, et al. Vardenafil, a new phosphodiesterase type 5 inhibitor, in the treatment of erectile dysfunction in men with diabetes: a multicenter double-blind placebo-controlled fixed-dose study. Diabetes Care 2003;26(3):777–83.

[43] Rendell MS, Rajfer J, Wicker PA, et al. Sildenafil for treatment of erectile dysfunction in men with diabetes: a randomized controlled trial. Sildenafil Diabetes Study Group. JAMA 1999;281(5):421–6.

[44] Lowentritt BH, Scardino PT, Miles BJ, et al. Sildenafil citrate after radical retropubic prostatectomy. J Urol 1999;162(5):1614–7.

[45] Montorsi F, Nathan HP, McCullough A, et al. Tadalafil in the treatment of erectile dysfunction following bilateral nerve sparing radical retropubic prostatectomy: a randomized, double-blind, placebo controlled trial. J Urol 2004;172(3):1036–41.

[46] Hong EK, Lepor H, McCullough AR. Time dependent patient satisfaction with sildenafil for erectile dysfunction (ED) after nerve-sparing radical retropubic prostatectomy (RRP). Int J Impot Res 1999; 11(Suppl 1):S15–22.

[47] Brock G, Nehra A, Lipshultz LI, et al. Safety and efficacy of vardenafil for the treatment of men with erectile dysfunction after radical retropubic prostatectomy. J Urol 2003;170(4 Pt 1):1278–83.

[48] McCullough AR. An update on the PDE-5 inhibitors (PDE-5i). J Androl 2003;24(6 Suppl):S52–8.

[49] Shabsigh R, Kaufman JM, Steidle C, et al. Randomized study of testosterone gel as adjunctive therapy to sildenafil in hypogonadal men with erectile dysfunction who do not respond to sildenafil alone. J Urol 2004;172(2):658–63.

[50] Sairam K, Kulinskaya E, McNicholas TA, et al. Sildenafil influences lower urinary tract symptoms. BJU Int 2002;90(9):836–9.

[51] McVary KT, Monnig W, Camps JL Jr, et al. Sildenafil citrate improves erectile function and urinary symptoms in men with erectile dysfunction and lower urinary tract symptoms associated with benign prostatic hyperplasia: a randomized, double-blind trial. J Urol 2007;177(3):1071–7.

[52] McVary KT, Roehrborn CG, Kaminetsky JC, et al. Tadalafil relieves lower urinary tract symptoms secondary to benign prostatic hyperplasia. J Urol 2007; 177(4):1401–7.

[53] Padma-Nathan H, Stecher VJ, Sweeney M, et al. Minimal time to successful intercourse after sildenafil citrate: results of a randomized, double-blind, placebo-controlled trial. Urology 2003;62(3):400–3.

[54] Carson CC 3rd, Hubbard JS, Wallen E. Erectile dysfunction and treatment of carcinoma of the prostate. Curr Urol Rep 2005;6(6):461–9.

[55] Bates MG, Thompson AA, Baillie JK. Phosphodiesterase type 5 inhibitors in the treatment and prevention of high altitude pulmonary edema. Curr Opin Investig Drugs 2007;8(3):226–31.

[56] Krymskaya VP, Panettieri RA Jr. Phosphodiesterases regulate airway smooth muscle function in health and disease. Curr Top Dev Biol 2007;79: 61–74.

[57] Kane LB, Klings ES. Present and future treatment strategies for pulmonary arterial hypertension: focus on phosphodiesterase-5 inhibitors. Treat Respir Med 2006;5(4):271–82.

[58] Reffelmann T, Kloner RA. Cardiovascular effects of phosphodiesterase 5 inhibitors. Curr Pharm Des 2006;12(27):3485–94.

[59] Gratzke C, Uckert S, Kedia G, et al. In vitro effects of PDE5 inhibitors sildenafil, vardenafil and tadalafil on isolated human ureteral smooth muscle: a basic research approach. Urol Res 2007;35(1):49–54.

[60] Salem EA, Kendirci M, Hellstrom WJ. Udenafil, a long-acting PDE5 inhibitor for erectile dysfunction. Curr Opin Investig Drugs 2006;7(7):661–9.

[61] Bayes M, Rabasseda X, Prous JR. Gateways to clinical trials. Methods Find Exp Clin Pharmacol 2006; 28(10):719–40.

ELSEVIER
SAUNDERS

Urol Clin N Am 34 (2007) 517–534

**UROLOGIC
CLINICS
of North America**

Peyronie's Disease

Frederick L. Taylor, MD*, Laurence A. Levine, MD

Department of Urology, Rush University Medical Center, Chicago IL, USA

Peyronie's disease is a psychologically and physically devastating disorder that is manifest by a fibrous inelastic scar of the tunica albuginea, resulting in palpable penile scar in the flaccid condition and causing penile deformity, including penile curvature, hinging, narrowing, shortening, and painful erections. Peyronie's disease remains a considerable therapeutic dilemma even to today's practicing physicians. Peyronie's disease (PD) is a psychologically and physically devastating disorder that is manifest by a fibrous inelastic scar of the tunica albuginea, resulting in palpable penile scar in the flaccid condition and causing penile deformity, including penile curvature, hinging, narrowing, shortening, and painful erections. In spite of multiple treatment options offered since Francois de la Peyronie described PD in 1743 [1], PD remains a considerable therapeutic dilemma even to today's practicing physicians.

History

Francois de la Peyronie was a French Barber Surgeon who practiced from 1693 until his death in 1747 [2]. His career was prolific; he acted as the commander of the medical corps under Louis XIV, founded the Royal Academy of Surgery in 1737, and became a famous surgeon in Paris, caring for prominent Parisians and the kings of Poland and Prussia [2]. His most famous

contribution to medical history is his classic paper on induratio penis plastica [1], describing "disfiguring knobs" [1] and "indurations" causing a bending of the penis. Other investigators throughout history have reported on PD, going as far back as Theoderic of Bologna in 1265 [3].

Etiology and molecular mechanisms

The etiology of PD is the subject of much scientific research. Historically described etiologies included the patient's sexual history or a history of "deviant behavior" [4,5]. Forceful penetration and penile trauma have long been thought to be causative factors [6], and although other investigators have questioned their causality [7], it is likely that they remain an important triggering or epigenetic event in the development of the disease. More contemporary thinking would consider PD as a disorder of wound healing and as such may be considered similar to the formation of hypertrophic scars. Recent investigations have focused on the mechanisms of wound healing, fibrosis, and scar formation and have correlated their findings to the Peyronie's population.

Normal wound healing can be divided into three distinct phases based on biochemical activity: the acute phase, characterized by hemostasis and inflammation; the proliferative phase, characterized by fibroblast and epithelial growth; and the remodeling phase, characterized by collagen breakdown and reorganization. An understanding of the typical biochemical events of each phase is necessary to approach a basic science study of this disorder of wound healing.

Tissue injury is inherent in the creation of wounds, and the body's response to blood vessel disruption is the central feature of the acute phase.

Dr. Levine is a Consultant with Pfizer, Lilly, American Medical Systems, Auxilium, Coloplast; Speaker for Pfizer, Lilly, Coloplast, Auxilium; Investigator with fsPhysioMed and Auxilium.

* Corresponding author.
E-mail address: frederick_taylor@rush.edu
(F.L. Taylor).

Exposure of subendothelial collagen to platelets from broken blood vessels leads to platelet aggregation and activation of the coagulation cascade. Platelets release granules containing several locally active and chemotactic agents, including platelet-derived growth factor, transforming growth factor–β (TGF-β), and platelet-activating factor. The end result is activation of the coagulation cascade, fibrin deposition, and clot formation. The clot functions not only to provide hemostasis but also as a physical scaffold for the movement of acute cellular response elements into the damaged area.

Cellular response follows a consistent pattern, with neutrophils arriving first, attracted by chemotactic agents including TGF-β, tumor necrosis factor alpha, and interleukin-1 [8].

Macrophages follow neutrophil arrival by approximately 48 hours. They function in a similar fashion to phagocytose dead or injurious material and by destroying bacteria or other foreign cells via oxygen free radical reactions. In addition, macrophages strongly recruit other cellular elements by releasing TGF-β [9] and stimulate local tissue repair through the release of vascular endothelial growth factor, insulin-like growth factor, and endothelial growth factor.

The proliferative phase spans days 4 through 12 after injury, and it is during this phase that scar initially forms. Fibroblasts migrate to the site of injury, particularly via the action of platelet-derived growth factor. Their role is the production of collagen and the recreation of the extracellular matrix lost during injury. Although there are many types of collagen in the body, types I and III dominate wound healing. Type I collagen is the primary collagen of skin, whereas type III becomes more important in wound healing. Collagen deposition is dependent on several cofactors, including adequate amino acid supply and vitamin C, which serves as an electron donor during key synthesizing steps. Fibroblasts also produce glycosaminoglycans, the principle elements of which in wound healing are chondroitan sulfate and dermatan. The interaction of collagen and glycosaminoglycans remains an active area of research in the science of wound healing. Endothelial cells proliferate to form new capillaries via the stimulus of vascular endothelial growth factor.

The remodeling phase of wound healing begins during the proliferative phase and results in the final production of a smaller, potentially contracted scar. This phase is marked by a balance between matrix metalloproteinases (MMPs),

which break down collagen, and the formation of collagen by fibroblasts. MMPs are induced by IL-1 and are inhibited by tissue inhibitors of metalloproteinases (TIMP), of which there are two identified molecules (TIMP-1 and TIMP-2), and by fibrinolytic inhibitors such as fibrin/plasminogen activator inhibitor–1 (PAI-1) [10].

Further study of the molecular etiology of PD has unearthed several important growth factors, which may be divided into profibrotic and anti-fibrotic groups. Profibrotic factors include TGF-β1, which is an activator of collagen I synthesis [11] and which is released by neutrophils and macrophages during the acute and proliferative phases of wound healing. El Sakka and colleagues [12] found that, in PD plaques, TGF-β1 protein expression, as measured by western blot, was over-expressed as compared with control subjects. In addition, TGF-β2 and TGF-β3 expression was not enhanced, suggesting that TGF-β1 overexpression may play a role in PD development. Subsequently, TGF-β1 was used to induce PD in a rat model, further solidifying its role as a central modulator of collagen deposition in PD [13].

A second group of profibrotic enzymes include the fibrin/PAI-1 system. Plasmin breaks down the extracellular matrix directly and by activating MMPs to break down collagen. PAI-1 inhibits MMPs and plasminogen activator, which is an activator of plasmin [14]. Fibrin has been studied as an inducer of PD [15,16] and has been used as an inducer of PD in an animal model [17]. It has also been found that levels of TGF-β1 and PAI-1 levels are increased in fibrin-induced PD plaques [16].

The major identified anti-fibrotic enzymes are the MMPs. Although many different MMPs have been discovered, there are a few that seem to be more relevant in PD research. Collagen I breakdown is mediated by MMPs 1 and 13, whereas for collagen III, MMPs 1, 3, 10, and 13 seem to be the most active. Studies are underway examining the possibility of fibrosis regression, particularly through the induction of the nitric oxide synthase pathway.

Recent work has further elucidated the molecular biology of PD and has unearthed potential targets for molecular-based therapies. Ryu and colleagues [18] evaluated the efficacy of a TGF-β1 inhibitor in the treatment of induced PD in a rat model. The rats were injected with TGF-β1 into the tunica albuginea, inducing a PD-like state. The rats were randomized into four groups: control, PD group without treatment, PD with saline injections, and PD with IN-1130 injections. IN-1130 is a small molecule inhibitor of activin receptor-like kinase 5 and is a receptor for TGF-β1. The rats with PD that were treated with IN-1130 showed significant improvement in curvature and fibrosis when compared with those receiving no injections or saline injections. The treatment group had a posttreatment curvature of 9.1° versus 23.0° and 32.6° for the no injection and saline injection groups, respectively.

Del Carlo and colleagues [19] investigated the role of MMPs and TIMPs in the pathogenesis of PD using harvested plaque from patients who have PD. PD tissue samples were found to have diminished or absent levels of MMP 1, 8, and 13 when compared with matched perilesional tunica. PD fibroblasts were cultured with soluble MMPs and TIMPs after treatment with TGF-β or IL-1β. They found that IL-1β stimulation increased the production of MMPs 1, 2, 8, 9, 10, and 13 in PD fibroblasts, whereas TGF-β increased the production of only MMP 10 and decreased the production of MMP-13, suggesting that the abnormal PD fibroblasts can be induced to make MMPs.

It is possible that a genetic predisposition toward impaired wound healing and PD exists. Qian and colleagues [20] compared gene expression profiles in samples taken from PD tunica albuginea plaques, Dupuytren's contractures, and normal palmar fascia and found several gene family similarities between the PD and Dupuytren's groups, including MMP-2, MMP-9, and thymosins TMβ10 and TMβ4.

Epidemiology

Epidemiologic data on PD are limited and inconsistent. The first published epidemiology report on PD was by Pokley in 1928 [21] and consisted of 550 patients. The historically accepted (although likely incorrect) prevalence of 1% in the American male population was popularized by studies from Ludvik and Wasserburger [22] and Devine [23]. In 1991, Lindsay and colleagues [24] reported an overall prevalence of 0.38% based upon hospital record review, estimating that at that time there were 423,000 men in the United States who had PD and that approximately 32,000 new cases occur annually. The mean age at diagnosis in their population was 53 years, with a highest incidence reported for the group 50 to 59 years of age. Sommer and colleagues [25] examined prevalence in the European population. Eight thousand men from Cologne, Germany were surveyed, and 3.2% reported a self-diagnosed palpable penile plaque. Their largest incidence (6.5%) was found among patients who were 70 years of age and older. In addition, 8.4% of men presenting for prostate cancer screening were found to have objective evidence for PD [26]. These studies suggest that the true prevalence of PD may be as high as 10%. Despite these more recent findings, many physicians, including urologists, believe incorrectly that 1% is the correct prevalence rate [27]. It is possible that reported rates of prevalence are falsely low, given patients' unwillingness to report such an embarrassing condition.

Controversy exists as to the age of presentation of PD. Although PD is thought to be a disease primarily of older men, there is research to suggest that PD occurs in younger men and may warrant more aggressive early therapy. PD has been reported in patients as young as 18 years [28]. In addition, in this study [28], patients presenting under the age of 40 were found to have a lower rate of concomitant erectile dysfunction (ED), were more likely to recall a specific traumatic event, were more likely to present during the acute phase of the disease, and were more likely to have multiple plaques and more complicated curvatures. Tefekli and colleagues [29] report an 8.2% prevalence of PD in men under 40 years of age. They also found that younger patients presented most often during the acute phase of the disease, had generally smaller curvatures (<60°), and had an ED rate of 21%. Briganti and colleagues [30] compared 20 patients under 40 years of age who had PD with 28 patients over 40 years of age who had PD and found that the younger patient group had significantly different International Index of Erectile Function scores and subjective loss of penile length. In addition, the younger patients were more likely to present during the acute phase of PD. More recently, Mulhall and colleagues [31] found that men younger than 40 years of age who had PD were more likely to present at earlier stages of the disease, were more likely to have diabetes, and were more likely to have multiple plaques as compared with patients over 40 years of age who had PD. These younger patients may benefit from treatment to minimize disease progression.

PD has historically been thought to be a disease with spontaneous resolution [32].More recent reports have disproved this theory. In 1990, Gelbard and colleagues [33] surveyed 97 men who had PD and found that, over a follow-up course of 3 months to 8 years, 47% felt that their disease had not changed, 40% felt that their disease was worse, and 13% felt that there was spontaneous gradual improvement. Similarly, in 2002 Kadioglu and colleagues [34] retrospectively reviewed 63 patients who presented with acute PD and were followed for 6 months without treatment. Thirty percent of patients felt that their disease worsened, whereas 67% felt that their disease was stable. Only two patients were found to have spontaneous improvement. In the largest published study looking at the natural history of untreated patients who had PD, Mulhall and colleagues [35] reviewed 246 men who presented within 6 months of the onset of PD and were followed for a minimum of 12 months without treatment. At a mean of 18 months of follow-up, 40% of patients who had curvature remained stable, 48% worsened, and only 12% improved. PD is a naturally progressive disease, with low rates of spontaneous resolution. In spite of this published information, survey data have revealed that primary care physicians and urologists believe that PD has a high rate of spontaneous resolution [27]. Men who present with active PD and compromising deformity should be managed with treatment that may offer deformity improvement or stabilization, not "watchful waiting," in contrast to those men who have disease that does not interfere with function because they can be reassured and followed expectantly.

Evaluation of the patient who has Peyronie's disease

Thorough evaluation of the patient who has PD is essential not only to diagnose the disease correctly but also to guide treatment. No universally accepted standardized evaluation for the PD man exists, nor has a validated questionnaire been developed. A suggested guideline for initial evaluation of the patient who has PD, including history, physical examination, and imaging analysis, has been published [36] and is outlined below. Subjective and objective data gathering remains discordant among clinicians and investigators, making the interpretation of clinical trial data confusing at best. The most efficacious mechanism for the evaluation of the patient who has PD may be via subjective and objective assessments specifically geared toward the application of known PD etiologies.

The subjective assessment begins with the patient interview. History should be focused on the onset and duration of symptoms, the patient's presenting signs and symptoms, and the presence or absence of pain. It is useful to elucidate whether the patient continues to experience pain at the time of the initial evaluation because this may represent acute phase of the disease. Pain may be present with palpation, erection, or during coitus and should be differentiated because this may indicate a different degree of acute inflammation. The patient's subjective curvature deformity should be noted. Up to 90% of men may present with ED as their presenting complaint, given that ED may be their most bothersome symptom. It is important to know what prior PD therapies the patient has undergone because such information may help guide future treatment.

A detailed past medical and sexual history should be part of the initial evaluation of every patient who has PD. Medical history should focus on personal or family history of wound-healing disorders, including Dupuytren's contracture, which is reported in up to 20% of patients who have PD. Any risk factors for ED, such as dyslipidemia, atherosclerotic disease, history of tobacco use, and diabetes, should be queried. Patient's baseline erectile function should be assessed using a validated questionnaire. Although a validated PD questionnaire is in development, the International Index of Erectile Function may be used to gauge the patient's baseline sexual function.

The objective evaluation begins with the physical examination. Although the focus should be on the genital examination, an examination of the hands or feet is appropriate given the patient's history. Measurement of penile length is critical because the loss of penile length is not only a known complication of PD but is also a source of great concern among patients. The penis should be measured stretched in its flaccid state dorsally from pubis to corona or meatus. The suprapubic fat pad should be compressed during measurement. Objective evaluation of curvature is best performed using penile duplex ultrasound after pharmacologic stimulation to produce a full erection equal to or better than the patient's at home. Simple erection induction in the office allows objective assessment of deformity. Duplex ultrasound allows assessment of vascular flow rates, the degree of curvature as measured with a protractor, the presence and location of Peyronie's plaque(s), and the presence of any hinge effect. In addition, the degree of plaque calcification can be assessed. Autophotography should not be used as the sole means for curvature measurement because this modality can be inconsistent and inaccurate.

The final portion of the PD evaluation is objective assessment of the patient's erectile capacity and penile sensation. During duplex ultrasound the patient should be asked to grade his pharmacologic erection as compared with home erections. Biothesiometry is recommended to assess penile sensation. Using the distal phalanx of the index fingers as positive control and the ventral surface of bilateral thighs as negative control, the point at which vibratory sensation is achieved should be measured on the mid shaft bilaterally and on the glans.

Nonsurgical therapy for Peyronie's disease

Since the first description of PD in the literature, physicians have been searching for medical therapy options with little confirmed success. Consistent successful medical therapies continue to evade the practicing urologist, although current research into the molecular pathophysiology of PD may lead to a medical cure. Several nonsurgical options are available and may stabilize or reduce deformity and improve sexual function. The evaluation of their efficacy has been compromised by small clinical trials and without, in most cases, placebo control. Data outcomes are difficult to interpret with an absence of a validated questionnaire and in a disease in which spontaneous improvement has been noted in 5% to 12% of patients [31–34]. The nonsurgical options for treatment of the pain and curvature of PD, including oral, topical, intralesional, external energy, and combination therapies are presented below and in Table 1.

Oral therapies

Vitamin E

Vitamin E was the first oral therapy to be described for the treatment of PD [37]. Vitamin E is a fat-soluble vitamin that is metabolized in the liver, excreted in bile, and is thought to have antioxidant properties in humans. Oxidative stress and the production of reactive oxygen species is known to be increased during the acute and proliferative phases of wound healing because neutrophils and macrophages produce these reactive oxygen species species [38], and the inflammatory phase of wound healing has been shown to be

prolonged in patients who have PD [39]. Thus, a biochemical mechanism does exist for vitamin E use. Gelbard and colleagues [33] compared vitamin E therapy with the natural history of PD in 86 patients. No significant differences were found between the two groups in terms of curvature, pain, or the ability to have intercourse. In 1983, Pryor and Farell [40] performed a double-blind, placebo-controlled crossover study evaluating vitamin E for the treatment of PD in 40 patients. No significant improvements were noted in plaque size or penile curvature. We do not recommend vitamin E for the treatment of PD because there is no evidence of benefit in placebo-controlled trials.

Colchicine

Colchicine is an antigout medication that inhibits fibrosis and collagen deposition primarily through its inhibition of the inflammatory response. Due to these factors, colchicine has been used as primary oral therapy for PD and in combination with other modalities. Akkus and colleagues [41] administered an escalating dose of colchicine in a nonrandomized, nonplacebo controlled fashion to 19 patients who had PD over a 3- to 5-month period. Thirty-six percent of patients noted a reduction in curvature, and 63% noted an improvement in the palpable plaque. Seventy-eight percent of those patients that experienced painful erections before treatment had resolution of their symptoms. Kadioglu and colleagues [42] treated 60 patients who had PD using 1 mg of colchicine twice daily, with a mean follow-up of 11 months. They found significant improvements in pain in 95% of men; however, 30% of patients reported improved curvature, whereas 22% of patients reported worsened curvature. Safarinejad performed a randomized, placebo-controlled trial of Colchicine in 2004 with 84 men [43] and found that Colchicine was no better than placebo at improvement of pain, curvature angle, or plaque size as measured by ultrasound. We do not recommend colchicine because of its lack of demonstrated efficacy in placebo-controlled trials. The agent is also associated with gastrointestinal distress, including diarrhea, and with rare aplastic anemia.

Potassium aminobenzoate

Potassium aminobenzoate is a member of the vitamin B complex that is believed to increase the activity of monoamine oxidase in tissues, thereby decreasing local levels of serotonin and thus

Table 1
Nonsurgical therapies for Peyronie's disease

Treatment	Mechanism of action	Comments
Oral		
Vitamin E	Antioxidant that theoretically reverses or stabilizes pathologic changes in the tunica albuginea.	Limited side effects, low cost. Efficacy not proven.
Colchicine	Inhibits fibrosis and collagen deposition.	Mixed reports of efficacy in noncontrolled trials. Single randomized controlled trial failed to show benefit. May cause GI disturbances including severe diarrhea.
Potassium aminobenzoate	Member of the vitamin B complex, thought to increase the activity of monoamine oxidase, thereby decreasing local serotonin levels, which may contribute to fibrogenesis.	Significant reduction in plaque size but not curvature. Expensive and difficult to tolerate due to GI side effects.
Tamoxifen	May reduce TGF-β release from fibroblasts and may block TGF-b receptors, resulting in diminished fibrogenesis.	Efficacy not proven. Side effects may include alopecia.
Carnitine	Believed to inhibit acetyl coenzyme-A.	Efficacy not proven. More investigation is needed.
L-Arginine	Amino acid substrate in the formation of nitric oxide, which is thought to be lacking in PD tissue.	Improvement in plaque size and collagen/fibroblast ratio in a rat model. Well tolerated.
Pentoxifylline	Nonspecific phosphodiesterase inhibitor that may reduce collagen levels in PD plaques.	Improvement in plaque size and collagen/fibroblast ratio in a rat model.
Topical		
Verapamil	Increases extracellular matrix collagenase secretion through fibroblast inhibition and decreases collagen and fibronectin synthesis and secretion. Decreases fibroblast proliferation	When administered topically the drug does not seem to penetrate into the tunica albuginea.
Intralesional		
Steroids	Anti-inflammatory and cause reduction in collagen synthesis.	Treatment with steroids is discouraged by the authors. Effects are unpredictable and may cause atrophy and distortion of tissue planes.
Collagenase	Breakdown of collagen.	Statistically significant improvement in curvature has been noted in men who have mild to moderate disease.
Verapamil	Same as topical verapamil.	Improvements in plaque volume, pain, and curvature have been reported in controlled and noncontrolled trials.
Interferons	Decrease the rate of proliferation of fibroblasts in Peyronie's plaques in vitro. Reduce production of extracellular collagen and increase production of collagenase.	Recent encouraging results with reports of improvement in curvature and pain. Dosing regimens and side effect profiles yet to be determined.

(*continued on next page*)

Table 1 (*continued*)

Treatment	Mechanism of action	Comments
External energy		
Penile ESWT	ESWT-induced inflammatory response with resultant plaque lysis, improved vascularity, and the creation of contralateral scarring.	No statistically significant improvement noted in curvature, plaque size, or pain.
Electromotively administered verapamil with or without dexamethasone	Electric current may have some beneficial effect on wound healing.	Objective improvements of plaque size and curvature have been noted. Adverse effects include erythema at electrode site.
Combination therapy		
Vitamin E and colchicine	Synergistic effect possible.	Improvements in curvature and plaque size have been noted.
ESWT with intralesional verapamil injection	Synergistic effect possible.	Significant improvement in plaque size compared with placebo.
Intralesional verapamil with oral carnitine or tamoxifen	Synergistic effect possible.	Statistically significant subjective improvement in curvature, plaque size, and erectile function in patients treated with carnitine and intralesional verapamil.
Penile traction devices		
fsPhysioMed penile extender	Stretching of contracted tissue may result in the formation of new connective tissue.	Early results demonstrate improvement in curvature, increase in length, and improvement in hinge effect. Side effects were limited to mild discomfort with the device.

Abbreviations: ESWT, electroshock wave therapy; GI, gastrointestinal; PD, Peyronie's disease.

possibly decrease fibrogenesis. This effect has been demonstrated in vitro with PD tissue. Potassium aminobenzoate is used for other conditions, including scleroderma, dermatomyositis, and pemphigus. Zarafonatis and Horrax [44] first described the use of potassium aminobenzoate for the treatment of PD, and a subsequent European study published in 1978 reported a 57% improvement rate with 9% complete resolution in a pooled cohort of 2653 patients [45]. This study did not include a control or placebo group. In 1999, Weidner and colleagues [46] published a randomized, placebo-controlled trial of potassium aminobenzoate given 3 g orally four times per day for 1 year in 103 men. The only significant difference found between the two groups was plaque size, which has not been shown to correlate with a decrease in penile curvature. A 2005 follow-up study by Weidner and colleagues [47] suggested that the use of potassium amionobenzoate may protect against progression of PD plaques. Potassium aminobenzoate is expensive and has low tolerability due to gastrointestinal side effects. It should be dosed at 3 g orally four times per day. We do not recommend the use of potassium

aminobenzoate because of its lack of evidence regarding its efficacy in the treatment of PD.

Tamoxifen citrate

Tamoxifen is a nonsteroidal antiestrogen that acts by competing with estrogen binding sites in target tissues. Tamoxifen affects the release of TGF-β from fibroblasts and blocks TGF-β receptors, thus potentially reducing fibrogenesis [48,49]. In 1992, Ralph and colleagues [48] investigated tamoxifen in 36 patients who had recent-onset PD (duration <4 months). Eighty percent of patients reported a reduction in pain, 35% reported a subjective reduction in curvature, and 34% reported a decrease in plaque size. A follow-up study in 1999 by Teloken and colleagues [50] failed to show any statistically significant difference between tamoxifen and placebo, and there was a reported increase of alopecia in the active treatment group. We do not recommend the use of tamoxifen.

Carnitine

Carnitine is a naturally occurring participant in metabolism. Carnitine facilitates the entry of long-chain fatty acids into muscle mitochondria, which are used as energy substrate. Carnitine is thought to inhibit acetyl coenzyme-A, which may aid in the repair of damaged cells. Biagiotti and Cavallini examined the use of carnitine for the treatment PD in 2001 [51]. Forty-eight men were divided into two groups to receive tamoxifen at 20 mg twice daily for 3 months or acetyl-L-carnitine 1 g twice daily for 3 months. The men taking carnitine saw greater improvement in curvature and had statistically significant improvement in pain. In addition, the patients taking carnitine reported far fewer side effects as compared with tamoxifen. More study is needed to elucidate the role of carnitine in the treatment of PD.

L-arginine

L-arginine is an amino acid that, when catalyzed by nitric oxide synthase, combines with oxygen to form nitric oxide. Inducible nitric oxide synthase is expressed in the fibrotic plaques of PD, and long-term suppression of nitric oxide synthase exacerbates tissue fibrosis [52]. In 2003, Valente and colleagues [52] reported that L-arginine, given daily in the drinking water of a rat model with TGF-β1–induced PD plaques, resulted in an 80% to 95% reduction in plaque size and in the collagen/fibroblast ratio. In addition, L-arginine was found to be antifibrotic in vitro. This suggests that L-arginine, as a biochemical precursor of nitric oxide, may be effective in reducing PD plaque size.

Pentoxifylline

Pentoxifylline is a nonspecific phosphodiesterase (PDE) inhibitor. Valente and colleagues [52] found that normal human and rat tunica albuginea and PD plaque tissue express PDE5A-3 and PDE4A, -B, and -D. In their in vitro study, PD fibroblasts were cultured with pentoxifylline and were found to have increased cAMP levels and reduced collagen I levels as compared with control subjects. Pentoxifilline given orally to a TGF-β1–induced PD rat model resulted in decrease in PD plaque size and collagen/fibroblast ratio. Brant and colleagues [53] reported a single case report of successful PD treatment using pentoxifylline alone. Further studies are required to definitively examine pentoxifylline for the treatment of PD; however, its known biochemical effect and early success in animal models make it an attractive option for oral therapy.

Topical therapies

Verapamil

Interest in topical verapamil for the treatment of PD has followed its success as an intralesional agent (see below). One study demonstrated that tunica albuginea tissue concentrations of verapamil are not achievable through topical application [54]. A recent three-arm trial without a known placebo demonstrated benefit with topical verapamil [55], but this study was significantly compromised [56]. Thus, the use of verapamil as a topical agent for PD is not recommended.

Intralesional therapies

Steroids

The powerful anti-inflammatory effect of steroids made them early investigated agents for intralesional therapy of PD. In 1954, Bodner and colleagues [57] reported improvement in 17 patients treated with intralesional hydrocortisone and cortisone. In 1975, Winter and Khanna [58] showed no difference between patients treated with dexamethasone injections and the natural history of the disease. In 1980, Williams and Green [59] published a prospective study using intralesional triamcinolone. All patients were observed for 1 year after study enrollment. During that time, only 3% of patients reported improvement. Triamcinolone was administered every 6 weeks for 36 weeks; 33% of patients reported improvement, particularly in pain and plaque size. The use of intralesional steroids is discouraged due to the side effects of local tissue atrophy, fibrosis, immune suppression, and lack of objective measures of benefit.

Collagenase

Collagenase was first studied in vitro by Gelbard and colleagues [60] in 1982. A subsequent clinical trial by that group [61] demonstrated subjective improvement in 64% of patients within 4 weeks of treatment. A decade after their initial study, they published their findings of a double-blind trial in 49 men [62]. Statistically significant improvement in curvature was noted in the collagenase treated group; however, improvement was seen only in patients who had less than 30° curvatures and plaques of less than 2 cm. Larger-scale controlled trials of collagenase are in development.

Verapamil

Verapamil is a calcium-channel blocker that has been shown in in vitro studies to inhibit local extracellular matrix production by fibroblasts, reduce fibroblast proliferation, increase local collagenase activity, and affect the cytokine milieu of fibroblasts [63,64]. In 1994, Levine and colleagues [65] reported on 14 men who underwent biweekly intralesional injections of verapamil for 6 months. Significant improvement in plaque-associated narrowing was noted in all patients, and curvature was improved in 42%. The first randomized, single-blind trial of intralesional verapamil was published in 1998 [66]. Significant differences were noted in terms of erection quality and plaque volume. A trend toward improvement in curvature was noted. As a follow up, Levine and Estrada reported on 156 men enrolled in a prospective, nonrandomized trial of patients who had PD with a mean follow up of 30.4 months [67]. A local penile block was performed with 10 to 20 mL 0.5% bupivicaine, followed by injection of 10 mg verapamil diluted in 6 mL sterile normal saline (total volume 10 mL) into the Peyronie's plaque using one to five skin punctures but with multiple passes through the plaque. The goal was to leave the drug in the needle tracks, not to tear or disrupt the plaque. Injections were administered every 2 weeks for 12 total injections. Eighty-four percent of patients with pain achieved complete resolution, 62% were found on objective measurement to have improved curvature ranging from 5° to 75° (mean 30°), and only 8% of patients had measured worsening of curvature. More recently, Bennett and colleagues [68] administered six intralesional injections (10 mg in 5 mL) every 2 weeks to 94 consecutive patients who had PD. Follow-up was at 5.2 months after completion of the sixth injection. Eighteen percent of patients (n = 17) were found to have improved curvatures (average improvement of 12°), 60% (n = 56) had stable curvature, and 22% (n = 21) had increased curvature (average increase of 22°). All patients who had pretreatment penile pain had improvement at follow-up. The authors suggest that these data support intralesional verapamil for the stabilization of PD. It may be that six injections provides stabilization but is insufficient to accomplish reduction of curvature. We recommend a trial of six injections with each injection occurring every 2 weeks. If no improvement is noted, the therapy may be terminated, the verapamil dose can be increased to 20 mg, or interferon (IFN) injections may be offered. We consider verapamil to be contraindicated in patients who have ventral plaques or extensive plaque calcification.

Interferons

Duncan and colleagues [69] reported in 1991 that IFNs decrease the rate of proliferation of fibroblasts in Peyronie's plaques in vitro, reduce the production of extracellular collagen, and increase the activity of collagenase. Initial studies performed by Wegner and colleagues [70,71] demonstrated low rates of improvement but a high incidence of side effects, including myalgia and fever. In 1999, Ahuja and colleagues [72] reported on 20 men who received 1×10^6 units of IFN-α–2b biweekly for 6 months. All patients reported softening of plaque, 90% of patients presenting with pain had improvement, and 55% had a subjective reduction in plaque size. Dang and colleagues [73] administered 2×10^6 units to 21 men biweekly for 6 weeks and found objective curvature improvements in 67% and improvement in pain in 80%. Seventy-one percent of patients reported improvement in ED symptoms. In 2006, Hellstrom and colleagues [74] reported on a placebo-controlled, multicenter trial of 117 patients who underwent biweekly injections of 5×10^6 units for a total of 12 weeks. Average curvature in the treatment group improved 13°, versus 4° in the placebo arm, and 27% of patients in the treatment group had measured improvement, versus 9% of saline group. Pain resolution was noted in 67% of the patients receiving treatment versus 28% for patients receiving placebo. IFN therapy requires further investigation to adequately determine efficacy, dosing regimens, and side-effect profiles before its routine use in patients who have PD.

External energy therapies

Penile electroshock wave therapy

Local penile electroshock wave therapy (ESWT) has been suggested to be helpful. Various hypotheses about its mechanism of action exist, including direct damage to the plaque resulting in an inflammatory reaction with increased macrophage reaction leading to plaque lysis, improved vascularity resulting in plaque resorption, and the creation of contralateral scarring of the penis resulting in "false" straightening [75]. Hauck and colleagues [76] randomized 43 men to ESWT or oral placebo for 6 months. No significant effect was noted in terms of curvature, plaque size, or subjective improvement in sexual function or rigidity. More recent work from a German group [77,78] randomized 102 men to ESWT or to receive placebo shocks.

There was no statistically significant difference found between the groups for plaque size, improvement of deformity, or sexual function post-treatment. ESWT cannot be recommended as therapy for PD.

Iontophoresis

Iontophoresis involves the transport of ions through tissue by means of an electric current. Several studies have investigated the efficacy of topically applied verapamil with or without dexamethasone with enhanced penetration using iontophoresis [79–82]. In 2002, Levine and colleagues [83] confirmed that verapamil was found within the exposed tunica albuginea by examining surgically retrieved tunica albuginea from patients after a single intraoperative exposure during plaque incision and grafting surgery. Di Stasi and colleagues [82] recently reported on a prospective, randomized study of 96 patients treated with 5 mg verapamil plus 8 mg dexamethasone using iontophoresis versus 2% lidocaine delivered electromotively. Forty-three percent of patients in the verapamil/dexamethasone group noted objective improvement in plaque size and curvature; no changes were noted in the lidocaine group. In 2007, Greenfield and colleagues [84] reported on the use of 10 mg verapamil versus saline iontophoresis. Patients were assessed using papavarine-induced erections before and 1 month after treatment. Sixty-five percent of patients in the verapamil group demonstrated improvement in curvature, versus 58% in the saline group. Mean curvature improvement was 9.1° in the treatment group versus 7.6° in the saline group, which is not as robust as intralesional verapamil injections. In addition, the electric current may have some beneficial effect on wound healing, which is supported in the dermatologic literature [85]. Further investigation into iontophoresis is ongoing.

Combination therapy

Vitamin E and colchicine

A placebo-controlled study by Preito Castro and colleagues [86] randomized 45 patients to receive vitamin E and colchicine or ibuprofen. Statistically significant improvements in curvature and plaque size were noted in the treatment arm. Patients in the treatment arm reported a greater decrease in pain, although this did not reach statistical significance.

Electroshock wave therapy with intralesional verapamil injection

In 1999, Mirone and colleagues [87] prospectively examined two groups of patients who had PD: one group was treated with ESWT, and the other group received ESWT and perilesional verapamil injections. A 52% improvement in plaque size by ultrasound was noted in the ESWT-only group compared with 19% for the combination therapy. A follow-up study by the same investigators involving 481 patients demonstrated a 49% improvement in plaque size among those treated with combination therapy [88].

Intralesional verapamil with oral carnitine or tamoxifen

In 2002, Cavallini and colleagues [89] randomized 60 men to receive intralesional verapamil plus oral carnitine or intralesional verapamil plus oral tamoxifen. Statistically significant subjective improvements in curvature, plaque size, and erectile function were found in the carnitine group. No difference in improvement of pain was found between the two groups.

Penile traction devices

The use of tissue expanders has long been a mainstay of treatment in the orthopedic, oral-maxillofacial, and plastic surgical fields. It is well documented that gradual expansion of tissue results in the formation of new bone and connective tissue. Recently, initial work was done to evaluate the efficacy of a penile extender device (fsPhysioMed; FastSize LLC, Aliso Viejo, CA) for the treatment of PD. An initial pilot study at our institution of 10 patients found that daily use of the fsPhysioMed device resulted in a 33% improvement in curvature (from an average curvature of 51° to 34°), an increase in penile length ranging from 0.5 to 2.0 cm, and an improvement in hinge effect in all those with advanced narrowing or indentation. No patients noted recurrence or worsening of curvature, and there was no incidence of local skin changes, ulceration, loss of sensation, or worsening of curvature. Long-term and larger studies are needed before penile extender devices can be recommended for all patients who have PD.

We favor a multimodal approach to nonsurgical therapy for PD. All patients are given pentoxifylline 400 mg orally three times a day, with L-arginine 1000 mg twice a day. Patients are encouraged to use the fsPhysioMed device 2 to 8 hours per day for 6 months and are offered verapamil injections as a means to improve curvature and pain.

Surgical treatment of Peyronie's disease

Surgery remains the gold standard treatment for PD. Surgery should be performed only when the disease is stable enough to ensure long-term efficacy. In general, surgery should be considered only when disease duration is 9 months to 1 year and when the disease has remained stable for at least 6 months.

Preoperative history, physical examination, and duplex ultrasonography are essential to formulating a treatment plan. A treatment algorithm was developed at Rush University Medical Center in Chicago, IL, based on the patient's erectile function, degree of curvature, and presence of hinge effect (Fig. 1) [90]. In brief, if rigidity is adequate for intromission with or without the use of pharmacotherapy and if the patient has a simple curve less than 60° and no hourglass or hinge effect, the patient is offered a plication procedure. If the patient has a complex curve greater than 60° or presence of destabilizing hourglass or hinge effect, he is offered a grafting procedure. Patients whose rigidity is inadequate for intromission despite oral pharmacotherapy are offered penile prosthesis with manual molding. Informed consent is critical before the initiation of any therapy for PD, particularly surgical correction. The risks of reduction of rigidity, diminished penile sensation, delayed ejaculation, shortening of the penis, and persistent or recurrent curvature should be carefully discussed with the patients and carefully documented in the medical record. It may also be wise to discuss with patients the expected changes in penile shape consistent with the early postoperative period.

PD – Surgical Algorithm

- When rigidity adequate +/- pharmacotherapy

1) Tunica plication techniques

 - Simple curve < 60 degrees

 - No destabilizing hourglass or hinge effect

2) Partial Excision and Grafting

 -Complex curve >60 degrees

 -Destabilizing hourglass or hinge effect

Fig. 1. Surgical algorithm for Peyronie's disease.

Surgery for PD generally falls into two categories: plication procedures for less severe disease and grafting procedures for significant ($>60°$) curves or the presence of hinge effect. It is beyond the scope of this article to detail all the available and practiced surgical techniques. Instead, the Rush University (Chicago) procedures of Tunica Albuginea Plication and plaque incision with Tutoplast (Coloplast, Minneapolis, MN) human pericardial grafting are detailed herein. Other published outcomes are presented in Tables 2 and 3 [91–105].

Tunica albuginea plication

An artificial erection is created in the operating room using 60 mg of papavarine and infusion of saline using an infusion pump. A circumcising incision is made 1.5 to 2 cm proximal to the corona, and the penis is degloved, exposing Buck's fascia to the base of the penis. Hemostasis is best achieved using bipolar current to avoid injury to the sensory nerves.

For ventral curves, the segment of Buck's fascia overlying the deep dorsal vein is opened, and the vein opposite the point of maximum curvature is excised. Circumflex and perforating veins are ligated using 4-0 silk ties, and the lateral neurovascular bundles are carefully elevated to expose the dorsum of the tunic. A pair of transverse incisions, each 1.0 to 1.0 cm in length and separated by 0.7 to 1.5 cm, is made directly over the septum. The incision is carried down sharply with the scalpel through the longitudinal tunical fibers, leaving the circular fibers intact. The intervening tunica is thinned to reduce the bulk of the plicated tissue. The tunica is plicated using 2-0 braided polyester suture (Tevdek; Teleflex Medical, Fall River, MA) in an inverting vertical mattress fashion, thus burying the knot; typically a single central plication suture is placed. The plication is reinforced with several 3-0 PDS sutures (Ethicon, Somerville, NJ) placed in a Lembert fashion. Penile straightness is rechecked by recreating an artificial erection using saline. Two to three plications are usually sufficient, although as many as six plications may be necessary.

For dorsal curves, Buck's fascia is opened longitudinally on both sides of the urethra, and the plication incisions include the thick ridge of tunica adjacent to the urethra bilaterally. Plication sutures are placed in the same fashion as for ventral curves.

Table 2
Published plication data

Author	Date of publication	Patient no.	Procedure type	% Straight	% with ED	Diminished sensation (%)	Mean follow-up duration (mo)
Montague et al [91]	1999	28	Modified corporoplasty (transverse closure of longitudinal corporal incisions)	89	4	Not reported	24.1
Gholami et al [92]	2002	132	16-dot plication technique	85	3	Not reported	31
Syed et al [93]	2003	50	Nesbit plication	90	Not reported	21	84
Savoca et al [94]	2004	218	Nesbit plication	86.3	13	11	89
Rolle et al [95]	2005	50	Nesbit plication	100	0	Not reported	Not reported
Brock et al [96]	2006	23	Minimally invasive intracorporeal plaque incision	91	Not reported	4	25
Greenfield et al [97]	2006	68	Tunica albuginea	99	7.3	4	29

Abbreviation: ED, erectile dysfunction.

Once satisfactory straightening has been reached, Buck's fascia is reapproximated using running 4-0 chromic suture, and the skin is reapproximated with 4-0 chromic sutures on a cutting needle in a horizontal mattress fashion. Xeroform (Tyco Health Care, Mansfield, MA) dressing is placed over the suture line and covered with sterile gauze. A Cobandressing (3M, St. Paul, MN) is lightly wrapped from the glans to the base of the penis.

The dressing is left in place for 3 days, at which time the patient is instructed to remove it at home. Patients are instructed to return for their initial follow-up visit 2 weeks after surgery. From weeks 2 to 6, patients are instructed in massage and stretch rehabilitation, which is undertaken for 5 minutes twice daily. Sexual activity is allowed 6 weeks postoperatively. Based upon the recent report by Moncada and colleagues [106], for patients undergoing surgical reconstruction, the use of an external penile traction device is recommended beginning 2 to 3 weeks postoperatively. It should be applied daily for up to 12 hours for 3 months to reduce postoperative shortening.

A review of long-term follow-up data for the Tunica Albuginea Plication procedure was recently performed [107]. Ninety patients were reviewed, with an average follow-up of 72 months.

Ninety-three percent of patients reported resolution of their curvature, with only 2% of patients reporting a recurrence of their curvature postoperatively. Twenty-eight percent of patients developed noted diminished rigidity, but 88% of patients were still capable of intromission with the use of oral phosphodiesterase-5 inhibitors. Sixty-eight percent of patients felt that their sensation was unchanged, and 98% report continued ability to achieve orgasm. In terms of penile shortening, which is a known complication of plication surgery, 74% of patients subjectively felt that their penis was shorter; however, objective, office-based data demonstrated that the majority (82%) of patients did not lose length.

Peyronie's plaque incision/partial excision and human pericardial tissue grafting

Penile reconstruction in the face of severe deformity demands plaque incision or partial excision with the placement of graft tissue over the resulting defect. Many different graft tissues are available, from autologous vein, dermal, or fascial transfer to commercially available "off-the-shelf" materials. Concerns regarding all grafting procedures include graft contracture, curvature recurrence, neurovascular injury, and impotence.

Table 3
Published graft data

Author	Date of publication	Patient no.	Procedure type	% Straight	% with ED	Diminished sensation (%)	Mean follow-up duration (mo)
Gelbard et al [98]	1996	69	Plaque incision and temporalis fascia grafting	74	14	Not reported	Not reported
Lue et al [99]	1998	112	Plaque incision with venous grafting	96	12	10	18
Hatzichristou et al [100]	2002	17	Tunica albuginea–free grafting	100	0	Not reported	39
Egydio et al [101]	2002	33	Tunica albuginea incision and bovine pericardial grafting	87.9	Not reported	Not reported	19
Levine et al [102]	2003	40	Tunica albuginea incision and human pericardial grafting	98	30	Not reported	22
Kalsi et al [103]	2005	113	Plaque incision with venous grafting	86	15	Not reported	12
Breyer et al [104]	2007	19	Porcine small intestine submucosa Graft	63	53	Not reported	15
Hsu et al [105]	2007	48	Plaque incision with venous grafting	90	5	Not reported	Not reported

Abbreviation: ED, erectile dysfunction.

The ideal graft material should be readily available, should possess enough compliance to function with erections, and should have a high rate of efficacy with a low complication rate [108]. Although the ideal graft material has yet to be confirmed, our preference is the Tutoplast processed human pericardium.

An artificial erection is created in the operating room using 6 mg of papavarine and a saline infusion pump. The penis is degloved via a circumcising incision initiated 1.5 cm proximal to the corona. When correcting a dorsal curvature, the neurovascular bundle is elevated over the area of maximum curvature, and Buck's fascia is incised bilaterally and longitudinal to the urethra. In the absence of hinge effect, a simple transverse incision should be made centered over the area of maximum curvature and performed to the 3 and 9 o'clock positions on the shaft bilaterally. Longitudinal extensions of this incision can be made at a 30° angle to the transverse incision, creating the modified "H" incision and thus resulting in a rectangular defect. In the presence of hinge effect, indentation, or extensive calcification, this tissue should be excised before graft placement.

Upon incision or partial excision of the plaque, the penis is placed on stretch, and 4-0 PDS (Ethicon, Somerville, NJ) stay sutures are placed in the four corners of the defect. The penis's stretched length should be remeasured at this point in the operation; it will likely be 1 cm longer than preoperatively. The stay sutures are used to stretch the defect to affect an accurate measurement of the defect in the longitudinal and transverse directions. Another stay suture is placed at the 12 o'clock position. The Tutoplast processed pericardial graft should be secured to the tunica in a running fashion, leaving approximately 10% extra to account for any minor graft shrinkage. The artificial erection is recreated, and the penis is inspected for residual deformity. Additional grafting or plication measures may be taken at this time. A recent analysis demonstrated that adding a plication does not compromise postoperative rigidity or cause significant shortening [109]. The graft is secured to septal fibers using two or three simple 4-0 PDS sutures. Buck's fascia is reapproximated using 4-0 chromic suture (Ethicon, Somerville, NJ), and the penile skin is reapproximated with horizontal mattress sutures of 4-0 chromic on a cutting needle. The same dressing as for the Tunica Albuginea Plication procedure is used, with Xeroform gauze, a dry sterile dressing, and Coban dressing.

The Coban dressing is removed on postoperative day 3, and the patient is seen in the office on postoperative day 14. At that time the patient is instructed on penile massage and stretch therapy as a means to aid in recovery. Small subgraft hematomas are not routinely aspirated unless they are a source of significant postoperative pain, and our experience is that the hematomas resorb with time, causing no residual effect. The use of penile traction devices is encouraged beginning 2 or 3 weeks postoperatively. These patients are encouraged to use a low-dose phosphodiesterase inhibitor nightly on postoperative days 10 to 50 as pharmacologic erectile rehabilitation [109].

A recent review of our long-term results of Tutoplast grafting for severe PD was recently performed [107]. One hundred eleven patients undergoing our grafting procedure were retrospectively reviewed, with an average follow-up of 58 months. Ninety-two percent of patients remained satisfactorily surgically straightened. There was some curvature recurrence in 12%. Thirty-five percent of patients noted diminished postoperative rigidity, but 76% of patients were able to achieve intromission with PDE-5 inhibitors. Ninety percent of these patients were taking PDE-5 inhibitors before their operation. Although 65% of patients felt that they lost length, flaccid stretched penile length measurements in the office demonstrated an average gain of 0.2 cm. Sensation remained intact in the majority of patients, with 89% reporting an ability to achieve orgasm.

Straightening with penile prosthesis

Patients presenting with PD and ED can achieve curvature straightening and definitive mechanical erections through the placement of a penile prosthesis. The risks of ED development after surgical correction of PD are well known and described, and all men who have baseline ED, vascular comorbidities, or severe curvatures likely requiring significant plaque excision and grafting should be counseled to consider penile prosthesis. Prosthesis choice depends on the patient and surgeon; the medical literature supports the use of semirigid implants [110,111], two-piece implants [112,113], and three-piece implants [114,115], although patient satisfaction seems to be best with inflatable devices [116]. Our treatment algorithm involves placement of penile prosthesis followed by manual molding and, if necessary, a relaxing tunical incision with or without patch grafting (Fig. 2). The prosthesis should be placed in the usual fashion.

PD – Prosthesis Algorithm

- When inadequate rigidity

Penile Prosthesis Placement
- IPP alone (not Ultrex)
- With modeling
- With incision
- With incision and grafting (when defect >2 cm)

Fig. 2. Prosthesis algorithm for Peyronie's disease.

After closure of the corporotomy incisions, the prosthesis should be inflated, demonstrating curvature. The cylinder tubing is clamped to protect the pump, and the penis should be bent in a direction opposite the curvature and held in that configuration for 60 to 90 seconds. The cylinders should be then filled with more saline, and the procedure should be repeated until adequate straightening (residual curve $\leq 30°$) is achieved. The cylinders should then be emptied and filled to approximately 75% rigidity, at which point penile straightness should be reassessed. If residual curve $> 30°$ persists, one option is to consider a relaxing tunical incision after elevating the overlying Buck's fascia. If the defect is 2 cm or greater, it should be grafted (we prefer Tutoplast processed pericardium) to prevent cylinder herniation or recurrent cicatrix contracture. Regular use of the prosthesis by the patient (once completely healed from surgery) helps to maintain penile straightness because the prosthetic cylinder acts like an internal tissue expander.

References

[1] La Peyronie F. Sur quelques obstaclesqui s'opposent à l'éjaculation nautrelle de la semence. Mem Acad Royale Chir 1743;1:337–42.

[2] Akkus E. Historical review of Peyronie's disease. In: Levine LA, editor. Peyronie's Disease: a guide to clinical management. Totowa (NJ): Humana Press; 2007. p. 1–8.

[3] Borgogni T. Cyrurgia edita et compilata. Venice 1498;1265–75.

[4] Murphy LJT. Miscellanea: peyronie's disease (fibrous cavernositis). In: Charles C, editor. The history of urology. 1st edition. Springfield (IL): Thomas; 1972. p. 485–6.

[5] Wesson MD. Peyronie's disease (plastic induration) cause and treatment. J Urol 1943;49:350–6.

[6] Devine, et al. Proposal: trauma as the cause of the Peyronie's lesion. J Urol 1997;157(1):285–90.

[7] Zargooshi, et al. Trauma as the cause of Peyronie's disease: penile fracture as a model of trauma. J Urol 2004;172(1):186–8.

[8] Feiken E, Romer J, Eriksen J, et al. Neutrophils express tumor necrosis factor-alpha during mouse skin wound healing. J Invest Dermatol 1995;105:120.

[9] DiPietro LA. Wound healing: the role of the macrophage and other immune cells. Shock 1995;4:233.

[10] Ravanti L, Kahari VM. Matrix metalloproteinases in wound repair. Int J Mol Med 2000;6:391–407.

[11] El Sakka AI, Hassoba HM, Chui RM. An animal model of Peyronie's like condition associated with an increase of transforming growth factor β mRNA and protein expression. J Urol 1997;158:2284–90.

[12] El Sakka AI, Hassoba HM, Pillarisetty RJ, et al. Peyronie's disease is associated with an increase in transforming growth factor-beta protein expression. J Urol 1997;158:1391–4.

[13] Bivalacqua TJ, Champion HC, Leungwattanakij S, et al. Evaluation of nitric oxide synthase and arginase in the induction of a Peyronie's like condition in the rat. J Androl 2001;22:497–506.

[14] Kucharewicz I, Kowal K, Buczko W, et al. The plasmin system in airway remodeling. Thromb Res 2003;112:1–7.

[15] Van de Water L. Mechanisms by which fibrin and fibronectin appear in healing wounds: implications for Peyronie's disease. J Urol 1997;157:306–10.

[16] Davila H, Magee TR, Rajfer J, et al. Peyronie's disease is associated with an increase of plasminogen activator inhibitor-1 in fibrotic plaque. Urology 2005;65:645–8.

[17] Davila H, Ferrini M, Rajfer J, et al. Fibrin induction of a Peyronie's-like plaque in the rat penile tunica albuginea. BJU Int 2003;91:830–8.

[18] Ryu JK, Piao S, Shin HY, et al. IN-1130, A novel transforming growth factor type 1 receptor kinase (ALK 5) inhibitor, regresses fibrotic plaque and corrects penile curvature in a rat model of Peyronie's disease [abstract 749]. In: Annual Meeting of the American Urological Association. Anaheim (CA), 2007.

[19] Del Carlo M, Levine LA, Cole AA. Differential regulation of matrix metalloproteinases (MMPs) and tissue inhibitors of matrix metalloproteinases (TIMPs) by interleukin-1beta (IL-1B) and transforming growth factor-beta (TGF-B) in Peyronie's fibroblasts [abstract 755]. In: Annual Meeting of the American Urological Association. Anaheim (CA), 2007.

[20] Qian A, Meals RA, Rajfer J, et al. Comparison of gene expression profiles between Peyronie's disease and Dupuytren's contracture. Urology 2004;64(2):399–404.

[21] Polkey HJ. ID induratio penis plastica. Urol Cutaneous Rev 1928;32:287–308.

[22] Ludvik W, Wasserburger K. Die Radiumbehandlung der induration penis plastica. Z Urol Nephrol 1968;61:319–25.

[23] Devine CJ. Introduction to Peyronie's Disease. J Urol 1997;157:272–5.

[24] Linday MB, et al. The incidence of Peyronie's disease in Rochester, Minnesota, 1950 through 1984. J Urol 1991;146:1007–9.

[25] Sommer F, et al. Epidemiology of Peyronie's disease. Int J Impot Res 2002;14:379–83.

[26] Mulhall JP, Creech SD, Boorjian SA, et al. Subjective and objective analysis of the prevalence of Peyronie's disease in a population of men presenting for prostate cancer screening. J Urol 2004;171:2350–3.

[27] La Rochelle JC, Levine LA. A Survey of primary-care physicians and urologists regarding Peyronie's disease. J Sex Med 2007;4:1167–73.

[28] Levine LA, Estrada CR, Storm DW, et al. Peyronie's disease in younger men: characteristics and treatment results. J Androl 2003;24:27–32.

[29] Tefekli A, Kandirali E, Erol H, et al. Peyronie's disease in men under 40: characteristics and outcome. Int J Impot Res 2001;13:18–23.

[30] Briganti A, et al. Clinical presentation of Peyronie's disease in young patients. Int J Impot Res 2003;15:S44–7.

[31] Deveci S, Hopps CV, O'Brien K, et al. Defining the clinical characteristics of Peyronie's disease in young men. J Sex Med 2007;4(2):485–90.

[32] Williams JL, Thomas GG. The natural history of Peyronie's disease. J Urol 1970;103:75.

[33] Gelbard MK, Dorey F, James K. The natural history of Peyronie's disease. J Urol 1990;144:1376–9.

[34] Kadioglu A, et al. A retrospective review of 307 men with Peyronie's disease. J Urol 2002;168:1075–9.

[35] Akin-Olugbade Y, Mulhall JP. The medical management of Peyronie's disease. Nat Clin Pract Urol 2007;4(2):95–103.

[36] Levine LA, Greenfield JM. Establishing a standardized evaluation of the man with Peyronie's disease. Int J Impot Res 2003;15(5):S103–12.

[37] Scott WW, Scardino PL. A new concept in the treatment of Peyronie's disease. South Med J 1948;41:173–7.

[38] Sikka SC, Hellstrom WJ. Role of oxidative stress and antioxidants in Peyronie's disease. Int J Impot Res 2002;14:353–60.

[39] Gholami SS, Gonzalez-Cadavid NF, Lue TF, et al. Peyronie's disease: a review. J Urol 2002;169:1234–41.

[40] Pryor JP, Farell CF. Controlled clinical trial of vitamin E in Peyronie's disease. Prog Reprod Biol 1983;9:41–5.

[41] Akkus E, Carrier S, Rehman J, et al. Is colchicine effective in Peyronie's disease? A pilot study. Urology 1994;44:291–5.

[42] Kadioglu A, Tefekli A, Koksal T, et al. Treatment of Peyronie's disease with oral colchicine: long term results and predictive parameters of successful outcome. Int J Impot Res 2000;12:169–75.

[43] Safarinejad MR. Therapeutic effects of colchicine in the management of Peyronie's disease: a randomized double-blind, placebo-controlled study. Int J Impot Res 2004;16:238–43.

[44] Zarafonetis CJ, Horrax TM. Treatment of Peyronie's disease with potassium para-aminobenzoate (POTABA). J Urol 1959;81:770–2.

[45] Hasche-Klunder R. Treatment of peyronie's disease with para-aminobenzoacidic potassium (POTOBA) (author's transl). Urologe A 1978;17:224–7.

[46] Weidner W, Schroeder-Printzen I, Rudnick J, et al. Randomized prospective placebo-controlled therapy of Peyronie's disease (IPP) with Potaba (aminobenzoate potassium). J Urol 1999;6:205.

[47] Weidner W, Hauck EW, Schnitker J. Potassium paraaminobenzoate (Potaba) in the treatment of Peyronie's disease: a prospective, placebo-controlled, randomized study. Eur Urol 2005;47:530–5.

[48] Ralph DJ, Brooks MD, Bottazzo GF, et al. The treatment of Peyronie's disease with tamoxifen. Br J Urol 1992;70:648–51.

[49] Colletta AA, Wakefield LM, Howell FV, et al. Anti-oestrogens induce the secretion of active transforming growth factor beta from human fetal fibroblasts. Br J Cancer 1990;62:405–9.

[50] Teloken C, Rhoden EL, Grazziotin TM, et al. Tamoxifen versus placebo in the treatment of Peyronie's disease. J Urol 1999;162:2003–5.

[51] Biagiotti G, Cavallini G. Acetyl-L-carnitine vs. tamoxifen in the oral therapy of Peyronie's disease: a preliminary report. BJU Int 2001;88:63–7.

[52] Valente EG, Vernet D, Ferrini M, et al. L-Arginine and phosphodiesterase (PDE) inhibitors counteract fibrosis in the Peyronie's fibrotic plaque and related fibroblast cultures. Nitric Oxide 2003;9:229–44.

[53] Brant WO, Dean RC, Lue TF. Treatment of Peyronie's disease with oral pentoxifylline. Nat Clin Pract Urol 2006;3:111–5.

[54] Martin DJ, Badwan K, Parker M, et al. Transdermal application of verapamil gel to the penile shaft fails to infiltrate the tunica albuginea. J Urol 2002;168:2483–5.

[55] Fitch WP, Easterling J, Talbert RL, et al. Topical verapamil HCl, topical trifluoperazine, and topical magnesium sulfate for the treatment of peyronie's disease—a placebo-controlled pilot study. J Sex Med 2007;4:477–84.

[56] Levine LA. Comment on topical verpamil HCl, topical trfluoperazine, and topical magnesium sulfate for the treatment of peyronie's disease—a placebo-controlled pilot study. J Sex Med 2007;4:1081–2.

[57] Bodner H, Howard AH, Kaplan JH. Peyronie's disease: cortisone-hyaluronidase-hydrocortisone therapy. J Urol 1954;400–3.

[58] Winter CC, Khanna R. Peyronie's disease: results with dermo-jet injection of dexamethasone. J Urol 1975;114:898–900.

[59] Williams G, Green NA. The non-surgical treatment of Peyronie's disease. Br J Urol 1980;52:392–5.

[60] Gelbard MK, Walsh R, Kaufman JJ. Collagenase for Peyronie's disease experimental studies. Urol Res 1982;10:135–40.

[61] Gelbard MK, Linkner A, Kaufman JJ. The use of collagenase in the treatment of Peyronie's disease. J Urol 1985;134:280–3.

[62] Gelbard MK, James K, Riach P, et al. Collagenase vs. placebo in the treatment of Peyronie's disease: a double blind study. J Urol 1993;149:56–8.

[63] Roth M, Eickelberg O, Kohler E, et al. Ca2+ channel blockers modulate metabolism of collagens within the extracellular matrix. Proc Natl Acad Sci U S A 1996;93:5478–82.

[64] Mulhall JP, Anderson MS, Lubrano T, et al. Peyronie's disease cell culture models: phenotypic, genotypic and functional analyses. Int J Impot Res 2002;14:397–405.

[65] Levine LA, Merrick PF, Lee RC. Intralesional verapamil injection for the treatment of Peyronie's disease. J Urol 1994;151:1522–4.

[66] Rehman J, Benet A, Melman A. Use of intralesional verapamil to dissolve Peyronie's disease plaque: a long term single-blind study. Urology 1998;51:620–6.

[67] Levine LA, Estrada CR. Intralesional verapamil for the treatment of Peyronie's disease: a review. Int J Impot Res 2002;14:324–8.

[68] Bennett NE, Guhring P, Mulhall JP. Intralesional verapamil Prevents the Progression of Peyronie's Disease. Urology 2007;69:1181–4.

[69] Duncan MR, Berman B, Nseyo UO. Regulation of the proliferation and biosynthetic activities of cultured human Peyronie's disease fibroblasts by interferons-α, β, and γ. Scand J Urol Nephrol 1991;25:89–94.

[70] Wegner HE, Andreson R, Knipsel HH, et al. Treatment of Peyronie's disease with local interferon-α-2b. Eur Urol 1995;28:236–40.

[71] Wegner HE, Andresen R, Knipsel HH, et al. Local interferon-α-2b is not an effective treatment in early-stage Peyronie's disease. Eur Urol 1997;32:190–3.

[72] Ahuja S, Bivalacqua TJ, Case J, et al. A pilot study demonstrating clinical benefit from intralesional interferon alpha 2B in the treatment of Peyronie's disease. J Androl 1999;20:444–8.

[73] Dang G, Matern R, Bivalacqua TJ, et al. Intralesional interferon-α-2b injections for the treatment of Peyronie's disease. South Med J 2004;97:42–6.

[74] Hellstrom WJ, Kendirici M, Matern R, et al. Single-blind, multicenter placebo-controlled parallel study to asses the safety and efficacy of intralesional

interferon-α-2b for minimally invasive treatment for Peyronie's disease. J Urol 2006;176:394–8.

[75] Levine LA. Review of current nonsurgical management of Peyronie's disease. Int J Impot Res 2003; 15:S113–20.

[76] Hauck EW, Altinkilic BM, Ludwig M, et al. Extracorporeal shock wave therapy in the treatment of Peyronie's disease. First results of a case-controlled approach. Eur Urol 2000;38:663–9.

[77] Hatzichristodoulou G, Meisner C, et al. Efficacy of Extracorporeal Shock Wave Therapy (ESWT) in patients with Peyronie's disease (PD)—first results of a prospective, randomized, placebo- controlled, single- blind study [abstract 993]. Annual Meeting of the American Urological Association, 2006.

[78] Hatzichristodoulou G, Meisner C, et al. Efficacy of extracorporeal shock wave therapy on plaque size and sexual function in patients with peyronie's disease—results of a prospective, randomized, placebo-controlled study [abstract 747]. Annual Meeting of the American Urological Association, 2007.

[79] Riedl CR, Plas E, Engelhard P, et al. Iontophoresis for treatment of Peyronie's disease. J Urol 2000; 163:95–9.

[80] Montorsi F, Salonia A, Guazzoni G, et al. Transdermal electromotive multi-drug administration for Peyronie's disease: preliminary results. J Androl 2000;21:85–90.

[81] Di Stasi SM, Giannantoni A, Capelli G, et al. Transdermal electromotive administration of verapamil and dexamethasone for Peyronie's disease. BJU Int 2003;91:825–9.

[82] Di Stasi SM, Giannantoni A, Stephen RL, et al. A prospective, randomized study using transdermal electromotive administration of verapamil and dexamethasone for Peyronie's disease. J Urol 2004;171:1605–8.

[83] Levine LA, Estrada CR, Show W, et al. Tunica albuginea tissue analysis after electromotive drug administration. J Urol 2003;169:1775–8.

[84] Greenfield JM, Shah SJ, Levine LA. Verapamil vs. saline in electromotive drug administration (EDMA) for Peyronie's disease: a double blind, placebo controlled trial. J Urol 2007;177:972–5.

[85] Ojingwa JC, Isseroff RR. Electrical stimulation of wound healing. J Invest Dermatol 2003;121:1–12.

[86] Preito Castro RM, Leva Vallejo ME, Regueiro Lopez JC, et al. Combined treatment with vitamin E and colchicines in the early stages of Peyronie's disease. BJU Int 2003;91:522–4.

[87] Mirone V, Palmieri A, Granata AM, et al. Ultrasound-Guided ESWT in Peyronie's disease plaques. Arch Ital Urol Androl 2000;72:384–7.

[88] Mirone V, Imbimbo C, Palmieri A, et al. Our experience on the association of a new physical and medical therapy in patients suffering from induration penis plastica. Eur Urol 1999;36:327–30.

[89] Cavallini G, Biagiotti G, Koverech A, et al. Oral propionyl-l-carnitine and intraplaque verapamil in the therapy of advanced and resistant Peyronie's disease. BJU Int 2002;89:895–900.

[90] Levine LA, Lenting EL. Experience with a surgical algorithm for Peyronie's disease. J Urol 1997;158: 2149–52.

[91] Daitch JA, Angermeier KW, Montague DK. Modified corporoplasty for penile curvature: long-term results and patient satisfaction. J Urol 1999;162: 2006–9.

[92] Gholami SS, Lue TF. Correction of penile curvature using the 16-dot plication technique: a review of 132 patients. J Urol 2002;167:2066–9.

[93] Syed AH, Abbasi Z, Hargreave TB. Nesbit procedure for disabling Peyronie's curvature: a median follow-up of 84 months. Urology 2003;61: 999–1003.

[94] Savoca G, Scieri F, Pietropaolo F, et al. Straightening corporoplasty for Peyronie's disease: a review of 218 patients with median follow-up of 89 months. Eur Urol 2004;6:610–4.

[95] Rolle L, Tamagnone A, Timpano M, et al. The Nesbit operation for penile curvature: an easy and effective technical modification. J Urol 2005; 173:171–3.

[96] Bella AJ, Beasley KA, Obied A, et al. Minimally invasive intracorporeal incision of Peyronie's plaque: initial experiences with a new technique. Urology 2006;68:852–7.

[97] Greenfield JM, Lucas S, Levine LA. Factors affecting the loss of length associated with tunica albuginea plication for correction of penile curvature. J Urol 2006;175:238–41.

[98] Gelbard MK. Relaxing incisions in the correction of penile deformity due to Peyronie's disease. J Urol 1995;154:1457–60.

[99] El-Sakka AI, Rashwan HM, Lue TF. Venous patch graft for Peyronie's disease. Part II: outcome analysis. J Urol 1998;160:2050–3.

[100] Hatzichristou DG, Hatzimouratidis K, Apostolidis A, et al. Corporoplasty using tunica albuginea free grafts for penile curvature: surgical technique and long-term results. J Urol 2002;167:1367–70.

[101] Egydio PH, Lucon AM, Arap S. Treatment of Peyronie's disease by incomplete circumferential incision of the tunica albuginea and plaque with bovine pericardium graft. Urology 2002;59:570–4.

[102] Levine LA, Estrada CR. Human cadaveric pericardial graft for the surgical correction of Peyronie's disease. J Urol 2003;170:2359–62.

[103] Kalsi J, Minhas S, Christopher N, et al. The results of plaque incision and venous grafting (Lue procedure) to correct the penile deformity of Peyronie's disease. BJU Int 2005;95:1029–33.

[104] Breyer BN, Brant WO, Garcia MM, et al. Complications of porcine small intestine submucosa graft for Peyronie's disease. J Urol 2007;177:589–91.

[105] Hsu GL, Chen HS, Hsieh CH, et al. Long-term results of autologous venous grafts for penile morphological reconstruction. J Androl 2007;28:186–93.

[106] Moncada I, Jara J, Marinez J. et al. Managing penile shortening after peyronie's disease surgery [abstract 750]. Annual Meeting of the American Urological Association, 2007.

[107] Taylor FL, Levine LA. Surgical correction of peyronie's disease via tunica albuginea plication or plaque partial excision with pericardial graft: long term follow-up [abstract 748]. Annual Meeting of the American Urological Association, 2007.

[108] Kadioglu A, Sanli O, Akman T, et al. Graft materials in Peyronie's disease surgery: a comprehensive review. J Sex Med 2007;4:581–95.

[109] Greenfield JM, Estrada CR, Levine LA. Erectile dysfunction following surgical correction of Peyronie's disease and a pilot study of the use of sildenafil citrate rehabilitation for postoperative erectile dysfunction. J Sex Med 2005;2:241–7.

[110] Carson CC, Hodge GB, Anderson EE. Penile prosthesis in Peyronie's disease. Br J Urol 1983;55:417–21.

[111] Ghanem HM, Fahmy I, El Meliegy A. Malleable penile implants without plaque surgery in the treatment of Peyronie's disease. Int J Impot Res 1998;10:171–3.

[112] Levine LA, Dimitriou RJ. A surgical algorithm for penile prosthesis placement in men with erectile failure and Peyronie's disease. Int J Impot Res 2000;12:147–51.

[113] Levine LA, Estrada CR, Morgentaler A. Mechanical reliability and safety of and patient satisfaction with the Ambicor inflatable penile prosthesis: results of a two center study. J Urol 2001;166:932–7.

[114] Montague DK, Angermeier KW, Lakin MM, et al. AMS 3-piece inflatable penile prosthesis implantation in men with Peyronie's disease: comparison of CX and Ultrex cylinders. J Urol 1996;156:1633–5.

[115] Dowalczyk JJ, Mulcahy JJ. Penile curvatures and aneurismal defects with the Ultrex penile prosthesis corrected with insertion of the AMS 700CX. J Urol 1996;156:398–401.

[116] Montorsi F, Rigatti P, Carmignani G, et al. AMS three-piece inflatable implants for erectile dysfunction: a long-term multi-institutional study in 200 consecutive patients. Eur Urol 2000;37:50–5.

ELSEVIER
SAUNDERS

Urol Clin N Am 34 (2007) 535–547

UROLOGIC
CLINICS
of North America

Updates in Inflatable Penile Prostheses

Gerard D. Henry, MD[a],*, Steven K. Wilson, MD, FACS[b]

[a]Regional Urology, Shreveport, LA, USA
[b]Department of Urology, University of Arkansas for Medical Sciences, Little Rock, AR, USA

Throughout history, many attempts to correct erectile dysfunction (ED) have been recorded. Early surgical approaches involved placing rigid devices outside of the corpora cavernosa, with high rates of erosion and infection. For the last 35 years, intracavernosal inflatable prostheses have been used, and these devices have undergone almost constant enhancement. The design and techniques of penile prostheses implantation have advanced such that now more complications are linked to medical causes (eg, infection and erosion) than to implant failure. Among virtually all medically implanted devices, the three-piece inflatable penile prosthesis (IPP) has the highest patient satisfaction rates (consistently > 90%) and lowest mechanical revision rates (96% at 5 years, > 60% at 15 years) [1].

In the decade before the introduction of sildenafil in 1998, annual sales of penile prostheses were approximately 30,000 worldwide. Penile implants had the distinction of being the most effective treatment for ED, with a high acceptance rate. The problem of ED became much more apparent with the introduction of oral medication and significant attendant publicity. Thus, more patients, over an ever-increasing age range, began requesting a solution for ED, and 65% of them responded to sildenafil. Less than 2 years after the introduction of sildenafil, sales of penile implants had plummeted by 50% [2]. A higher percentage of implants were being provided to patients for replacement and revision than to first-time recipients. Also, patients receiving first-time implants had more comorbidities.

Despite the introduction of two additional phosphodiesterase inhibitors, current implant sales exceed the presildenafil era as more patients have become refractory to the oral medications. Most of these patients have tried the so-called "second-line" therapies (intracorporeal injections, intraurethral therapy, and vacuum devices) but opted for implant surgery instead.

Types of penile implants

There are three classes of penile implants: hydraulic, semi-rigid, and soft silicone. Although malleable, semi-rigid, and positional penile prostheses are available and used, this article focuses on the three-piece IPP. In the United States, hydraulic prostheses outsell the paired semi-rigid type by a ratio of 4 to 1. Composed of paired cylinders, a scrotal pump, and a reservoir, these devices have been available for almost 30 years. Many improvements and changes in design have produced an IPP with less than 5% mechanical failure rates at 5 years. Two companies manufacture the three-piece IPP: American Medical Systems (AMS) and Coloplast (formerly Mentor) Corporation, both offering two widths of cylinders. The AMS standard sized cylinders are the CX and LGX, and the narrow cylinders are the CXM and CXR (Fig. 1). The Mentor standard cylinder is the Titan, and its narrow model is the Titan NB (Fig. 2).

The critical determinant for inflatable cylinder size is the proximal dilation. The narrow cylinders expand to 14 mm, and the standard cylinders expand to 18 mm (AMS 700 CX) or more (Titan). Placement of the base of the standard size cylinder for AMS and Mentor cylinders requires dilation to at least 12 mm and optimally to 13 mm. The newer AMS 700

* Corresponding author.

E-mail address: gdhenry@hotmail.com (G.D. Henry).

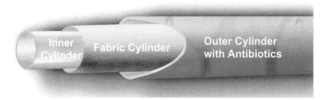

Fig. 1. Paralyne coating (*light blue areas*) on the surfaces of the silicone in the AMS 700 cylinders, which is not in contact with the body tissues. (*Courtesy of* American Medical Systems Corporation, Minneapolis, MN; with permission.)

MS cylinders require dilation to 10 mm proximally. If it is not possible to pass the 11 mm dilator to the ischial tuberosity, a downsized cylinder is recommended. The Mentor NB requires dilation to 10 mm, the AMS CXM to 11 mm, and the AMS CXR to 9 mm. The 700 CXM prostheses were originally introduced by AMS in 1990 as a narrower version for use in smaller girth penises, although now they are used most often in patients who have corporal fibrosis. The CXR, designed specifically for patients who have corporal fibrosis, requires corporal dilation to 9 mm, as compared with 11 mm for the CXM.

Cylinder construction is different for the two manufacturers. AMS cylinders are composed of three layers. The inner layer is silicone, the middle layer is a fabric of woven Dacron and Lycra, and the outer layer is silicone. The CX and CXR have a unidirectional weave to their fabric allowing only girth expansion, whereas the LGX has a bidirectional weave permitting expansion in length and girth. In 2001, AMS added a Paralyne coating to the surfaces of the silicone not in contact with the body tissues (see Fig. 1). This micropolymer increases the lubricity of the silicone and, in lab testing by the manufacturer, makes the silicone much more wear resistant.

The Titan cylinders and reservoir are made of Bioflex, a material similar to polyurethane. Silicone is the material used for the pump and the tubing to connect the components. It apparently is not possible to make tubing from Bioflex because it is formulated as a dispersion, whereas tubing construction requires extrusion. Bioflex and silicone do not bond to each other chemically; the process used to bond the components to the silicone tubing is proprietary and undisclosed. Mentor cylinders in testing are more abrasion resistant than silicone cylinders. Clinical studies before Paralyne introduction bore this out: The recent studies showed non-Paralyne AMS devices had worse 5-year rates for freedom from mechanical revision than did the Mentor implants [3]. A large series of Mentor devices had virtually no failures from Bioflex; most revisions were caused by silicone tubing failure adjacent to the pump [4].

The only two-piece penile prosthesis available in the United States is the AMS Ambicor (Fig. 3). This device has cylinders similar to the obsolete AMS self-contained implant, the Dynaflex. In this two-piece model, the pump mechanism has been moved from the tip of each cylinder to a separate scrotal pump attached to the two cylinders. Depression of the pump causes fluid to move from a 3- to 5-ml reservoir in the base of the cylinder into a cylinder in the middle of the penile shaft that is distensible to a fixed width to achieve rigidity. Detumescence is obtained by bending the penis 90° from the horizontal position for 12 seconds. Relative to the three-piece IPP, flaccidity and erection are compromised with this model because the reservoir volume is severely restricted.

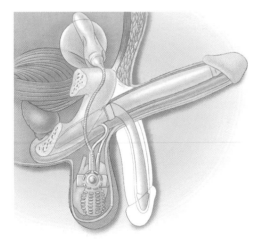

Fig. 2. A rendering of the Momentary Squeeze Pump (*Courtesy of* American Medical Systems Corporation, Minneapolis, MN; with permission.)

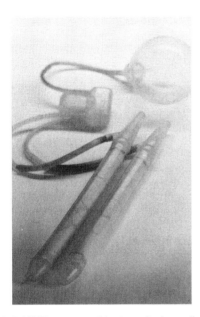

Fig. 3. InhibiZone, a combination of minocycline and rifampin, is impregnated into the external silicone surfaces of the inflatable penile prosthesis. (*Courtesy of* American Medical Systems Corporation, Minneapolis, MN; with permission.)

The device is not available with Paralyne or Inhibi-Zone coatings but has a popular following and good short-term mechanical reliability [5]. Nevertheless, in a recent unpublished study that used a five-point satisfaction survey, patients with the three-piece IPPs seem to be much more satisfied than those with two-piece IPPs. Mentor previously marketed a two-piece device called Mentor Mark II. This device had an egg-shaped pump/reservoir that contained 25 ml normal saline but delivered approximately 15 to 20 ml to Bioflex standard-sized cylinders. The device was not popular, and Mentor withdrew it from the marketplace. Mentor has a similar device in clinical trials, the Excel, which has narrow-based cylinders attached to a smaller (20 ml) combined pump/reservoir. This device is approved in a number of markets outside the United States.

The three-piece IPPs are somewhat complex to insert because they require a reservoir placed in the abdominal cavity. They give the best rigidity because they fill every part of the corporal bodies, just as an inner tube fills a bicycle tire. Because reservoir capacity is capacious, stretching of pliant tunica and compression of erectile tissue does not cause deterioration of the erection in time, as commonly occurs with self-contained or two-piece devices, which have no reserve fluid volume for future needs [6]. The three-piece IPP also gives the best flaccidity because all fluid can be drained out of the cylinders into the reservoir for a non-erect state. The pumping and deflating mechanisms of the Coloplast and AMS devices require some manual dexterity, and some patients may find it difficult to work these devices.

Recent design developments

A recent improvement to the AMS three-piece is the tactile pump. Compared with their previous pump design, this larger pump delivers more volume per squeeze and has a much larger deflation zone with "ribs and pads" that facilitate grasping, activating, and deactivating the device. Early clinical reports indicate a marked reduction in the amount of time required for patient instruction [7] and minimized finger slippage during inflation and easier patient identification of the deflation portion [8]. Another new pump design from AMS is the Momentary Squeeze (MS) Pump, a one-touch button designed for easier deflation (see Fig. 1). This pump features a lock-out valve designed to resist auto-inflation (data on file at AMS). The pump volume is much smaller, and with the lock-out valve feature in the pump, some patients have difficulty inflating the MS pump to the desired rigidity.

Additional developments with the MS pump include an optimized pump tubing angle to ease placement into proximal corpora (to 11 mm), new isodiametric snap-on rear tip extenders to provide a more secure connection, and a new Paralyne-coated reservoir designed to improve reservoir durability (data on file at AMS). Coloplast is developing a one-touch release pump for their Titan IPP, which is likely to be launched in 2007. Coincident with the introduction of the new-coated Titan prosthesis in 2002, the distal tips of the cylinders were changed to a more appropriate tapered shape rather than the former blunt appearance.

Biofilm and infection control

Postoperative infection is the most feared complication of genitourinary prosthetic surgery. It is believed that in most cases of infection associated with primary implantation, the bacteria are introduced at the time of surgery [9,10]. A capsule of tissue is presumed to envelope the implant, effectively sealing off the prosthesis, within 72 hours [11–13].

538   HENRY & WILSON

Although the incidence of infection during the original implant is only 1% to 3%, traditionally revision surgery carries a 7% to 18% risk [3, 14–17]. Increased incidence of infection with revision/replacement may be due to decreased host resistance, impaired antibiotic penetration due to capsule formation, and decreased wound healing related to scarring. Infection may be induced by contamination at surgery, as suggested by preoperative nasal swab cultures of staphylococci that significantly correlate to postoperative infection rates [18]. Hematogenous late infections rarely occur [9].

Staphylococcus epidermidis is the most common organism found at removal of penile prostheses for infection [19]. Licht and colleagues [14] found that 40% of clinically uninfected penile prostheses had low colony counts of *S. epidermidis*. Three of the culture-positive patients in the study became infected with higher colony counts at explantation. None of the IPP patients who had a negative culture at reoperation developed an infection. Ensuring a sterile environment at the time of revision/replacement surgery may lower the rate of reoperation infection.

Many bacteria produce a protective mucin coat or biofilm, which allows bacteria to survive at a lowered metabolic rate, causing no overt symptoms [10]. Occasionally, bacteria are released from the biofilm, becoming free-floating or "planktonic" and causing symptoms [10]. Antibiotics or the body's defense mechanisms can kill planktonic bacteria, but within a biofilm associated with an implant, the bacteria cannot be eradicated except by implant removal and lavage of the implant spaces. Recent studies have confirmed that most implants removed for noninfectious reasons have bacteria/biofilm on them at the time of revision surgery [11,12].

Revision washout

In 1996, Brant and colleagues [20] reported salvage success with removal of infected penile implants and sequential antiseptic lavage to sterilize the implant space followed by immediate reimplantation. Henry and associates applied this washout principle to revision surgery for mechanical reasons, with a resultant decrease in infection rate after removal of a clinically noninfected device [11]. Many believe the success of this revision washout technique is predicated on removal of the biofilm by the vigorous lavage. Theoretically, some aspect of the revision surgery may stimulate

the quiescent bacteria living in their lowered metabolic state in the biofilm, causing them to become clinically active and causing symptoms of an infection. The increased infection rate seen in clinically uninfected revisions may be due to such activation of biofilm-protected bacteria present since the original surgery.

As further proof, the authors have shown that revision washout reduces bacterial load on the capsule that forms around the implant in a study of 148 patients who had IPPs who had had revision surgery for noninfectious reasons conducted at four institutions [21]. From 65 patients, a wedge of tissue was removed from the capsule that forms around the pump and sent for culture. After removal of the implant, a revision washout of the implant spaces was performed, and a second wedge of tissue was obtained for culture. Twenty-eight (43%) of the 65 implant capsule tissue cultures obtained before washout were positive for bacteria. Sixteen (25%) tissue cultures obtained after revision washout were positive.

Although washout solutions are antiseptic, it is possible that the most important part of the washout is the mechanical debridement of the bacteria/biofilm in the implant space. For example, Povidone-iodine becomes bactericidal when it dries, making debridement a critical feature of efficacy. Further, it is possible that some irrigants (ie, hydrogen peroxide) cause tissue irritation or disruption, making patients more susceptible to infection. A future study comparing antiseptic solutions WITH normal saline as the irrigant in the washout would be helpful.

During revision surgery for noninfectious reasons, if the entire implant is not removed, there is a possibility of reactivating biofilm-protected bacteria existing on the original implant's retained components. Although it is theoretically optimum to remove reservoirs at the time of revision surgery, our experience is that reservoirs may be placed in more than one location. Because of the difficulty involved in removing some reservoirs, removal of the reservoir is not standard of care during revision surgery for reasons other than infection. If removal of the reservoir proves difficult and if there is no evidence of biofilm on the pump and cylinders, then the original reservoir could be retained. In our experience, the reservoir can be emptied of fluid and a new reservoir placed on the opposite side. If the old reservoir becomes infected, the component could be removed without compromising the new system. Our practice is supported by a recent study that noted no added incidence of subsequent infection in a large series of retained reservoirs [22].

Antibiotic-coated prostheses

AMS introduced a significant innovation in 2000 with InhibiZone, in which minocycline and rifampin are impregnated into the external silicone surfaces of the IPP (see Fig. 3). The antibiotics disperse in vivo, creating a zone of bacterial growth inhibition. The antibiotics elute into the implant spaces over 7 to 10 days, and all traces are gone by 12 days. In a 2004 study of 700 series prostheses, Carson [23] reported on 2261 men who had the InhibiZone-coated IPP and 1944 men who had uncoated prostheses. Infection incidence was 0.28% in the treated group and 1.59% in the control group ($P = .0034$) after 60 days and 0.68% and 1.61%, respectively ($P = .0047$), after 180 days. InhibiZone conferred an 82.4% lower infection rate than the control group after 60 days and a 57.8% lower rate after 180 days. This study did not report a similar reduction of infection in revision procedures using the InhibiZone-coated implants, probably because the washout technique had not been popularized.

Mentor introduced the Titan prosthesis in 2002, which is coated with a hydrophilic substance that reduces bacterial adherence and absorbs and diffuses antibiotics, into which the implant is immersed intraoperatively into the implant spaces (Fig. 4). The Titan IPP allows the surgeon to choose the preferred antibiotic for each individual. In 2004, Wolter and Hellstrom published a study comparing 1-year infection rates from the Titan IPP to Mentor's previous Alpha 1 prostheses. Infection rates were 1.06% (25/2357) for the Titan IPP and 2.07% (10/482) for the Alpha 1 noncoated prostheses [24]. The Carson and Wolter studies used manufacturer-supplied retrospective data for the conclusion of infection reduction with their respective coated devices. There has been no large prospective series published that confirms reduction of infection rates with coated implants. Our group has such an article in press confirming infection reduction with InhibiZone coating in virgin implantations but not in revisions without washout [25].

Although the InhibiZone coating has been shown to reduce infection rates for primary surgeries, the effect is less dramatic among revision cases [13]. The amount of antibiotic used to coat the InhibiZone IPP is less than a single oral pill, potentially enough to lower infection rates in primary surgeries but apparently not enough to combat established biofilm. Combining revision washout with replacement with an antibiotic-coated IPP seems to lower infection rates, and most authorities strongly suggest incorporating this technique into a regimen for clinically uninfected revision/replacement cases [13,26].

Preoperative preparation

Because infection of the prosthesis can be the worst possible complication, avoidance of an infected prosthesis is of paramount importance. Despite the availability of infection-retardant coatings on today's prosthetics, good surgical technique must not be neglected. Most IPP infections are from skin organisms. The patient

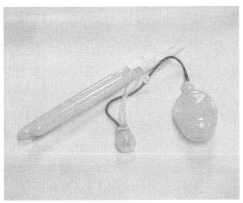
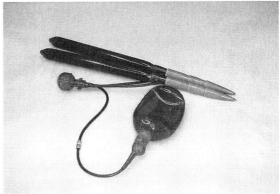

Fig. 4. The Titan three-piece penile prostheses: before and after soaking the hydrophilic coating in a blue solution. (*Courtesy of* Coloplast Corporation, Minneapolis, MN; with permission.)

should be screened to exclude active infection, including open skin lesions or dermatitis in the lower abdominal/genital area, and urine should be sterile. Preoperative antibiotics before skin incision targeting gram-positive bacteria are recommended. Many operating theater techniques for surgical implantation have been suggested over the 30-year history of IPP implantation: (1) all staff wearing face masks and disposable gowns; (2) minimal movement into and out of the theater; (3) double-gloving, with frequent changing of the outer pair; (4) laminar flow or positive pressure ventilation systems; and (5) low ambient temperature, as long as the patient is fitted with a hot-air warming system. Preoperative preparation of the patient is important and includes the following suggested regimens: (1) shaving immediately before the incision; (2) broad-spectrum antibiotics; (3) alcohol-based skin preparation; and (4) draping for scrotal incision, with extremity (orthopedic) drape and self-adhesive u-drape.

Surgical considerations

There are five surgical approaches for penile prosthesis implantation; two are historical: the midline umbilicus to pubis suprapubic incision and the perineal approach, described by Small and colleagues [27]. The subcoronal approach is still used for malleable and semi-rigid implants. Three-piece IPPs may be implanted via an infrapubic or penoscrotal approach. The infrapubic approach permits implanting the reservoir under direct vision; however, the risk of dorsal nerve injury remains a major pitfall. In the early 1990s, approximately 80% of three-piece IPPs were placed via infrapubic incision. Now, an estimated 85% are placed penoscrotally, which allows better corporeal exposure, easier anchoring of the pump in the scrotum, and avoidance of dorsal nerve injury. Although "blind placement" of the reservoir is a disadvantage, tens of thousands of successful implantations attest to the safety of the penoscrotal technique.

Update on the corpora cavernosa

Although the most frequently implanted penile prostheses are multicomponent IPPs, surgeons who implant rods may benefit from guidance on dilation of the corpora cavernosa because more than half of the iatrogenic complications occur during this critical step. Several new, unpublished techniques for surgically implanting the cylinders

are being discussed, with short-term follow-up success. At the 2007 meeting of the American Urological Association, Moncada [28] showed that he no longer dilates the corpora beyond passing the Metzenbaum scissors and the Furlow inserter. Another new technique, advocated by Dr. Paul Perito, is to hydrodistend the corpora with a dilute lidocaine mixture before incision that apparently makes it easier to pass dilators. Less postoperative pain is reported with this technique.

Corporal fibrosis is the transformation of supple erectile tissue into sheets of scar tissue. Segmental corporal fibrosis can occur from vascular insufficiency. Extensive corporal fibrosis is caused by priaprism or removal of an infected implant. In affected individuals, there is no readily discernible cavity to dilate in which to place the cylinders. Corporal fibrosis is worse distally after priaprism and worse proximally after removal of an implant for infection. These scarred corporal bodies frequently result in penile shortening by as much as 2 to 3 in. These patients represent the most difficult surgical challenge in prosthetic urology. There is no authoritative published article on the surgical management of corporal fibrosis, mainly due to insufficient numbers of patients or inadequate follow-up. Many of the articles on corporal fibrosis are anecdotal and opinion based [29–41]. In addition, with the reduction in infection rates associated with antibiotic-coated IPPs, there may never be a significant article on corporal fibrosis because the bulk of severe fibrosis cases result from implant infection. If corporal fibrosis is expected, a wide, transverse, penoscrotal incision is the best approach for proximal exposure of the tunica albuginea [29,30]. With careful, deliberate dilation of the corpora cavernosa, most complications can be avoided. If distal corporal perforation is identified during dilation (eg, a distally placed dilator comes out the meatus or, while irrigating the distal corpora, the fluid is visible out of the meatus), the safest course of action is to abort the case. No good techniques have been published on how to handle distal perforation of the urethra. Proximal laceration of the urethra during scrotal exposure can be repaired, and the implant may proceed.

Proximal perforation of the corporal body is common during implantation into scarred corporal bodies. A sling of nonabsorbable suture through the rear tip extender has been shown to be effective for proximal perforation (Box 1). With the rear tip extender sling keeping the cylinder base out of the damaged tunica, the

---

Box 1. Rear tip sling placement for perforation of the proximal tunica albuginea

1. Using a large permanent monofilament stitch (the sling), go outside-in of the tunica albuginea at the corporotomy site.
2. Drive the stitch through the rear tip extender (the outermost one if more than one rear tip extender is used) at the proximal end of the extender.
3. Take the stitch inside-out the corporotomy.
4. Fire the Furlow inserter and secure the strings.
5. Carefully place the cylinder base with rear tip extender proximally.
6. Pull on the secured strings to bring the cylinder's distal tip out as far distally as it will go.
7. Close the corporotomy.
8. Maximally inflate the cylinders with the secured strings pulled with constant force.
9. Meticulously tie down the sling stitch while the inflated cylinder is pulled out distally.

---

perforation heals without the necessity of surgical repair. Even if the rear tip extender is positioned outside the tunica albuginea at the crus level, this repair works well because by 6 months postoperatively, the rear tip extender is encased in fibrous scar tissue. Most authorities advocate that the patient cycle his implant but avoid the thrusting trauma of intercourse for 3 months.

Traditional correction for proximal perforation involved the use of synthetic graft material to form a "windsox." The use of synthetic grafts resulted in infection rates as high as 30% [40,42], purportedly because bacteria are able to grow in the protected environment between two synthetic surfaces (ie, the graft and the penile implant) [13]. Organic tissue grafts, such as cadaver pericardium, have been shown to be good grafting material [43,44], avoiding this increased risk of infection [42]; however, in our opinion, they are not necessary with stabilization of the cylinder base out of the perforation as outlined previously.

Delayed perforation of the tunica distally resulting in chronic impending cylinder erosion can occur. If the problem is not addressed, skin perforation by the cylinder tip and resultant prosthesis infection can occur. Mulcahy has shown that the tough fibrous capsule that develops around the penile implant can be used for distal corporoplasty in cases of lateral tunica albuginea weakness [45]. The IPP of choice for patients who have tunica albuginea defects is the AMS 700 CX (controlled expansion) or the AMS 700 CXR because the controlled expansion limits the chance of subsequent aneurysm formation. If an aneurysm is encountered during revision/replacement surgery, a "belt and suspenders" repair should be attempted. Here the tunica albuginea is dissected back to stronger tissue, and a layer of simple interrupted 2-0 braided absorbable sutures (the belt) is placed, followed by a second layer of horizontal mattress sutures (the suspenders) to close up the defect. If the repair seems to be inadequate to the prosthetic surgeon, an organic tissue graft can add strength to the repair. Again, the recommended cylinder for repairs of tunical weakness of any location is one that has restriction of expansion.

During implantation of the cylinders, crossover may be detected. Crossovers are rarely complete with the tip of both cylinders in one corporal body. The corporal septum has windows, and the typical crossover is an over-and-back movement that is subtle at the time of surgery. Use of the scrotal incision and placing the penis on stretch in the Scott retractor helps the operator avoid this over-and-back movement. If crossover is suspected, both cylinders should be removed, and the corpora cavernosa should be redilated proximally and distally with a size 11 or 12 Hegar dilator in the opposite corpora. If the active dilator hits the opposite stationary Hegar, a crossover situation needs to be rectified. Typically, a dilator tracts over the midline into the contralateral corpora cavernosa, with the angle of the dilators indicating the side that crosses over. The Hegar dilator should be placed on the side in which both cylinders resided, whether proximal or distal. The operator carefully rechannels the crossover side, staying lateral and using the stationary Hegar as a point of reference. The cylinder should be implanted with the stationary Hegar in place; if it goes in correctly, the stationary Hegar is removed, and the contralateral cylinder is implanted. It is not necessary to repair the crossover because the septum of the corpora is variable, has windows, and occasionally is filamentous.

Finger rake dissection

Traditionally, sharp dissection has been favored to expose the tunica albuginea after skin incision, especially when using the SKW Lone Star Retractor Kit [46]. The optimum incision location was to avoid scrotal fat inferiorly and poorer healing penile skin superiorly. Less experienced urologists (eg, residents) found correctly placing the retractor and clearing off Buck's fascia to be tedious and time consuming. Moreover, injuring the urethra was a risk. The new "skin rake" method is a safe and quick alternative.

A small transverse incision is made 1 to 2 cm inferior to the penile scrotal junction, deep enough to free the separate skin edges with the penis on retractor stretch. Two fingers are inserted inside the incision until the tips are firmly on Buck's fascia. The fingertips are forcefully pushed down along the course of the corpora cavernosa, "sweeping" away the scrotal fat and connective tissue caudally. The fingers work like a rake, cleaning off the tunica albuginea with repeated sweeps in multiple locations along the horizontal line below the incision. Both hands can be used in opposite directions for more direct power, continuing until the tunica albuginea and urethra are cleaned off anteriorly. Six stay hooks for the retractor are applied, and additional dissection can be used to finely clean Buck's fascia. Frequently, the surgeon may proceed to cylinder implantation without additional exposure.

The finger rake dissection has several advantages over the traditional sharp dissection technique, especially for less experienced prosthetic surgeons. Even surgeons doing IPPs for the first time can clean off the tunica and set the retractor within 2 minutes. We believe this technique is safer; with this technique there is less bleeding, and it is virtually impossible to damage the urethra. The finger rake method allows the surgeon to get a more proximal placement of his corporotomy by sweeping away connective tissue and scrotal fat caudally. A more proximal corporotomy can help avoid "tail pipe" penis (whereby cylinder tubing is visible under penile skin because the tubing exited the corporotomy too far distally). It also facilitates placement of longer cylinders with fewer rear tips.

Ectopic reservoir placement

Many prospective implant patients have had previous abdominal surgery that makes traditional reservoir placement problematic.

Individuals who have had a cystectomy, kidney transplant, bilateral hernias, or radical prostatectomies fit into this category. The traditional location for reservoir placement has been obliterated by the previous surgery. Surgeons have experimented with alternate or ectopic placement of reservoirs out of need. Ectopic placement of the reservoir is done through infrapubic incision by staying anterior to the transversalis fascia and finger dissecting underneath the rectus muscle until a space is created that holds the filled reservoir. The same space is created via scrotal incision by displacing the incision over the inguinal area. The pubic tubercle is palpated and the finger inserted into the inguinal ring. The finger is then forcibly passed cephalad, piercing the back wall of the inguinal canal. A space anterior to the transversalis fascia and posterior to the muscle layers is fashioned by sweeping the fingers back and forth.

A major disadvantage of ectopic reservoir placement is that the reservoir is frequently palpable, and a bulge may be visible in thin individuals. For patients who have complex issues, such as kidney transplant or neobladder, a surgeon might consider a simpler prosthesis than the three-piece IPP. Another solution is to place the reservoir outside its usual location behind the pelvic bone in the space of Retzius. In this technique, the surgeon makes a second incision and places the reservoir intra-abdominally or in the retroperitoneal space beneath the kidney. Three months after implantation, the tissue capsule around the reservoir usually prevents increased abdominal pressure from milking fluid from reservoir to cylinder. In 2000, Mentor enhanced their reservoir with a "lock-out valve," preventing fluid from exiting when pressure is applied to the reservoir (Fig. 5). Previous reservoirs allowed fluid to flow in and out with abdominal pressure, potentially causing autoinflation. The Titan reservoir with Lock-Out Valve allows placement of the reservoir in locations that would be subject to considerable autoinflation (eg, anterior to the transversalis fascia) but posterior to the abdominal wall muscles. In 2002, Wilson and colleagues [47] published a study comparing 160 patients undergoing the lock-out design with 339 patients undergoing the original design. Only two patients (1.3%) with a lock-out valve complained of autoinflationinitially, with the problem resolved on further instruction. Among patients who had original reservoirs, 11% reported autoinflation, with 2% requiring operative correction.

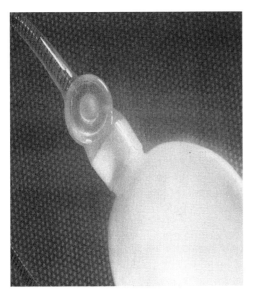

Fig. 5. The Lock-Out Valve on the Titan Reservoir. (*Courtesy of* Coloplast Corporation, Minneapolis, MN; with permission.)

The AMS new 700 MS pump (2006) has a similar enhancement, thus allowing ectopic reservoir placement with both company's devices in patients whose abdominal anatomy is challenging. In our opinion, ectopic reservoir placement could be enhanced if the reservoir design were changed from spherical (AMS) or cylindrical (Mentor) to one resembling a hot water bottle.

Many skilled surgeons use the traditional reservoir position even in anatomically compromised patients and tailor prosthetic components to fit the challenging clinical picture. The tubing caliber for the AMS and Mentor products is similar, permitting the surgeon to mix manufacturer's components. On occasion (eg, in anatomically compromised patients who have had previous infection), we have combined AMS InhibiZone CXR cylinders, the new AMS Tactile pump, and a Mentor Lock-Out Valve reservoir. Mixing components from different vendors voids the warranty.

Treatment of Peyronie's disease

For patients who have Peyronie's disease (PD) without ED, we tend to use simple plication procedures. It is well known that elliptical excision or the more extensive surgery of plaque excision and grafting—essentially any procedure that interrupts tunical integrity—may lead to ED. Furthermore, because 70% of Peyronie's plaques occur on the dorsum of the penis, plaque resection requires elevation of the neurovascular bundle. Dorsal nerve injury and consequent decreased penile sensation have no effective treatment. In our opinion, plaque excision and grafting is a formidable exercise. Thus, for complex repair, we suggest penile prostheses.

Men who have ED and PD should be considered candidates for prostheses [48]. Curvature with flaccidity distal to the plaque resulting in flail penis is a typical presentation. Because surgical interventions without prosthesis placement can result in penile shortening and subsequent exacerbation or development of ED, the pool of candidates for prostheses can be expanded to include men who have short penises and partially impaired erections. In our practice, all patients who have PD who are over 50 years old are counseled to consider prostheses. Many of these older men demonstrate poor axial rigidity distal to the plaque after a penile injection of vasoactive material. Additionally, penile duplex Doppler may demonstrate nonsymptomatic impairment of penile blood flow (arterial or venous) in older men. This restriction increases the possibility that ED will result from any straightening procedure that does not include prosthesis placement.

Chaudhary and colleagues [49] conducted a retrospective study of 46 patients to evaluate the impact of penile modeling over IPP and the subsequent improvement in erectile function. Modeling of the penis over the penile implant was performed in 28 patients (61%). The other 18 patients (39%) did not need additional modeling because their curvature was corrected by inflation alone. Other than two infected cases, all patients were satisfied with the penile correction, and none of them needed additional straightening operations.

Long-term follow up for PD modeling over inflatable penile prostheses was conducted on 104 patients by Wilson and colleagues [50]. Maximum follow-up was over 12 years, and average follow-up was over 5 years. Their results show that implantation and modeling provided permanent straightening without increased revisions. In modeled cases, the Mentor Alpha 1 seemed less likely to fail mechanically than the AMS 700 CX when followed more than 5 years.

Postoperative care

Traditionally, many prosthetic surgeons advocate a complicated, compressive tape dressing applied with the patient in frog-leg position [46].

Application of this dressing creates an abundance of tape, the removal of which is painful for the patient. Moreover, if the IPP is left inflated at the end of surgery (to minimize corporal bleeding with compression), the doctor has to deflate the prosthesis, with resultant discomfort for some patients. A patient satisfaction study found that for many patients, the most negative experience of the surgery was the dressing removal/deflation of the IPP on the morning after surgery [51].

Experts have disagreed on whether or not to place a drain. In an attempt to avoid postoperative hematoma, Sadeghi-Hejad and colleagues [52] conducted a multi-institutional study on the efficacy of closed-suction drainage of the scrotum in three-piece IPP surgery. This study of 425 patients was used to put an end to the debate of whether closed suction drainage increased the incidence of infection. The results demonstrate a 3.3% infection rate and 0.7% hematoma rate during an average 18-month follow-up period. They concluded that short-term, closed-suction drainage decreased hematoma formation after implantation surgery without demonstrable increased risk of prosthesis infection.

Some experts worry that a drain placed next to an implant can result in more infections. A multi-institutional study recently showed that putting on the compressive "spider web" tape dressing and placing a drain seems to reduce the rate of significant hematomas to about 1% [52]. Some frequent implanters adopt another approach to avoid hematomas. Because the occurrence of scrotal hematoma is thought to result from corporal bleeding, another approach is closing the corporal incision with a running water-tight closure; however, in our opinion, this running suture takes considerably longer and risks inadvertent cylinder puncture.

The Henry Soft Cast wrap

The complicated compressive "spider web" tape dressing or placement of a drain may require the patient to stay over night in the hospital. With reimbursement changes forcing many cases to become outpatient surgeries, a quandary remained for using dressing to prevent hematomas. This predicament inspired creation of the Henry Soft Cast. Compressive penile wraps had been used in the past, most using a sticky-type dressing wrap like Coban. Rarely, IPP patients' penises developed necrosis postoperatively, leading to the abandonment of this dressing wrap.

The Henry Soft Cast wrap uses a nonsticky dressing. Initially the dressing is wrapped loosely. Only after winding the dressing around the base of the entire genitalia a couple of times is the dressing wrapped more tightly, and it is wrapped only moderately tightly where dressing already exists. A key element is getting the wrap underneath both testicles with the pump positioned where the surgeon desires it to be located long-term. A major benefit to this dressing is that the pump is held in this position for as long as the dressing is left on, causing the body to start to form a capsule around the pump in the desired long-term position. In our experience, a high-riding or low-riding (perineal) pump position seems to be used less frequently. The soft cast that develops at the end of the wrap procedure resembles an orthopedic extremity cast. After the dressing is placed, a soft cloth surgical tape is applied around the soft cast, with a minimum of the tape adhering to the patient's skin. The Foley catheter is left in place as long as the wrap is on because some patients have difficulty voiding with the soft cast. Obese patients or patients who have a small tight scrotum can require several circumferential wraps around the base of the whole genitalia to ensure that the testicles and pump are pushed forward into the cast.

The day-surgery IPP patient returns to clinic the next day for Foley catheter and dressing removal. For patients on anticoagulant therapy, or for other reasons, the wrap may be left on for 2 days. Because there is no tape on the patient and no drain, removing the dressing is easy. If the IPP was left inflated, it is easy and much less painful to deflate because there is essentially no swelling (the soft cast does not allow for expansion of the scrotum as did the old compressive dressing), and the pump is easily palpated. Without expansion of the scrotum, there should be no hematoma while the dressing is in place. The IPP is left about 40% inflated, and only stay sutures (not a running closure) are used on the corporotomy. Although no prospective studies of the dressing's effectiveness have been instituted, our initial feeling is enthusiastic regarding lack of scrotal hematoma without the necessity of closed suction drainage.

Additional instruction

Patients should be instructed at discharge from the hospital to wear brief-type underwear for the first month with their penis up, pointing cephalad in their shorts. This encourages capsule formation around the cylinders, permitting normal physiologic upward deflection of the erect penis. Instruction is particularly important for patients who have a lock-out valve because there is little transfer of fluid from reservoir to penis, and the patient may be tempted to wear his flaccid penis down against the scrotal wall. Subsequent capsule formation with the flaccid penis in a head-down position will influence the erection in a similar downward direction.

Summary

In the era of increased availability of medical information from the marketing of drugs and the Internet, patients have never been so well informed. Outcome studies indicate higher satisfaction from penile implants than from pills, injections, or vacuums [22]. Nevertheless, 94% of American urologists treat ED, but only 7% include IPP implantation in their treatment armamentarium. An unfortunate recent occurrence is hospitals' claim that they are losing money on IPP procedures, leading several hospitals to discontinue their urologic prosthetic surgery programs. Essentially, the patient must be treatable by same-day surgery unless there is a serious medical reason for admission for the hospital not to lose money on the procedure, at least in the United States. Conversion of the IPP patient from being a 24-hour observation/overnight stay surgery to a same-day surgery has forced several new issues to be addressed, including pain control, postoperative dressing/drain placement, and return visits.

Inflatable penile prostheses have been available for over 35 years and have had an important role in the treatment of ED. Although penile implants are the least chosen and most invasive treatment option, they provide a predictable, reliable, and durable result. When compared with other devices implanted into humans, the penile implant is one of the least likely to require revision surgery. Virtually any patient who is motivated and medically suitable to continue with sexual activity can be a candidate for placement of these devices with subsequent improvement in his quality of life.

References

[1] Wilson SK, Delk JR Jr, Salem EA, et al. Long-term survival of inflatable penile prostheses: single surgical group experience with 2,384 first-time implants spanning two decades. J Sex Med 2007;4: 1074–9.

[2] Stanley GE, Bivalacqua TJ, Hellstrom WJ. Penile prosthetic trends in the era of effective oral erectogenic agents. South Med J 2000;76:1153–6.

[3] Govier FE, Gibbons RP, Correa RJ, et al. Mechanical reliability, surgical complications and patients partner satisfaction of the modern three-piece inflatable penile prosthesis. Urology 1998; 52:282–6.

[4] Wilson SK, Cleves MA, Delk JR Jr. Comparison of mechanical reliability of original and enhanced Mentor Alpha 1 penile prosthesis. J Urol 1999;162: 715–8.

[5] Levine LA, Estrada CR, Morgentaler A. Mechanical reliability, safety and patient satisfaction with the Ambicor inflatable penile prosthesis: results of a two-center study. J Urol 2001;166:932–7.

[6] Raad I, Darouiche R, Hachem R, et al. Antibiotics and prevention of microbial colonization of catheters. Antimicrob Agents Chemother 1995;39: 2397–400.

[7] Henry GD, Wilson SK, Delk JR Jr. Early results with new ribs and pads AMS 700 pump: device instruction easier. J Sex Med 2004;1(Suppl 1):81.

[8] Delk JR Jr, Knoll LD, McMurray J, et al. Early experience with the American Medical Systems new tactile pump: results of a multicenter study. J Sex Med 2005;2(2):266–71.

[9] Carson CC. Infections in genitourinary prostheses. Urol Clin North Am 1988;16:139–47.

[10] Stewart PS, Costerton JW. Antibiotic resistance of bacteria in biofilms. Lancet 2001;358:135–8.

[11] Henry GD, Wilson SK, Delk JR Jr, et al. Penile prosthesis cultures during revision surgery: a multicenter study. J Urol 2004;172:153–6.

[12] Silverstein AD, Henry GD, Evans B, et al. Biofilm formation on clinically non-infected penile prostheses. J Urol 2006;176(3):1008–11.

[13] Henry GD, Wilson SK, Delk JR Jr, et al. Revision washout reduces penile prosthesis infection in revision surgery: a multicenter study. J Urol 2005; 173(1):89–92.

[14] Licht MR, Montague DK, Angermeier KW, et al. Cultures from genitourinary prostheses at reoperation: questioning the role of Staphylococcus epidermidis in periprosthetic infection. J Urol 1995; 154(2):387–90.

[15] Wilson SK, Delk JR II Jr. Excessive periprosthetic capsule formation of the penile prosthesis reservoir: incidence in various prostheses and a simple surgical solution. J Urol 1995;153:358A.

[16] Jarow JP. Risk factors for penile prosthetic infection. J Urol 1996;156:402–6.

[17] Lotan Y, Roehrborn CG, McConnell JD, et al. Factors influencing the outcomes of penile prosthesis surgery at teaching institution. Urology 2003;62(5): 918–21.

[18] Casewell MW. The nose: an underestimated source of *Staphylococcus aureus* causing wound infection. J Hosp Infect 1998;40:S3–11.

[19] Wilson SK, Delk JR Jr, Terry T. Improved implant survival in patients with severe corporal fibrosis: a new technique without the necessity of grafting. J Urol 1995;153:359A.

[20] Brant MD, Ludlow JK, Mulcahy JJ. Prosthesis salvage operation: immediate replacement of infected penile prostheses. J Urol 1996;155:155–7.

[21] Henry GD, Carson CC, Wilson SK, et al. Revision washout reduces implant capsule tissue culture positivity: a multicenter study. J Urol, in press.

[22] Rajpurkar A, Dhabuwala CB. Comparison of satisfaction rates and erectile function in patients treated with sildenafil, intracavernous prostaglandin E1, and penile implant surgery for erectile dysfunction in urology practice. J Urol 2003;170:159–63.

[23] Carson CC. Efficacy of antibiotic impregnation of inflatable prostheses in decreasing infection in original implants. J Urol 2004;171:1611–4.

[24] Wolter CE, Hellstrom WJG. The hydrophilic-coated inflatable penile prosthesis: one-year experience. J Sex Med 2004;1(2):221–4.

[25] Wilson SK, Delk JR Jr, Cleves MA. InhibiZone in the reduction of primary and revision surgical infection rates for three-piece penile prostheses. Urology, in press.

[26] Abouassaly R, Angermeier KW, Montague DK. Risk of infection with an antibiotic coated penile prosthesis at device replacement for mechanical failure. J Urol 2006;176:2471–3.

[27] Small MP, Carrion HM, Gordon JA. Small-Carrion penile prosthesis: new management of impotence. Urology 1974;2:80–2.

[28] Moncada I, Jara J, Martinez J, et al. Implantation of IPP without dilatation of the corpora: a cavernosal-tissue sparing technique. J Urol 2007;177(4):313.

[29] Carbone DJ Jr, Daitch JA, Angermeier KW, et al. Management of severe corporeal fibrosis with implantation of prosthesis via a transverse scrotal approach. J Urol 1998;159(1):125–7.

[30] Mooreville M, Adrian S, Delk JR Jr, et al. Implantation of inflatable penile prosthesis in patients with severe corporeal fibrosis: introduction of a new penile cavernotome. J Urol 1999;162(6):2054–7.

[31] Montorsi F, Salonia A, Maga T, et al. Reconfiguration of the severely fibrotic penis with a penile implant. J Urol 2001;166(5):1782–6.

[32] Herschorn S. Penile implant success in patients with corporal fibrosis using multiple incisions and minimal scar tissue excision. Urology 2000;55(2):299–300.

[33] Rajpurkar A, Li H, Dhabuwala CB. Penile implant success in patients with corporal fibrosis using multiple incisions and minimal scar tissue excision. Urology 1999;54(1):145–7.

[34] Knoll LD, Fisher J, Benson RC Jr, et al. Treatment of penile fibrosis with prosthetic implantation and flap advancement with tissue debulking. J Urol 1996;156(2 Pt 1):394–7.

[35] George VK, Shah GS, Mills R, et al. The management of extensive penile fibrosis: a new technique of 'minimal scar-tissue excision'. Br J Urol 1996; 77(2):282–4.

[36] Knoll LD. Use of penile prosthetic implants in patients with penile fibrosis. Urol Clin North Am 1995;22(4):857–63.

[37] Herschorn S, Ordorica RC. Penile prosthesis insertion with corporeal reconstruction with synthetic vascular graft material. J Urol 1995;154(1): 80–4.

[38] Knoll LD, Furlow WL, Benson RC Jr, et al. Management of nondilatable cavernous fibrosis with the use of a downsized inflatable penile prosthesis. J Urol 1995;153(2):366–7.

[39] Kabalin JN. Corporeal fibrosis as a result of priapism prohibiting function of self-contained inflatable penile prosthesis. Urology 1994;43(3):401–3.

[40] Knoll LD, Furlow WL. Corporeal reconstruction and prosthetic implantation for impotence associated with non-dilatable corporeal cavernosal fibrosis. Acta Urol Belg 1992;60(1):15–25.

[41] Mireku-Boateng A, Jackson AG. Penile prosthesis in the management of priapism. Urol Int 1989; 44(4):247–8.

[42] Carson CC, Noh CH. Distal penile prosthesis extrusion: treatment with distal corporoplasty or gortex windsock reinforcement. Int J Imp Res 2002;14: 81–4.

[43] Hellstrom WJ, Reddy S. Application of pericardial graft in the surgical management of Peyronie's disease. J Urol 2000;163:1445–7.

[44] Palese MA, Burnett AL. Corporoplasty using pericardium allograft (Tutoplast) with complex penile prosthesis surgery. Urology 2001;58:1049–52.

[45] Mulcahy JJ. Distal corporoplasty for lateral extrusion of penile prosthesis cylinders. J Urol 1999;161: 193–5.

[46] Wilson SK, Henry GD. Penoscrotal approach for the three-piece and two-piece hydraulic implants. In: Mulcahy JJ, editor. Surgical atlas: impotence therapy. Atlas Urol Clin 10 2002. p. 169–80.

[47] Wilson SK, Henry GD, Delk JR, et al. Mentor Alpha 1 penile prosthesis with reservoir lock-out valve: effective prevention of auto-inflation with improved capability for ectopic reservoir placement. J Urol 2002;168:1475–8.

[48] Wilson SK, Delk JR Jr. A new treatment for Peyronie's disease: modeling the penis over an inflatable penile prosthesis. J Urol 1994;152:1121–3.

[49] Chaudhary M, Sheikh N, Asterling S, et al. Peyronie's disease with erectile dysfunction: penile modeling over inflatable penile prostheses. Urology 2005; 65(4):760–4.

[50] Wilson SK, Cleves MA, Delk JR Jr. Long-term follow-up of treatment of Peyronie's disease: modeling

the penis over an inflatable penile prosthesis. J Urol 2001;165:825–9.

[51] Brinkman MJ, Henry GD, Wilson SK, et al. A survey of patients with inflatable penile prostheses for satisfaction. J Urol 2005;174:253–7.

[52] Sadeghi-Hejad H, Ilbeigi P, Wilson SK, et al. Multi-institutional outcome study on the efficacy of closed suction drainage of the scrotum in three piece inflatable penile prosthesis surgery. Int J Impot Res 2005; 17:535–8.

ELSEVIER
SAUNDERS

Urol Clin N Am 34 (2007) 549–553

UROLOGIC
CLINICS
of North America

The Role of Testosterone Replacement Therapy Following Radical Prostatectomy

Mohit Khera, MD*, Larry I. Lipshultz, MD

Scott Department of Urology, Baylor College of Medicine, Houston, TX, USA

Hypogonadism is associated with a decreased serum testosterone level and numerous signs and symptoms, such as decreased libido, erectile dysfunction, decreased muscle mass, increased fat deposition, decreased ability to concentrate, and decreased bone mineral density [1–3]. Hypogonadism affects nearly 13 million Americans, with the incidence increasing with age [4,5]. Mulligan and colleagues [4] found that roughly 39% of men between the ages of 45 and 85 years had low testosterone levels. Despite its prevalence, many men who have this condition do not seek treatment.

Unlike women, who have a sudden loss of estrogen during menopause, men experience a gradual 1% to 2% decline in testosterone every year starting at age 30. There are several reasons for decreasing testosterone levels with age. As men age, they have a decline in Leydig cell numbers (primary failure), a decrease in gonadotropin-releasing hormone pulse amplitude (secondary failure), and an increase in sex hormone–binding globulin, all of which result in the reduction of available free or total testosterone [6,7].

Testosterone replacement therapy (TRT) is effective in treating the signs and symptoms of hypogonadism. These benefits include improvements in sexual function, muscle mass and strength, fat distribution, bone density, cognition, and mood [2,3,8,9]. Although hypogonadism also was shown to have an increased association with obesity and diabetes [10], TRT improves insulin resistance and weight loss. Pitteloud and colleagues [11] demonstrated that insulin resistance significantly improved after human chorionic gonadotropin stimulation. Wang and colleagues [12] found a significant increase in lean body mass and decrease in fat composition in hypogonadal men who were treated with transdermal testosterone replacement.

Hypogonadism occurs frequently among men who have prostate cancer. Yamamoto and colleagues [13] found that among men scheduled for a radical prostatectomy, approximately 18% had low testosterone levels. Mulligan and colleagues [4] found that 20% of men who had prostate disease or disorders were hypogonadal. Because prostate cancer and hypogonadism are much more common in men as they age, patients who have prostate cancer are a subset of men who are more likely to be hypogonadal.

The association between testosterone replacement therapy and the development of prostate cancer

In 1941, Huggins and Hodges [14] first demonstrated that a reduction in testosterone by castration caused metastatic prostate cancer to regress and that administration of exogenous testosterone promoted prostate cancer growth; however, current data have demonstrated that low testosterone levels are more likely to be associated with prostate cancer [15]. Morgantaler and Rhoden [15] found that cancer was detected in 21% of men with a low testosterone level of 250 ng/dL or less compared with 12% of men with a testosterone level greater than 250 ng/dL. Hoffman and colleagues [16] demonstrated that men with low testosterone values (<300 ng/dL) had a 47% chance of having prostate cancer on transrectal ultrasound biopsy compared with only 28% of men with normal testosterone levels ($P = .018$). Recently, Yamamoto and colleagues [13] showed that preoperative testosterone serum levels were

* Corresponding author.

E-mail address: mkhera@bcm.tmc.edu (M. Khera).

an independent and significant predictor of PSA failure after radical prostatectomy in patients who had clinically localized prostate cancer. In this study, 5-year prostate-specific antigen (PSA) failure-free survival rates of the patients with pre-operative low testosterone levels were significantly lower than those with normal testosterone values (67.8% versus 84.9%, respectively; $P = .035$). These findings suggest that low circulating testosterone levels may not have a protective effect against the development of prostate cancer. In fact, several studies showed that low testosterone levels were associated with more aggressive and higher-grade prostate cancer [16,17].

There is further evidence to support the belief that increased testosterone levels do not increase the risk for prostate cancer and growth. PSA values have not been shown to increase significantly after TRT [18–20]. In addition, prostate cancer exerts an inhibitory effect on testosterone synthesis, with studies demonstrating a significant increase in testosterone after a radical prostatectomy [21]. Finally, TRT in hypogonadal and eugonadal men has not been shown to increase prostate volume significantly [20,22].

Studies also report that TRT is a safe treatment for patients who are at high-risk for prostate cancer development. Rhoden and Morgentaler [23] treated 55 men with benign prostate biopsies and 20 men who had high-grade prostatic intraepithelial neoplasia (HGPIN) with TRT. The investigators followed these men for 1 year and found that there was no significant change in PSA in either group. Testosterone values improved significantly in both groups. A single patient who had HGPIN was diagnosed with prostate cancer based upon a biopsy after an abnormal digital rectal examination. Rhoden and Morgentaler concluded that men who have prostatic intraepithelial neoplasia (PIN) do not have a significantly greater risk for developing prostate cancer than do men without PIN after 1 year of TRT. If TRT is safe in treating men who have HGPIN, then administration of TRT to selected men following a radical prostatectomy (with negative margins and no biochemical recurrence) may be safe as well.

Marks and colleagues [24] studied the effect of TRT on prostate tissue in men who had late-onset hypogonadism. In this randomized, double-blinded, control trial, 40 hypogonadal men were treated with 150 mg of testosterone enanthate or placebo intramuscularly every 2 weeks. Prostate biopsies were performed at baseline and at the end of 6 months. Serum testosterone increased from 282 ng/dL to 640 ng/dL in the treated men. In contrast, there was no significant change in testosterone levels within the placebo-treated group (282 to 273 ng/dL). Testosterone and dihydrotestosterone (DHT) concentrations within the prostate did not change significantly in either group. Treatment-related changes in prostate histology, PSA, tissue biomarkers, gene expression, or cancer incidence or severity were not evident. In a related study, Heracek and colleagues [25] found no significant correlation between intraprostatic and serum testosterone levels in patients who had benign prostatic hyperplasia or prostate cancer. In this study, serum samples were analyzed for testosterone and DHT in 75 patients who had prostate cancer and 51 patients who had BPH. Significantly higher intraprostatic dihydroepiandrosterone concentrations were found in patients who had prostate cancer than in men who had BPH (8.9 ng/dL versus 6.4 ng/dL, respectively; $P < .01$). Similarly, there were higher intraprostatic concentrations of testosterone in men who had prostate cancer as compared with men who had BPH (4.6 ng/dL versus 3.4 ng/dL, respectively; $P < .05$); however, no differences were found in serum levels between the two groups of patients. Furthermore, there was no correlation between tissue and serum testosterone and DHT levels in either group of patients. These data support the safety of TRT in hypogonadal patients and demonstrate that there is no association between serum and intraprostatic levels of testosterone. There seems to be a threshold at which the prostate becomes saturated with testosterone and higher levels of serum testosterone do not affect intraprostatic levels.

TRT is withheld from many patients after surgery for prostate cancer for fear of exacerbating latent cancer cells; however, in each of the three small published series of TRT after a radical prostatectomy, there was not a single documented PSA increase [26–28]. In all three series, testosterone values increased significantly after initiation of TRT with an average follow-up of 21 months. Similarly, Sarosdy [29] evaluated TRT in patients with prostate cancer who were treated with brachytherapy. In this study, 31 men were followed for a median of 5 years after starting TRT. Although testosterone levels increased significantly, no patient stopped TRT because of cancer recurrence, and no patient experienced cancer progression. Although there are limited data in the literature evaluating the long-term safety of TRT in men who are treated for prostate cancer, early results suggest that TRT is safe within this population.

The importance of testosterone replacement therapy in erectile preservation following radical prostatectomy

Androgens play an important role in penile rehabilitation and overall erectile function. Nonresponders to phosphodiesterase type 5 inhibitors (PDE5i) often are hypogonadal men. TRT in these men converts PDE5i nonresponders to PDE5i responders [30–32]. Guay and colleagues [33] demonstrated that hypogonadal men not treated with androgens had a lower response rate to sildenafil citrate than did men receiving TRT (75% versus 85%, respectively). Similar findings were observed by Shabsigh and colleagues [31]. They conducted a randomized, placebo-controlled trial in 75 men who had hypogonadism (testosterone <400 ng/dL) who failed to respond to sildenafil citrate. Half of these patients received 5 g/d of transdermal testosterone gel. Testosterone-treated subjects had greater improvements in erectile function at 4 weeks than did those who received placebos. The results of these two studies can be explained by the fact that increased testosterone levels have been associated with greater phosphodiesterase type 5 and nitric oxide synthase activity within cavernosal tissue [34–37]. Enhancement in erectile dysfunction treatment response may reflect the actions of testosterone on the up-regulation of NOS isoenzymes in the corpora cavernosa [35]. Thus, testosterone plays an important role in erectile function and in augmenting the effects of PDE5i.

Testosterone also has an important role in cavernosal nerve function and growth. Schirar and colleagues [38] demonstrated that androgen receptors were present in approximately 40% of neurons of the major pelvic ganglion innervating the corpora cavernosa of the rat penis. They also showed that in the major pelvic ganglion, 87% of the neurons contained nitric oxide synthase. These results suggest that androgens, which are known to modulate penile erections, may do so by regulating nitric oxide synthase within the major pelvic ganglia by way of direct interaction with ganglionic neurons. In another study, Baba and colleagues [39] demonstrated that there was a significant reduction in nerve fibers in the corpora cavernosa and both dorsal nerves in castrate rats. Rogers and colleagues [40] found that in castrated rats, the diameter of the myelinated and nonmyelinated axons of the dorsal penile nerve were significantly smaller than were those of the sham-operated rats. When these animals were given testosterone, the nerve fibers and myelin sheath size appeared similar to those in the sham-operated group. Finally, Syme and colleagues [41] studied 45 rats that underwent bilateral cavernosus nerve neurotomy, followed by unilateral nerve graft using the genitofemoral nerve. Then rats were randomized to castrate, intact, and testosterone-treated arms. At 3 months, grafts were explored, and electrostimulation was performed with intracavernous pressure responses recorded. Then grafted nerves were harvested for immunohistochemical analysis. Castration resulted in a decreased erectile response to electrostimulation following nerve grafting, and castrate animals had lower neuronal nitric oxide synthase axon counts than did intact animals. It is clear from these several studies that androgens play an important role in cavernosal nerve function and growth.

There is substantial evidence to support that DHT, not testosterone, is the more active and potent androgen in preventing erectile impairment [42–44]. Lugg and colleagues [42] found that DHT was the active androgen in the prevention of erectile failure seen in castrated rats and that this effect may be mediated, at least partially, by changes in nitric oxide synthase levels within the penis. DHT may be more effective in improving erectile function because of its higher affinity for binding with the androgen receptor [45]. The prostate is a major source of DHT in men; thus, it is not surprising that there is a significant reduction in DHT following radical prostatectomy. Because DHT has been shown to be the major source for maintenance of erectile function, it seems likely that patients who have undergone radical prostatectomy may be more susceptible to experiencing erectile dysfunction than are men who still have their prostates.

Summary

Hypogonadism is highly prevalent in older men and men who have prostate cancer. The symptoms of hypogonadism, such as depression, decreased libido, erectile dysfunction, and decreased bone mineral density, can impair a man's quality of life significantly. Moreover, we know that testosterone plays an important role in erectile preservation by improving the effects of PDE5i and in the growth and function of cavernosal and penile nerves. There are now compelling data to suggest that TRT in normal and high-risk men does not increase the risk for prostate cancer. In the few studies of men treated with TRT after a radical prostatectomy, there have been no biochemical recurrences. Based on these data, it is difficult to justify withholding TRT in men following a radical prostatectomy. If we do not lower the testosterone levels of eugonadal men after a radical prostatectomy, how can we justify not replacing testosterone levels in hypogonadal men to make them eugonadal following a radical prostatectomy?

References

[1] Kelleher S, Conway AJ, Handelsman DJ. Blood testosterone threshold for androgen deficiency symptoms. J Clin Endocrinol Metab 2004;89:3813–7.

[2] Sih R, Morley JE, Kaiser FE, et al. Testosterone replacement in older hypogonadal men: a 12-month randomized controlled trial. J Clin Endocrinol Metab 1997;82:1661–7.

[3] Snyder PJ, Peachey H, Berlin JA, et al. Effects of testosterone replacement in hypogonadal men. J Clin Endocrinol Metab 2000;85:2670–7.

[4] Mulligan T, Frick MF, Zuraw QC, et al. Prevalence of hypogonadism in males aged at least 45 years: the HIM study. Int J Clin Pract 2006;60:762–9.

[5] Harman SM, Metter EJ, Tobin JD, et al. Longitudinal effects of aging on serum total and free testosterone levels in healthy men. Baltimore Longitudinal Study of Aging. J Clin Endocrinol Metab 2001;86: 724–31.

[6] Morley JE, Kaiser FE, Perry HM III, et al. Longitudinal changes in testosterone, luteinizing hormone, and follicle-stimulating hormone in healthy older men. Metabolism 1997;46:410–3.

[7] Neaves WB, Johnson L, Porter JC, et al. Leydig cell numbers, daily sperm production, and serum gonadotropin levels in aging men. J Clin Endocrinol Metab 1984;59:756–63.

[8] Snyder PJ, Peachey H, Hannoush P, et al. Effect of testosterone treatment on body composition and muscle strength in men over 65 years of age. J Clin Endocrinol Metab 1999;84:2647–53.

[9] Snyder PJ, Peachey H, Hannoush P, et al. Effect of testosterone treatment on bone mineral density in men over 65 years of age. J Clin Endocrinol Metab 1999;84:1966–72.

[10] Guay A, Jacobson J. The relationship between testosterone levels, the metabolic syndrome (by two criteria), and insulin resistance in a population of men with organic erectile dysfunction. J Sex Med 2007;4:1046–55.

[11] Pitteloud N, Hardin M, Dwyer AA, et al. Increasing insulin resistance is associated with a decrease in Leydig cell testosterone secretion in men. J Clin Endocrinol Metab 2005;90:2636–41.

[12] Wang C, Swerdloff RS, Iranmanesh A, et al. Transdermal testosterone gel improves sexual function, mood, muscle strength, and body composition parameters in hypogonadal men. J Clin Endocrinol Metab 2000;85:2839–53.

[13] Yamamoto S, Yonese J, Kawakami S, et al. Preoperative serum testosterone level as an independent predictor of treatment failure following radical prostatectomy. Eur Urol 2007;52:696–701.

[14] Huggins C, Hodges CV. Studies on prostate cancer. 1. The effect of castration, of estrogen and androgen injection on serum phosphatase in metastatic carcinoma of the prostate. Cancer Res 1941;293–7.

[15] Morgentaler A, Rhoden EL. Prevalence of prostate cancer among hypogonadal men with prostate-specific antigen levels of 4.0 ng/mL or less. Urology 2006;68:1263.

[16] Hoffman MA, DeWolf WC, Morgentaler A. Is low serum free testosterone a marker for high grade prostate cancer? J Urol 2000;163:824.

[17] Ribeiro M, Ruff P, Falkson G. Low serum testosterone and a younger age predict for a poor outcome in metastatic prostate cancer. Am J Clin Oncol 1997; 20:605.

[18] Rhoden EL, Morgentaler A. Influence of demographic factors and biochemical characteristics on the prostate-specific antigen (PSA) response to testosterone replacement therapy. Int J Impot Res 2006;18:201.

[19] Svetec DA, Canby ED, Thompson IM, et al. The effect of parenteral testosterone replacement on prostate specific antigen in hypogonadal men with erectile dysfunction. J Urol 1997;158:1775.

[20] Behre HM, Bohmeyer J, Nieschlag E. Prostate volume in testosterone-treated and untreated hypogonadal men in comparison to age-matched normal controls. Clin Endocrinol (Oxf) 1994;40:341.

[21] Miller LR, Partin AW, Chan DW, et al. Influence of radical prostatectomy on serum hormone levels. J Urol 1998;160:449.

[22] Marks LS, Hess DL, Dorey FJ, et al. Tissue effects of saw palmetto and finasteride: use of biopsy cores for in situ quantification of prostatic androgens. Urology 2001;57:999.

[23] Rhoden EL, Morgentaler A. Testosterone replacement therapy in hypogonadal men at high risk for prostate cancer: results of 1 year of treatment in men with prostatic intraepithelial neoplasia. J Urol 2003;170:2348.

[24] Marks LS, Mazer NA, Mostaghel E, et al. Effect of testosterone replacement therapy on prostate tissue in men with late-onset hypogonadism: a randomized controlled trial. JAMA 2006;296:2351.

[25] Heracek J, Richard H, Maratin H, et al. Tissue and serum levels of principal androgens in benign prostatic hyperplasia and prostate cancer. Steroids 2007;72:375–80.

[26] Agarwal PK, Oefelein MG. Testosterone replacement therapy after primary treatment for prostate cancer. J Urol 2005;173:533.

[27] Kaufman JM, Graydon RJ. Androgen replacement after curative radical prostatectomy for prostate cancer in hypogonadal men. J Urol 2004;172: 920.

[28] Khera M. The efficacy and safety of testosterone replacement therapy following radical prostatectomy. J Urol 2007.

[29] Sarosdy MF. Testosterone replacement for hypogonadism after treatment of early prostate cancer with brachytherapy. Cancer 2007;109:536–41.

[30] Rosenthal BD, May NR, Metro MJ, et al. Adjunctive use of AndroGel (testosterone gel) with sildenafil to treat erectile dysfunction in men with acquired androgen deficiency syndrome after failure using sildenafil alone. Urology 2006;67:571.

[31] Shabsigh R, Kaufman JM, Steidle C, et al. Randomized study of testosterone gel as adjunctive therapy to sildenafil in hypogonadal men with erectile dysfunction who do not respond to sildenafil alone. J Urol 2004;172:658–63.

[32] Shabsigh R. Testosterone therapy in erectile dysfunction and hypogonadism. J Sex Med 2005;2:785–92.

[33] Guay AT, Perez JB, Jacobson J, et al. Efficacy and safety of sildenafil citrate for treatment of erectile dysfunction in a population with associated organic risk factors. J Androl 2001;22:793–7.

[34] Baba K, Yajima M, Carrier S, et al. Delayed testosterone replacement restores nitric oxide synthase-containing nerve fibres and the erectile response in rat penis. BJU Int 2000;85:953–8.

[35] Marin R, Escrig A, Abreu P, et al. Androgen-dependent nitric oxide release in rat penis correlates with levels of constitutive nitric oxide synthase isoenzymes. Biol Reprod 1999;61:1012–6.

[36] Traish AM, Park K, Dhir V, et al. Effects of castration and androgen replacement on erectile function in a rabbit model. Endocrinology 1999;140:1861–8.

[37] Traish AM, Munarriz R, O'Connell L, et al. Effects of medical or surgical castration on erectile function in an animal model. J Androl 2003;24:381–7.

[38] Schirar A, Chang C, Rousseau JP. Localization of androgen receptor in nitric oxide synthase- and vasoactive intestinal peptide-containing neurons of the major pelvic ganglion innervating the rat penis. J Neuroendocrinol 1997;9:141–50.

[39] Baba K, Yajima M, Carrier S, et al. Effect of testosterone on the number of NADPH diaphorase-stained nerve fibers in the rat corpus cavernosum and dorsal nerve. Urology 2000;56:533–8.

[40] Rogers RS, Graziottin TM, Lin CS, et al. Intracavernosal vascular endothelial growth factor (VEGF) injection and adeno-associated virus-mediated VEGF gene therapy prevent and reverse venogenic erectile dysfunction in rats. Int J Impot Res 2003;15:26–37.

[41] Syme DB, Corcoran NM, Bouchier-Hayes DM, et al. The effect of androgen status on the structural and functional success of cavernous nerve grafting in an experimental rat model. J Urol 2007;177:390–4.

[42] Lugg JA, Rajfer J, Gonzalez-Cadavid NF. Dihydrotestosterone is the active androgen in the maintenance of nitric oxide-mediated penile erection in the rat. Endocrinology 1995;136:1495–501.

[43] Park KH, Kim SW, Kim KD, et al. Effects of androgens on the expression of nitric oxide synthase mRNAs in rat corpus cavernosum. BJU Int 1999;83:327–33.

[44] Schultheiss D, Badalyan R, Pilatz A, et al. Androgen and estrogen receptors in the human corpus cavernosum penis: immunohistochemical and cell culture results. World J Urol 2003;21:320–4.

[45] Grino PB, Griffin JE, Wilson JD. Testosterone at high concentrations interacts with the human androgen receptor similarly to dihydrotestosterone. Endocrinology 1990;126:1165–72.

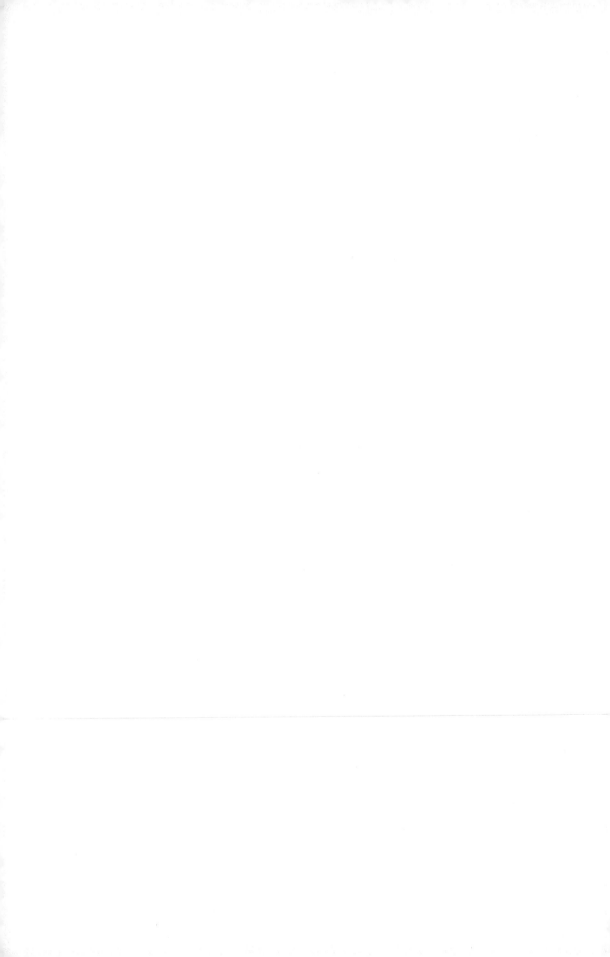

ELSEVIER
SAUNDERS

UROLOGIC
CLINICS
of North America

Urol Clin N Am 34 (2007) 555–563

Testosterone Replacement Therapy and Prostate Cancer

Abraham Morgentaler, MD, FACS[a,b]

[a]Men's Health Boston, Brookline, MA, USA
[b]Harvard Medical School, Boston, MA, USA

For the past 65 years, it has been axiomatic that higher serum testosterone (T) levels cause increased prostate cancer (PCa) growth and that T supplementation carries the risk for converting occult PCa into a clinical PCa. This theory originated with the work of Huggins and his coworkers [1,2], who, in 1941, published the landmark papers establishing the androgen dependence of PCa. They reported that reducing serum T to castrate levels caused PCa to regress and that T administration caused enhanced PCa growth.

During this author's training in the 1980s, this relation between T and PCa was unassailable. The arguments supporting the concept that T caused PCa growth were multiple: lowering of T to castrate levels caused PCa to regress (and remains a mainstay of treatment for advanced disease to this day), men castrated early in life never developed PCa, and the occasional new diagnosis of PCa in a patient receiving testosterone replacement therapy (TRT) confirmed the danger of T for men with occult PCa. No wonder, then, that we learned to describe the relation between T and PCa as "fuel for a fire" or "food for a hungry tumor."

This concern regarding PCa and T has led to the lifetime prohibition against TRT for any man diagnosed with PCa, regardless of disease status. It has even been suggested that men at higher risk for development of PCa, such as those with a family history of PCa, be excluded from TRT

trials because of the concern that higher T may cause growth of occult cancer in these men [3].

If T truly caused significant PCa growth, however, there should be observable evidence for it, such as increased PCa rates in men receiving TRT or among men with high endogenous T. Yet, multiple reviews have failed to identify any such supporting evidence [4–7]. A report on T and aging by the Institute of Medicine concluded, "In summary, the influence of T on prostate carcinogenesis and other prostate outcomes remains poorly defined..." [3].

This relation between TRT and PCa is important because of the large number of symptomatic hypogonadal men who might potentially benefit from treatment. TRT has been shown to improve erectile dysfunction and diminished libido and to have a wide range of nonsexual benefits as well, including positive effects on mood, fatigue, sense of well-being, muscle strength and mass, bone mineral density, glucose metabolism, and markers of the metabolic syndrome [4,8]. In addition, there is a substantial and growing population of men who have been successfully treated for PCa and who are symptomatic from low serum T and desire TRT. This population, in particular, has caused urologists and oncologists to re-examine the old concern regarding TRT and PCa.

Arguments made to support the belief that testosterone causes prostate cancer growth

Huggins: testosterone administration caused "enhanced growth" of prostate cancer

In 1941, Huggins and his coworkers [1,2] published two articles establishing the hormonal responsiveness of PCa. In the first, it was noted that acid phosphatase declined after lowering of

Dr. Abraham Morgentaler has received lecture honoraria, research funding, or served on clinical advisory boards for the following companies with relevant interests: Solvay, Auxilium, Indevus, and Schering.

E-mail address: amorgent@bidmc.harvard.edu

T by castration or estrogen treatment and that acid phosphatase levels rose with T administration [1]. Although it was reported that T administration was given to three men, results were only provided for two men, and one of these men had been previously castrated. In the second article, T was also administered to three men, and it was reported that acid phosphatase values rose. All men in this study had previously undergone orchiectomy, however [2].

We know today that normalization of T levels after a reduction to castrate levels causes PCa regrowth and also that the serum acid phosphatase test used by Huggins in this study would turn out to perform erratically [9]. The issue at hand, however, is whether T administration causes increased PCa growth in a previously untreated man. In a review 25 years after his original work, Huggins [10] reasserted the concept that T administration in previously untreated men caused enhanced PCa growth, citing only his first article. It is simply astounding to discover that the origin of this long-standing near-universal belief was based on a single patient [11].

"Testosterone is a growth factor for prostate cancer"

This statement has generally been used to imply that there exists a concentration-dependent rate of growth of PCa for T, without an upper limit. A more accurate statement is that the presence of androgens is necessary for the growth of most but not all human prostate cancer and under many but not all laboratory conditions [12,13].

There is strong evidence that a saturation level exists for prostate tissue with regard to T, with T levels greater than this saturation point not associated with additional growth. For example, TRT in hypogonadal men caused prostate volume to increase to the size of age-matched eugonadal controls but no higher [14]. Further, administration of supraphysiologic doses of T to a group of healthy men resulted in no change in prostate-specific antigen (PSA) or prostate volume [15].

The saturation for T in prostate tissue likely occurs at relatively low serum concentrations, because TRT in hypogonadal men causes only a minor increase in PSA and prostate volume of approximately 15% [16]. This compares with a 13% increase in PSA at 48 weeks among men aged 50 to 60 years in the placebo arm of an unrelated clinical trial [17]. In contrast, these parameters

increase several fold in healthy volunteers when castrate T levels are allowed to normalize after discontinuation of luteinizing hormone-releasing hormone (LHRH) agonists [18]. Finally, there is recent evidence that the effects of dutasteride, a 5α-reductase inhibitor, on PSA, prostate volume, and voiding symptoms were no different for men even with substantially reduced endogenous serum T levels [19]. These results suggest that maximal or near-maximal prostate growth (and its potential for reversal with 5α-reductase inhibitors) occurs at low circulating levels of T.

"Prostate cancer does not occur in eunuchs"

Although often mistakenly attributed to Huggins, the source for this statement is a 1948 article by Hovenanian and Deming [20], in which they report on growth characteristics of human PCa tumors transferred to guinea pigs. In an unreferenced comment, they wrote, "...human clinical experiences have revealed that cancer of the prostate has not been found in eunuchs" [20].

The assertion was made during a time when prostate examinations were not routinely performed, there was no accurate blood test for PCa, and there was no existing large population of men castrated early in life who had been followed for 40 to 50 years to determine whether or not they ever developed PCa. Moreover, PCa has indeed been reported in anorchic men [21], and one series reported 25 men with PCa and testicular atrophy at the time of therapeutic orchiectomy [22].

Testosterone administration caused high rate of unfavorable responses among men with metastatic prostate cancer

In 1981, Fowler and Whitmore [23] reported on the experience at Memorial Sloan Kettering Cancer Center, in which 67 men with a history of PCa with bony metastases received T injections. In this review of cases accumulated from 1949 through 1967, T administration had been attempted as a possible therapeutic measure because of a lack of additional treatment options in advanced cases. Of 52 evaluable cases, 45 men had an "unfavorable response," defined broadly to include subjective symptoms, such as worsening of bone pain, and objective measures, such as an increase in acid phosphatase or clinical progression.

This high rate of unfavorable responses has been offered as proof that T causes rapid PCa growth and progression. However, all but four of these men had previously been castrated or treated with estrogen, however. Within this small untreated group, one man had an unspecified unfavorable response within 30 days of beginning daily T injections, another had a subjective "beneficial response," and the remaining two eventually developed unfavorable responses at 56 and 310 days. Given the advanced stage of PCa in these men, and the lack of a control group, it must be considered that the unfavorable responses seen in this population may have been attributable entirely to the natural history of their disease and were unrelated to T administration.

Intrigued by the apparent lack of T-related clinical progression in this previously untreated group, Fowler and Whitmore [23] postulated that "near maximal stimulation of prostate cancer occurred at physiologic T levels." This statement represents an early and prescient articulation of the saturation model for PCa and T.

Testosterone flare

LHRH agonists are known to increase T levels substantially for 7 to 10 days before they decline to castrate levels [24]. This "testosterone flare" has been associated with adverse events, such as increased bone pain, urinary retention, and vertebral collapse with paraplegia, and it has been assumed that these adverse events occurred because of T-driven PCa growth [24]. Several clinical strategies have thus been developed to prevent the consequences of this flare phenomenon, such as the addition of antiandrogens or the use of LHRH antagonists that do not cause a transient increase in T levels.

Surprisingly, in the two studies that measured PSA during the period of elevated T, PSA values never rose to greater than baseline [25,26]. Because PSA levels have been shown to correlate with PCa progression [27], the failure of PSA to increase during the T flare suggests that higher serum T levels do not cause increased PCa growth even in men with stage D disease.

Case reports

Several anecdotal reports have described development of PCa some time after initiation of TRT [28,29]. Because the diagnoses of PCa and TRT are common occurrences in urology practices, however, it is to be expected that some men receiving TRT are eventually likely to be diagnosed with PCa. This is no different

than reporting cases of PCa in men with blue eyes. Because association does not equal causality, these types of reports are of value only if they bring to light an unrecognized relation. In this case, if TRT truly increased PCa rates in the short term, there should be an observable increased rate of PCa in men receiving TRT, an effect that has not been demonstrated. These reports and their cautions regarding TRT are examples of confirmation bias, in which an observation seems to confirm a previously held belief without being subject to standard scientific rigor.

Racial variation in prostate cancer prevalence corresponds with serum testosterone levels

It has been argued in the past that the greater prevalence of PCa in African-American men can be explained by higher serum T levels in African-American men compared with US men of European descent [30]. Multiple studies have shown the magnitude of this difference to be nonexistent or small ($<10\%$) for men older than 30 years of age, however [30]. Moreover, several studies have also shown higher serum T levels in low-risk Asian populations compared with white men [31,32]. Ethnic or racial variation in serum T levels thus seems to be highly unlikely to account for observed racial differences in PCa prevalence.

Prostate Cancer Prevention Trial

The Prostate Cancer Prevention Trial (PCPT) trial was a placebo-controlled study of the effects of finasteride on the risk for PCa development [33]. Finasteride is a 5α-reductase inhibitor that markedly reduces the conversion of T to dihydrotestosterone (DHT) the primary androgen for the prostate. A 25% reduction in PCa risk was observed for men taking finasteride, suggesting that androgens are indeed involved in the development or growth of PCa [33].

It is important to emphasize here that there is no dispute that the presence of androgens is important for PCa growth or that severe reduction of androgens causes PCa regression. The question at hand is whether higher concentrations of T cause increasingly greater PCa growth, especially beyond the near-castrate range. The PCPT did not address this question.

Review of historical and current evidence regarding the relation of testosterone and prostate cancer

Historical experience with testosterone administration in men with prostate cancer

Several reports before 1980 described the results of T administration in previously untreated men with advanced PCa, most of whom had bony metastases. The largest of these was by Prout and Brewer [9], who described daily T injections in 26 men, 20 of whom were previously untreated, and other investigators reported smaller experiences [34,35]. The behavior of acid phosphatase in response to T administration was highly variable. Pearson [36], noting that Huggins and Hodges had described only one hormonally intact patient who developed an increase in acid phosphatase with T administration, offered a case report of another individual with metastatic PCa who received daily T injections without an appreciable increase in acid phosphatase until he developed clinical progression 9 months later.

Although these reports were not controlled, it is noteworthy that none of the investigators described clinical progression attributable to T administration. On the contrary, several men treated with T experienced subjective improvement, including prompt resolution of bone pain, increased appetite, weight gain, and improved sense of well-being [10]. Some of these men with metastatic disease were treated with daily T injections for as long as 1 year without adverse results.

These reports, largely lost to history, suggest a lack of apparent clinical progression with T administration, even in men with far-advanced disease.

Testosterone replacement therapy trials

Although no large-scale long-term studies of TRT have been performed, several smaller TRT trials of greater than 6 months' duration have revealed an annual cancer detection rate of approximately 1% [4]. The longest of these trials was 42 months [8]. This 1% cancer rate is similar to cancer detection rates in prostate screening trials [4].

Testosterone replacement therapy in a high-risk population

Men with high-grade prostatic intraepithelial neoplasia (PIN) have been reported to develop frank PCa at a rate 25% or greater over 3 years [37]. In one study, TRT was provided to 20 hypogonadal men with PIN and 55 hypogonadal men with benign biopsies [38]. At the end of 12 months, PCa was identified in 1 man in the PIN group and none in the benign group. This represents a 5% cancer rate in the PIN group and a 1.3% cancer rate for the entire group. These results do not suggest a precipitous increase in the risk for PCa in this high-risk population.

Longitudinal studies

The relation of T and other sex hormones to subsequent development of PCa has been extensively studied in at least 16 population-based longitudinal studies [39–44]. In these studies, a health history is obtained and blood samples at baseline are then frozen for the duration of the study, up to 20 years or longer in some cases. At the end of the study, men who have developed PCa are identified, and a matched set of men without PCa serves as a control group.

A total of greater than 430,000 men have been included in these studies, including 1400 men with PCa and 4400 men identified as controls. Not one study has shown a direct correlation between total T levels and PCa. Isolated associations have been reported with some measures and PCa: minor androgens [42] in one study, calculated free T [43] in another study, and with quartile analysis of hormone ratios or controlling for multiple variables in a third study [44]. None of these positive associations have been supported by later studies. It is worth noting that the largest study of this type actually noted reduced PCa risk in men with higher T levels [41].

The importance of these studies is that they provide a sophisticated method of investigation to determine the long-term effects of hormone levels, especially T, on the subsequent risk for development of PCa. Although such studies cannot entirely replace the value of a prospective, long-term, controlled study of TRT, they do address the question as to whether high levels of T (or other hormones) predispose men to a greater risk for later development of PCa. On this question, these prospective longitudinal studies provide two uniform and convincing answers: first, that men who develop PCa do not have higher baseline T levels and, second, that men with higher T levels are at no greater risk for developing PCa than men with lower T concentrations.

Prostate cancer rates in men with low testosterone

If high T is believed to be associated with an increased risk for PCa, it follows that low T should be associated with a reduced risk. Sextant prostate biopsy in 77 hypogonadal men with normal digital rectal examination results and PSA of 4.0 ng/mL or less revealed cancer in 11 men, however [45]. A more recent study in 345 hypogonadal men found a similar overall cancer rate of 15.1% in men with PSA of 4.0 ng/mL or less, with an odds risk that was doubled for men with the lowest tertile of serum T compared with the upper tertile [46]. The overall cancer rate was similar to the 15.2% PCa rate noted by Thompson and colleagues [47] in the placebo arm of the PCPT but in a population that was a decade younger.

Other work has shown that low T is associated with high-grade Gleason scores, advanced stage at presentation, and worse survival [48–52]. These associations between low T and PCa risk constitute a new and emerging area of interest in oncology research [53].

Epidemiology of prostate cancer and testosterone

A major shortcoming of the theory that T causes enhanced PCa growth is the natural history of PCa. Clinical PCa almost never occurs when men are in their 20s, when T levels are at their lifetime peak. Conversely, it becomes highly prevalent when men are older and T levels have declined. If T truly behaved as fuel for a fire for PCa, one should expect to see a substantial number of PCa cases in extremely young men, especially because autopsy studies have identified the presence of PCa microfoci in as many as 2% of men in their 20s and 29% in their 30s [54]. In addition, because one in seven hypogonadal men has biopsy-detectable PCa [45,46], why is it that the cancer rate in clinical TRT trials is only 1% [4]?

Resolving the paradox: saturation

Because castration causes PCa to regress, how is it possible that T administration would fail to cause PCa to grow? The resolution of this apparent paradox was recognized at least a quarter of century ago by Fowler and Whitmore [23], who suggested that near-maximal stimulation of PCa occurred at physiologic T levels. This suggests a model of saturation in which existing PCa tumors have access to all the androgens they can use at fairly low serum concentrations, with

higher amounts representing a surfeit without impact on further growth.

This saturation model is supported by the landmark article by Marks and colleagues [55], in which intraprostatic levels of T and DHT were determined before and after 6 months of TRT. Although serum levels of both hormones increased substantially in the treatment arm, intraprostatic T and DHT did not change significantly and were no different from intraprostatic T and DHT in the placebo arm. Moreover, markers of cellular proliferation also did not change with therapy. These results indicate that changes in serum androgen levels in hypogonadal men are not reflected within the prostate itself. Another implication of the study is that the prostate seems able to create for itself a homeostatic environment with regard to androgens, at least within the range of serum T included in the study.

The traditional model regarding the relation of T and PCa is that PCa growth is tied to serum T concentration, such that low levels cause low rates of growth (or even negative growth in the case of castration) and higher levels cause enhanced growth, as originally described by Huggins. A graphic representation of this traditional model is shown in Fig. 1 and is represented by curves a and b, with an unquantified positive correlation between T and PCa growth, without apparent

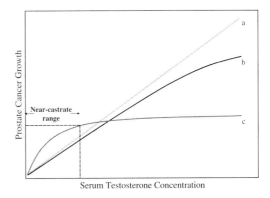

Fig. 1. Proposed saturation model for the relation of PCa growth and serum T concentration. The traditional belief has been that higher T concentrations caused increasing rates of PCa growth, as represented by curves a and b. All available evidence demonstrates a powerful effect of T on PCa growth at low T concentrations, however, but little or no effect beyond the near-castrate range. The proposed model for the relation between T and PCa is thus shown as curve c and is consistent with a saturation model, as seen in many other biologic systems.

limit. This approach can be summarized as "more T, more PCa growth."

Yet, all available evidence fails to demonstrate any significant relationship between T and PCa beyond the castrate or near-castrate range. Without question, there is a powerful effect of T concentration on PCa at the low extreme of serum T concentration. However, this effect clearly plateaus at some low concentration of T. This saturation model is represented by curve c in the Fig. 1.

This type of saturation curve is common in biology and oncology. A similar curve c would apply to nearly any tumor and glucose or calcium. Both chemicals are metabolically required for growth; however, at some concentration, the cellular requirement for these agents is satisfied and higher concentrations do not have an impact on tumor growth.

This saturation model for T and PCa suggests that our old analogy of T being like food for a hungry tumor is false and misleading. An analogy that fits the available evidence far better is that "T is like water for a thirsty tumor." Once the thirst has been quenched by adequate (and relatively low) T concentrations, additional amounts serve as nothing more than an excess.

Testosterone replacement therapy after treatment for prostate cancer

There are now several publications reporting no ill effects from administration of TRT in hypogonadal men previously treated for PCa. These included two small series in men with an undetectable PSA level after radical prostatectomy, with no recurrences noted in the 17 men followed for up to 12 years [56,57]. A more recent study of 31 hypogonadal men receiving TRT after brachytherapy for a mean of 4.5 years revealed that 100% maintained PSA levels less than 1.0 ng/mL, with a mean follow-up of 5 years [58]. No biochemical or clinical recurrences occurred. These results are consistent with the previously mentioned historical studies before 1980 in which T was administered to men with metastatic and advanced local disease without clinical evidence of harmful effects.

Discussion

The theory that higher T leads to enhanced PCa growth has been widely held for more than two thirds of a century and continues to inform current medical behavior and recommendations. As reviewed previously, however, arguments offered over the years to support this theory lack substance, scientific rigor, or relevance. It is critical to acknowledge that the original assertion by Huggins that T causes greater PCa growth in untreated men was based on a single patient [1].

The persistence of this unsupported theory seems to owe its appeal and longevity to the confounding of three concepts regarding the relationship of T and PCa:

1. T is important for PCa growth (True).
2. Reducing androgens to castrate levels causes PCa regression (True).
3. Raising T in noncastrated men leads to enhanced PCa growth (Alleged, despite all evidence to the contrary).

The indisputable evidence supporting the first two does not necessarily make the third true. Yet, there has been little attempt in the past to tease apart these various points, and they have thus been accepted together as a general "truth" regarding the relation of T and PCa.

Evidence for a lack of a growth-enhancing effect of T beyond the near-castrate level includes the following: longitudinal studies show no correlation of PCa risk with serum T levels, no precipitous increase in PCa is seen in high-risk men receiving TRT, PCa risk does not seem to be reduced in men with low T, and the natural history of PCa is that clinical disease is almost nonexistent when T levels are at their lifetime peak and only becomes highly prevalent when T levels have declined. In addition, among men with known PCa, studies have failed to show any correlation between higher T levels and tumor grade, stage of presentation, or survival.

The assumption that T causes enhanced growth of PCa in otherwise untreated men represents the persistence of an unexamined historical belief [11]. This historical model is overly simplistic, suggesting that T provides a stimulus to PCa growth as a continuous variable (ie, more T, more growth). Available evidence supports a different model in which PCa growth is stimulated at near-castrate serum T concentrations but then soon reaches a saturation point greater than which higher T concentrations provide no increased stimulus to growth. This saturation model would explain why PCa occurs rarely in young men despite the simultaneous presence of PCa microfoci and high T levels and also why PCa behavior and characteristics do not seem to correlate with T levels within the physiologic range. Although this saturation model accounts for much of what is known regarding T and PCa, its validity remains to be confirmed. If confirmed, might it be possible that TRT could be offered to men with untreated or even metastatic PCa?

At a minimum, it is time to acknowledge that our behavior regarding T and PCa is inconsistent and illogical. For example, we allow serum T levels to increase within the normal range after discontinuation of LHRH agonist treatment with radiation therapy, yet we generally withhold TRT from those who are symptomatic from failure of T levels to normalize, citing concerns of PCa progression. Some have suggested that TRT should not be offered to hypogonadal men at risk for PCa, yet there is no serious discussion of reducing T as prophylaxis for these men.

Although there is yet to be a large, long-term, controlled study on the effect of TRT on PCa risk, it should be abundantly clear that raising T in hypogonadal men has little, if any, impact on PCa risk or growth in the short to medium term. The withholding of TRT in men because of the fear of PCa risk or progression is no longer tenable in an age of evidence-based medicine, because neither evidence nor theory supports this position. It is time for a more sophisticated rethinking of the relation between T and PCa, one that is internally consistent, scientifically based, and accounts for all the rich and varied set of clinical and research data regarding PCa and hormones. Most importantly, physicians should be freed of antiquated and unscientific restrictions that inhibit optimal treatment of their patients.

Summary

The long-standing belief that higher T leads to greater PCa growth in noncastrated men is contrary to all accumulated evidence and should be discarded. The relation of T and PCa seems most consistent with a saturation model in which there is a powerful impact of serum T on PCa growth at castrate or near-castrate concentrations but little or no effect at higher T concentrations. Although there are no large long-term studies on the safety of TRT with regard to PCa, there does exist a wealth of evidence suggesting that TRT does not increase PCa risk. With proper medical monitoring, TRT can be safely offered to men with T deficiency.

References

[1] Huggins C, Hodges CV. Studies on prostatic cancer. I. The effect of castration, of estrogen and of androgen injection on serum phosphatases in metastatic carcinoma of the prostate. Cancer Res 1941; 1:293–7.

[2] Huggins C, Stevens RE Jr, Hodges CV. Studies on prostatic cancer. II. The effects of castration on advanced carcinoma of the prostate gland. Arch Surg 1941;43:209–23.

[3] Institute of Medicine. Testosterone and aging: clinical research directions. In: Liverman CT, Blazer DG, editors. Washington, DC: National Academies Press; 2004. p. 56.

[4] Rhoden EL, Morgentaler A. Risks of testosterone-replacement therapy and recommendations for monitoring. N Engl J Med 2004;350:482–92.

[5] Morgentaler A. Testosterone replacement therapy and prostate risks: where's the beef? Can J Urol 2006;13(Suppl 1):S40–3.

[6] Bhasin S, Singh AB, Mac RP, et al. Managing the risks of prostate disease during testosterone replacement therapy in older men: recommendations for a standardized monitoring plan. J Androl 2003;24: 299–311.

[7] Barqawi AB, Crawford ED. Testosterone replacement therapy and the risk of prostate cancer: a perspective view. Int J Impot Res 2005;17: 462–3.

[8] Wang C, Cunningham G, Dobs A, et al. Long-term testosterone gel (AndroGel) treatment maintains beneficial effects on sexual function and mood, lean and fat mass, and bone density in hypogonadal men. J Clin Endocrinol Metab 2004;89:2085–98.

[9] Prout GR, Brewer WR. Response of men with advanced prostatic carcinoma to exogenous administration of testosterone. Cancer 1967;20:1871–8.

[10] Huggins C. Endocrine-induced regression of cancers. Cancer Res 1967;27:1925–30.

[11] Morgentaler A. Testosterone and prostate cancer: an historical perspective on a modern myth. Eur Urol 2006;50:935–9.

[12] Isaacs JT, Heston WD, Weissman RM, et al. Animal models of the hormone-sensitive and insensitive prostatic adenocarcinomas, Dunning R-3327-H, R-3327-HI, and R-3327-AT. Cancer Res 1978;38: 4353–9.

[13] Chuu C, Hipakka RA, Fukuchi J, et al. Androgen causes growth suppression and reversion of androgen-independent prostate cancer xenografts to an androgen-stimulated phenotype in athymic mice. Cancer Res 2005;65:2082–4.

[14] Behre HM, Bohmeyer J, Nieschlag E. Prostate volume in testosterone-treated and untreated hypogonadal men in comparison to age-matched normal controls. Clin Endocrinol 1994;40:341–9.

[15] Bhasin S, Woodhouse L, Casaburi R, et al. Testosterone dose-response relationships in healthy young

men. Am J Physiol Endocrinol Metab 2001;281: E1172–81.

[16] Rhoden EL, Morgentaler A. Influence of demographic factors and biochemical characteristics on the prostate-specific antigen (PSA) response to testosterone replacement therapy. Int J Impot Res 2006;18:201–5.

[17] D'Amico AV, Roehrborn CG. Effect of 1 mg/day finasteride on concentrations of serum prostate-specific antigen in men with androgenic alopecia: a randomised controlled trial. Lancet Oncol 2007;8:21–5.

[18] Peters CA, Walsh PC. The effect of nafarelin acetate, a luteinizing-hormone-releasing hormone agonist, on benign prostatic hyperplasia. N Engl J Med 1987;317:599–604.

[19] Marberger M, Roehrborn CG, Marks LS, et al. Relationship among serum testosterone, sexual function, and response to treatment in men receiving dutasteride for benign prostatic hyperplasia. J Clin Endocrinol Metab 2006;91:1323–8.

[20] Hovenanian MS, Deming CL. The heterologous growth of cancer of the human prostate. Surg Gynecol Obstet 1948;86:29–35.

[21] Sharkey DA, Fisher ER. Carcinoma of the prostate in the absence of testicular tissue. J Urol 1960;83: 468–70.

[22] Daniell HW. A worse prognosis for men with testicular atrophy at therapeutic orchiectomy for prostate carcinoma. Cancer 1998;83:1170–3.

[23] Fowler JE, Whitmore WF Jr. The response of metastatic adenocarcinoma of the prostate to exogenous testosterone. J Urol 1981;126:372–5.

[24] Bubley GJ. Is the flare phenomenon clinically significant? Urology 2001;58(Suppl 2A):5–9.

[25] Kuhn JM, Billebaud T, Navratil H, et al. Prevention of the transient adverse effects of a gonadotropin-releasing hormone analogue (Buserelin) in metastatic prostatic carcinoma by administration of an antiandrogen (Nilutamide). N Engl J Med 1989;321:413–8.

[26] Tomera K, Gleason D, Gittelman M, et al. The gonadotropin-releasing hormone antagonist Abarelix depot versus luteinizing hormone releasing hormone agonists leuprolide or goserelin: initial results of endocrinological and biochemical efficacies in patients with prostate cancer. J Urol 2001;16:1585–9.

[27] Freeland SJ, Partin AW. Prostate-specific antigen: update 2006. Urology 2006;67:458–60.

[28] Loughlin KR, Richie JP. Prostate cancer after exogenous testosterone treatment for impotence. J Urol 1997;157:1845.

[29] Gaylis FD, Lin DW, Ignatoff JM, et al. Prostate cancer in men using testosterone supplementation. J Urol 2005;174:534–8.

[30] Bosland MC. The role of steroid hormones in prostate carcinogenesis. J Natl Cancer Inst Monogr 2000;27:39–66.

[31] Ross RK, Bernstein L, Lobo RA, et al. 5-alpha-reductase activity and risk of prostate cancer among Japanese and US white and black males. Lancet 1992;339:887–9.

[32] Wu AH, Whittemore AS, Kolonel LN, et al. Serum androgens and sex hormone-binding globulins in relation to lifestyle factors in older African-American, white and Asian men in the United States and Canada. Cancer Epidemiol Biomarkers Prev 1995; 4:735–41.

[33] Thompson IM, Goodman PJ, Tangen CM, et al. The influence of finasteride on the development of prostate cancer. N Engl J Med 2003;349:215–24.

[34] Brendler H, Chase WE, Scott WW. Prostatic cancer: further investigations of hormonal relationships. Arch Surg 1950;61:433–40.

[35] Trunnel JB, Duffy BJ Jr. The influence of certain steroids on the behavior of human prostatic cancer. Trans N Y Acad Sci 1950;12:238–41.

[36] Pearson OH. Discussion of Dr. Huggins' paper "Control of cancers of man by endocrinological methods." Cancer Res 1957;17:473–9.

[37] Lefkowitz GK, Taneja SS, Brown J, et al. Followup interval prostate biopsy 3 years after diagnosis of high grade prostatic intraepithelial neoplasia is associated with high likelihood of prostate cancer, independent of change in prostate specific antigen levels. J Urol 2002;168:1415–8.

[38] Rhoden EL, Morgentaler A. Testosterone replacement therapy in hypogonadal men at high risk for prostate cancer: results of 1 year of treatment in men with prostatic intraepithelial neoplasia. J Urol 2003;170:2348–51.

[39] Hsing AW. Hormones and prostate cancer: what's next? Epidemiol Rev 2001;23:42–58.

[40] Eaton NE, Reeves GK, Appleby PN, et al. Endogenous sex hormones and prostate cancer: a quantitative review of prospective studies. Br J Cancer 1999; 80:930–4.

[41] Stattin P, Lumme S, Tenkanen L, et al. High levels of circulating testosterone are not associated with increased prostate cancer risk: a pooled prospective study. Int J Cancer 2004;108:418–24.

[42] Barrett-Connor E, Garland C, McPhillips JB, et al. A prospective, population-based study of androstenedione, estrogens, and prostatic cancer. Cancer Res 1990;50:169–73.

[43] Parsons JK, Carter HB, Platz EA, et al. Serum testosterone and the risk of prostate cancer: potential implications for testosterone therapy. Cancer Epidemiol Biomarkers Prev 2005;14:2257–60.

[44] Gann PH, Hennekens CH, Ma J, et al. Prospective study of sex hormone levels and risk of prostate cancer. J Natl Cancer Inst 1996;88:1118–26.

[45] Morgentaler A, Bruning CO III, DeWolf WC. Incidence of occult prostate cancer among men with low total or free serum testosterone. JAMA 1996;276: 1904–6.

[46] Morgentaler A, Rhoden EL. Prevalence of prostate cancer among hypogonadal men with

prostate-specific antigen of 4.0 ng/ml or less. Urology 2006;68:1263–7.

[47] Thompson IM, Pauler DK, Goodman PJ, et al. Prevalence of prostate cancer among men with a prostate-specific antigen level ≤4 ng per milliliter. N Engl J Med 2004;350:2239–46.

[48] Hoffman M, DeWolf WC, Morgentaler A. Is low serum free testosterone a marker for high grade prostate cancer? J Urol 2000;163:824–7.

[49] Schatzl G, Madersbacher S, Thurridl T, et al. High-grade prostate cancer is associated with low serum testosterone levels. Prostate 2001;47:52–8.

[50] Massengill JC, Sun L, Moul JW, et al. Pretreatment total testosterone level predicts pathological stage in patients with localized prostate cancer treated with radical prostatectomy. J Urol 2003;169:1670–5.

[51] Teloken C, Da Ros CT, Caraver F, et al. Low serum testosterone levels are associated with positive surgical margins in radical retropubic prostatectomy: hypogonadism represents bad prognosis in prostate cancer. J Urol 2005;174:2178–80.

[52] Ribeiro M, Ruff P, Falkson G. Low serum testosterone and a younger age predict for a poor outcome in metastatic prostate cancer. Am J Clin Oncol 1997; 20:605–8.

[53] Morgentaler A. Testosterone deficiency and prostate cancer: emerging recognition of an important and troubling relationship. Eur Urol 2007;52:623–5.

[54] Sakr WA, Grignon DJ, Crissman JD, et al. High grade prostatic intraepithelial neoplasia (HGPIN) and prostatic adenocarcinoma between the ages of 20–69: an autopsy study of 249 cases. In Vivo 1994;8:439–43.

[55] Marks LS, Mazer NA, Mostaghel E, et al. Effect of testosterone replacement therapy on prostate tissue in men with late-onset hypogonadism: a randomized controlled trial. JAMA 2006;296:2351–61.

[56] Kaufman JM, Graydon RJ. Androgen replacement after curative radical prostatectomy for prostate cancer in hypogonadal men. J Urol 2004;172:920–2.

[57] Agarwal PK, Oefelein MG. Testosterone replacement therapy after primary treatment for prostate cancer. J Urol 2005;173:533–6.

[58] Sarosdy MF. Testosterone replacement for hypogonadism after treatment of early prostate cancer with brachytherapy. Cancer 2007;109:536–41.

ELSEVIER
SAUNDERS

Urol Clin N Am 34 (2007) 565–574

UROLOGIC
CLINICS
of North America

Depression and Erectile Dysfunction

Antoine Makhlouf, MD, PhD[a],*, Ashay Kparker, MD[b],
Craig S. Niederberger, MD[b]

[a]Department of Urologic Surgery, University of Minnesota, Minneapolis, MN, USA
[b]Department of Urology, University of Illinois at Chicago, Chicago, IL, USA

Depression and erectile dysfunction (ED) clearly are associated [1–3]. In the landmark Male Massachusetts Aging Study (MMAS), men who had untreated depression were almost twice as likely to report ED than were men who did not have depression [1]. Although urologists and psychiatrists have long recognized that antidepressant medications affect erectile function negatively [4], the interplay between the two conditions remains underappreciated. Psychiatrists may be reluctant to question a patient in detail about ED [5], and urologists seldom perform a formal assessment of the presence of depression in patients who have ED. This article gives a quick overview of the relationship between these two conditions and provides the clinician with the knowledge required to effectively manage ED with comorbid depression.

Epidemiologic association

Depression is an affective disorder with a heterogeneous manifestation and multifactorial etiology. Excluding bipolar (manic-depressive) disorders, clinical depression generally is classified as major depressive disorder (MDD) or dysthymia, depending on severity. In this article we use depression to refer to both conditions. The hallmark symptoms of depression include feelings of sadness and hopelessness, loss of interest in pleasurable activities (anhedonia), changes in appetite, disturbance of sleep, fatigue, and inability to concentrate [6]. There is a strong overlap between depression and anxiety symptomatology. Depression is a major health problem, with a lifetime prevalence of 16% [7]. It has been estimated that 18 million Americans currently are treated with antidepressants for depression or anxiety [6–8].

Depression, libido, and orgasmic dysfunction

Many studies have documented an association between depression and ED. Because loss of interest in pleasurable activities, including sex, is a diagnostic criterion of depression, it is not surprising that sexual dysfunction is common in men who have depression. Of sexual complaints among depressed men, low libido is most prevalent, followed by orgasmic difficulty and finally ED, which generally is considered an arousal disorder [9]. Poor sexual satisfaction also is invariably present. Early studies using the Derogatis Sexual Function Inventory, a 200-item inventory of 10 psychologic areas affecting sexual function, examined the correlation between depression and sexual function [10]. Compared with controls, depressed men had lower sexual desire, a poorer self-image, and less sexual satisfaction, despite no significant difference in the frequency of sexual episodes in which they engaged [11]. Similar findings were reported by Nofzinger and colleagues [12], who found no decrease in the frequency of sexual activity in men who had depression, yet detected a significant decrease in sexual satisfaction. Finally, during validation of the Brief Sexual Function Questionnaire, men who had a known organic etiology for ED were compared with men who had clinical depression [13]. Both groups reported low satisfaction and scored similarly on several measures; however, depressed men

* Corresponding author.
  E-mail address: makhl001@umn.edu (A. Makhlouf).

reported a lower frequency of sexual activity, but more confidence in obtaining erections [13].

Depression and erectile dysfunction

Early studies

Reports dating back to the late 1970s have suggested that arousal, including erectile function, is affected negatively by depression [14,15]. In one of the earliest surveys that examined depression and ED, Derogatis and colleagues [16] enrolled more than 400 men and women who had sexual dysfunction, including 137 men who had ED. They found a significant elevation in the depression score on the multidimensional Symptom Checklist-90-Revised (SCL-90-R) inventory among the men who had ED. Nocturnal penile tumescence (NPT) testing showed that men who had depression had decreased nocturnal erections [17]. This corroborated with a self-reported decrease in the frequency of awakenings with an erect penis in men who had depression [13]. Normalization of NPT with resolution of depression also was reported [18,19]. It is not clear, however, if the loss of NPT in depression is a generalized finding, or if it is more restricted to a subset of depressed men who have other sleep disturbances, as argued by Nofzinger and colleagues [12]. These studies in men who had depression were complemented by Shabsigh and colleagues [3], who looked at the prevalence of depression symptomatology in a urology clinic population. In a survey of 100 men who had ED, benign prostatic hyperplasia (BPH), or both, the presence of ED increased the odds of having depression by 2.6 fold, again confirming a link between the two. More importantly, men who had depression were more likely to discontinue ED treatment than were men who did not have depression, although this was before the introduction of phosphodiesterase 5 inhibitors (PDE5i).

The Male Massachusetts Aging Study and later studies

All of the studies mentioned so far have suffered from referral and selection bias because they mostly used convenience clinic samples. Analysis of the MMAS, however, finally established a robust link between ED and depression [1,20]. In the MMAS, depression was assessed using the Center for Epidemiologic Study Depression scale (CES-D), a validated depression screening tool [21,22]. The prevalence of ED correlated strongly with advancing age [20], whereas the prevalence of depression remained constant

(10%–15%). In all age groups, ED was more common in the upper quintiles of depression scores. In a multivariate model that corrected for copredictors (eg, the association of heart disease with both ED and depression), as well as confounders (eg, income, education level), depression remained strongly associated with ED, and men who had depression symptoms were 1.8 times more likely to report moderate to severe ED than were their counterparts with normal mood [1]. More studies have since supported the epidemiologic linkage between depression and ED [2,23]. In an analysis of a health plan claims database encompassing 28 million men, depression was a common comorbidity associated with ED. The crude prevalence of clinically diagnosed depression in men who had ED was around 11.1%, with the prevalence peaking at 15% in the 35- to 46-year-old age group [2]. Similar conclusions can be drawn from the Multinational Men's Attitudes to Life Events and Sexuality study; depression symptomatology was a prevalent comorbid condition, being detected in 25% of men who had ED compared with 13% of men who did not [23]. In a random survey of 199 patients attending outpatient clinics, moderate and severe ED was found in 36%, depression symptoms were in 12%, and both conditions were found in 5% [24].

Causality

Epidemiologic data and common sense suggest that the relationship between ED and depression is bidirectional. In the model proposed by the authors of the MMAS study, ED and depression are depicted as two conditions that reinforce each other in a downward spiral [1]. Additional factors, such as lifestyle, social context, and medical interventions, can hasten or reverse this interaction [1]. The underlying mechanism of the link between ED and depression, however, has not been established. In general, there are two models for how depression exacerbates ED: the "behavior-based" model and the "biologic-based" model.

The behavior-based model postulates that men who have depression engage in behavior or thoughts that cause performance anxiety, which, in turn, negatively affects erectile function. Being more self-conscious, depressed men are believed to engage in "spectatoring" (focusing on oneself from a third-person perspective during sexual activity) [1,17]. The loss of libido and the decrease in enjoyment of sexual activity are believed to lead to more passive participation, less stimulation, and, consequently, ED [16]. The behavior model is supported by the experiments of Meisler and Carey [25], who showed that mood could affect sexual arousal. They reported that subjective arousal in response to erotica was affected negatively by induction of depressed mood in sexually functional men [25]. Although objectively measured tumescence was not changed in the same experiment, poststimulation mood correlated with tumescence [25]. Attention and emotional factors also affect sexual arousal in response to stimulation [26]. When volunteers were exposed to a series of erotic movies, they exhibited variable degrees of arousal that correlated well with how much they perceived the material as entertaining versus repulsive and whether they were distracted by extraneous stimuli [26]. Despite advances in mapping the neurocircuitry of male arousal [27], much remains to be learned before a full understanding of the effects of mood on erections can be elucidated.

The biologic model has been described best by Goldstein [28], who added cardiovascular disease to the bidirectional model to come up with a "triad model" of mutually reinforcing conditions. Depression is a known risk factor for the development of cardiovascular disease, and its presence increases the risk for mortality after a first infarction [29]. This is ascribed to the effect of mental stress on the hypothalamic-pituitary-adrenocortical axis, leading to excess catecholamine production. This, in turn, leads to poor cavernosal muscle relaxation and ED [28].

Hypogonadism, depression, and erectile dysfunction

Hypogonadism and depression share several symptoms, such as loss of libido, fatigue, poor appetite, and dysphoria [6,30]. They also may be linked epidemiologically. In a study of 856 men in southern California, depressed mood (measured by the Beck Depression Inventory questionnaire) correlated with lower bioavailable testosterone levels, independent of age [31]. In a cohort of 278 men attending a single hospital, the 2-year incidence of depression was 21% in men who had hypogonadism (defined as $T < 200$ ng/dL), compared with only 7% in eugonadal men, a threefold increase [32]. We showed recently that men with hypogonadal testosterone levels (< 300 ng/dL)

were 1.94 times more likely to have significant depressive symptomatology compared with their eugonadal counterparts [33]. Conversely, the much larger MMAS survey did not detect a relationship between low testosterone and depression [1]. Also, a comparative study of men who had MDD, dysthymia, or no affective disorder found lower testosterone levels in the dysthymic group but not in the men who had MDD, which does not support a dose-effect relationship between low testosterone and depression [34].

The link between hypogonadism and ED is much stronger. Experimental androgen ablation in animals leads to loss of erectile function through structural changes (eg, smooth muscle cell loss) or down-regulation of nitric oxide synthase [35,36]. A large nonplacebo-controlled trial showed that testosterone supplementation improved mood and sexual function (including erection strength) in hypogonadal men [37]. A later randomized, placebo-controlled trial in hypogonadal men confirmed these results. It showed that 30- or 90-day treatment with testosterone gel was superior to placebo in improving sexual desire, frequency of intercourse, and nocturnal tumescence [38]. Furthermore, testosterone treatment also was shown to rescue sildenafil failures in men who had hypogonadism and ED [39].

Taken together, the above studies suggest that, in a subset of men, low testosterone may be a link between depression and ED. Still, this does not determine whether hypogonadism or depression is the primary disease. This linkage has prompted studies of testosterone supplementation as a treatment for depression with concomitant ED. An early trial in eugonadal men who had depression showed testosterone injections to be ineffective in enhancing mood [40]. Most other studies focused on hypogonadal men or men who had refractory depression. In asymptomatic (ie, nondepressed) hypogonadal men, testosterone injections improved self-reported mood ratings of anger, irritability, fatigue, sadness, irritability, nervousness, and sense of well-being [41]. This was followed by a promising pilot study using testosterone injections in men who had depression refractory to selective serotonin reuptake inhibitors (SSRIs) [42]. A later double-blind, placebo-controlled trial by the same group, however, failed to find an effect of testosterone injections superior to placebo on the Hamilton Rating Scale for Depression (HAM-D) [43]. That trial, however, suffered from low power (30 patients) and a strong placebo effect. It did show a statistical improvement in sexual function in response to testosterone, however. In contrast, a later trial, also with small numbers (23 men), looked at men who had refractory depression; testosterone gel treatment led to a significant change in the HAM-D scale compared with placebo [44]. While we await a larger randomized trial, these results can be reconciled by the theory that chronic depression (eg, dysthymia or refractory MDD) leads to blunting of the hypothalamic-pituitary-gonadal axis and to hypogonadism [34,44], whereas more acute forms of MDD may not be associated with hypogonadism. Part of the problem in assessing the contribution of hypogonadism to depression or ED continues to be the absence of a standardized assessment of testosterone bioactivity [45].

Antidepressants and erectile dysfunction

Sexual dysfunction is associated often with depression. Antidepressant therapy is highly effective in treating depression. Unfortunately, improvement of sexual function as a result of antidepressant therapy is seldom seen (with the notable exception of premature ejaculation) [46,47]. Rather, exacerbation of *de novo* development of sexual dysfunction can occur as an untoward side effect of antidepressants [48], and the incidence of sexual dysfunction in men who are on antidepressant therapy is higher than in untreated men [9,49–51]. In fact, several investigators have warned that treatment-emergent sexual side effects that are seen with various of antidepressants are much higher than indicated in drug inserts, and range from 20% to 70% [9,50–52].

The inhibitory effect of serotonin (5-hydroxytryptamine [5-HT]) on orgasm is well known, and it forms the basis of the off-label use of SSRIs in the treatment of premature ejaculation [53–55]. It is less clear how SSRIs affect erections. A generalized increase in serotonin in the brain is believed to counter the proarousal effects of dopamine and lead to a global depression of sexual functions, including arousal, orgasm, and erections [53,56]. This theory, however, does not take into account the presence of at least seven distinct serotonin receptors in the brain and the fact that stimulation of certain subtypes, such as the 5-HT2c, actually promotes erections [57]. Other evidence points to a peripheral effect of SSRIs on erectile function. Paroxetine is an inhibitor of nitric oxide synthase [58]. Acute and chronic treatment with paroxetine or fluoxetine

in rats decreases penile production of nitric oxide and depresses the erectile response in response to electrical stimulation of cavernosal nerves [59,60]. This inhibitory effect is not seen with citalopram [59], and this may correlate with the lower incidence of ED seen with citalopram [61]. The inhibitory effect in rats is countered by the action of PDE5i [60,62].

Several studies have attempted to define the rate of sexual dysfunction with various antidepressants. Most of them, however, did not focus specifically on ED. The landmark study by Clayton and colleagues [52,63] prospectively studied changes in sexual function in 1763 men (and 4534 women) taking a "newer" antidepressants. It revealed a prevalence rate for sexual dysfunction of 7% to 30% in a population with no obvious predisposing factors. Unfortunately, results were not broken down by gender or by type of sexual dysfunction, and the questionnaire used (Changes in Sexual Functioning Questionnaire, CSFQ) does not focus specifically on ED. Comparison of the various antidepressants revealed that, in general, pure SSRIs fared the worst, whereas agents that enhance dopamine and norepinephrine (eg, bupropion) fared best. Agents that affect serotonin and norepinephrine (eg, nefazodone) fell in between. This agreed with the results of a similar study conducted in Spanish patients, in which SSRIs had the highest rate of sexual dysfunction (generally between 60%–70%) compared with the tetracyclic antidepressant mirtazapine and the 5HT2-blocker nefazodone (rates of 24% and 8%, respectively). Looking at ED in particular, paroxetine was the worst offender, with a reported rate of 40%. This was followed by sertraline, fluvoxamine, and fluoxetine. In contrast, the tetracyclic nefazodone and atypical tricyclic antidepressant amineptine (not available in the United States) had virtually no ED side effects [50]. SSRIs are prescribed to more than 50% of patients who have depression, and patients on SSRIs do not accommodate to the sexual side effects, with only 9% reporting spontaneous resolution [64,65]. Thus, these rates translate to a high number of patients with unsatisfactory sexual function. Patients discontinue paroxetine, which has the highest rate of sexual side effects, much more often than sertraline or citalopram [66].

The sexual dysfunction associated with SSRIs may be used for beneficial purposes. Dapoxetine is an SSRI with short time to peak concentration and short elimination time. Using the SSRI's sexual dysfunction in a controlled short period of time, dapoxetine may be an effective therapy against premature ejaculation. In a recently reported controlled trial, over a 12-week period, 874 men were assigned randomly to receive dapoxetine, 30 mg; 870 men received dapoxetine, 60 mg; and 870 men received placebo. The medication was taken 1 to 3 hours before sexual intercourse. After 12 weeks, both doses were better than placebo ($P<.001$), with time to ejaculation increased threefold to fourfold [67].

Management of antidepressant-associated erectile dysfunction

The management of the sexual side effects of SSRIs has been reviewed extensively in the psychiatric literature [68–70]. This falls into two general categories: manipulation of psychotropic drugs and ED-directed therapy.

Antidepressant manipulation

Higher doses of antidepressants tend to be associated with more sexual dysfunction [48,51,52]. Thus, reducing the drug dose is one possible approach. This has to be done gradually, however, and under the close supervision of the treating psychiatrist because patients are at increased risk for relapse and symptoms of antidepressant withdrawal [71]. In the same vein, some patients may benefit from a brief "drug holiday," typically lasting 48 hours (eg, a weekend) [72]. This is only feasible in drugs with a short half-life (eg, not fluoxetine) and has to be undertaken with care because of the risk for withdrawal as well.

Awaiting the spontaneous resolution of sexual side effects is a strategy that is seldom effective. Adaptation rates generally have been low, with only 9% to 19% reporting abatement of sexual side effects [50,65]. Generally, this is a viable strategy only when the initial symptoms are mild. If they are not, or if they persist beyond 4 to 6 months, this approach should be abandoned [69].

Switching antidepressants is an attractive strategy because the various classes differ in the severity of their sexual side effects [50,52]. Thus, several trials have directly examined the question of whether sexual dysfunction improves upon changing medication [50,73,74]. In one of the first promising trials, Ferguson and colleagues [75] randomized 75 patients (including 38 men) who

responded to sertraline to continue sertraline or to switch to nefazodone. They reported a three times higher rate of sexual side effects in those continuing on sertraline as opposed to nefazodone. Furthermore, there seemed to be no loss of antidepressant efficacy in patients who switched to nefazodone. Unfortunately, nefazodone has been withdrawn from the United States market because of concerns about hepatotoxicity [76]. In a small pilot study, 5 patients were switched from fluoxetine to the reversible monoamine oxidase inhibitor moclobemide (not approved in the United States). They all showed improvement in the sexual side effect profile, including resolution of ED in one man [77]. A similar pilot study suggested that switching to mirtazapine could help to resolve sexual dysfunction side effects [78,79]. In a retrospective review of patients (including 27 men) who switched from an SSRI to citalopram, most reported improvement in sexual side effects [80]. This promising result awaits confirmation in a randomized trial. One caveat to this approach is the risk for relapse, because patients who respond to one class of antidepressants may not respond to another [69]. In fact, in one such trial in which patients were switched from the SSRI to bupropion (a norepinephrine and dopamine reuptake inhibitor), 64% reported improvement in sexual side effects, but 36% experienced a significant loss of antidepressant treatment efficacy [69].

Antidote medications

Addition of a second medication is the most common approach taken by clinicians. PDE5i recently gained recognition as effective adjuncts to antidepressants in managing SSRI-induced ED and are discussed separately. Other medications may still be used, particularly when decreased libido and orgasmic dysfunction are present as well. In a randomized trial of 117 patients (37 men), addition of the anxiolytic buspirone led to an improvement in sexual function in 58%, compared with 30% with placebo [81]. This effect was more pronounced in women and did not achieve statistical significance in men [81]. Bupropion, which is known to have a low rate of sexual side effects, is another agent that has been added to SSRIs [82]. In a series of 47 patients (including 7 men who had arousal disorder), bupropion was efficacious in improving sexual function [83]. Unfortunately, a later randomized trial of 31 patients did not confirm these findings [84]. Although another trial in 41 patients (7 men) showed improvement in the CSFQ, these were mostly in the desire and satisfaction domains, not in the arousal (which includes the question "Do you get erections easily?") domain [85]. Other interventions, such as the use of stimulants (ephedrine, methylphenidate) or herbal supplements (*Ginkgo biloba*), showed promise in uncontrolled studies [69], but have not been confirmed in randomized trials [54,86].

Phosphodiesterase 5 inhibitors

Sildenafil, the first PDE5i approved for treatment of ED, was introduced in 1998 [87]. Shortly thereafter, its use in treating SSRI-related side effects was reported [88]. This was followed by a retrospective analysis of premarket trial data on the efficacy of sildenafil in men concomitantly treated with an SSRI [89]. Men taking sildenafil and an SSRI had significant improvements in their ability to achieve an erection, maintain an erection, and reach orgasm and ejaculation compared with their counterparts receiving placebo and an SSRI. The magnitude of improvement was not significantly different compared with men not taking SSRIs. Not surprisingly, there was no effect of sildenafil on desire [89]. A prospective, randomized trial in men treated for depression confirmed these findings [90]. These results were refined further in a slightly larger study [91] that showed improvements in all domains of the International Index of Erectile Function (IIEF) (erection, orgasm, desire, and satisfaction). A General Efficacy Questionnaire showed that 70% of treated men reported improvement in erections compared with 28% in the placebo arm. These results are in line with what is expected of sildenafil in a general population of patients who have ED [92]. The adverse events reported in these trials generally were no different from the expected side effects of sildenafil treatment (headache, dyspepsia, abnormal vision) [87,92]. Despite these excellent results, we should caution that trial patients might be more motivated and, therefore, less susceptible to treatment discontinuation compared with real-life clinic patients. Shabsigh and colleagues [3] found that patients who had ED and concomitant depression were more likely to discontinue vacuum or penile injection therapy than were their counterparts who did not have depression. It has not been studied extensively whether these findings translate to patients on PDE5i.

Another trial assessed the efficacy of sildenafil in men who had untreated depressive symptoms [93]. Men presenting with ED were assessed for depressive symptoms using the CES-D questionnaire with a cutoff of at least 16, which was confirmed by interview with a psychologist and administration of the HAM-D (cutoff ≥ 12). Most men had mild to moderate symptoms of depression. The response to sildenafil was unusually high—90% on the global assessment questions versus 11% for placebo. Using a more rigid efficacy criterion (IIEF-ED domain ≥ 21), 42% of men were considered responders. Overall improvements in mood, measured by the HAM-D, in response to sildenafil were not as dramatic; however, when responders with IIEF-ED scores greater than 21 were considered separately, a significant improvement in HAM-D scores was noted, with scores decreasing a mean of 10.6 points, an improvement similar to that seen with traditional antidepressant therapy [94]. Thus, it seems that sildenafil is particularly efficacious in men who have untreated comorbid depression.

These results were essentially confirmed in a similar study comparing flexible-dose vardenafil to placebo in men who had ED and comorbid untreated mild depression [95]. Two hundred and eighty men who had ED and mild depression (HAM-D score of 11 to 17) were randomized to vardenafil or placebo. As expected, vardenafil led to a robust improvement in IIEF scores (from 13.2 at baseline to 22.9 at 12 weeks), whereas placebo did not. On the global efficacy question, improvement was noted in 83% of treated men versus 30% of those who took placebo. More importantly, HAM-D scores declined more in the vardenafil group (from 14.4 to 7.9) compared with the placebo group (from 14.3 to 10.1), a difference that was statistically significant. Thus, this study confirmed that, as a class, PDE5i are effective in treating comorbid ED and mild depression and that some degree of improvement in depression symptoms is to be expected with treatment.

Prospective studies of the efficacy of the third PDE5i, tadalafil, in comorbid ED and depression have not been published. Retrospective analysis of past trials, however, suggests that it also would be efficacious in treating ED in the presence of depression [96]. To our knowledge, no head-to-head trials comparing the three agents in men who have depression has been performed. A direct comparison of the vardenafil and sildenafil studies described previously cannot be performed either, because the vardenafil study excluded previous sildenafil nonresponders, which would be expected to give favorable results and may explain the presence of an effect on HAM-D score in that study and not in the sildenafil study. Until further data are published, we would presume that all three agents are equally efficacious, although sildenafil and vardenafil have the benefit of supporting prospective studies. In fact, in a survey of patient prescription filling patterns in the United Kingdom, the presence of depression was not a factor in switching from one PDE5i to another [97]. The effectiveness of PDE5i in men who have depression is such that addition of these agents to an antidepressant regimen is cost-effective when depression relapse and a switch in medications are taken into account [98].

Summary

Comorbid ED and depression are seen commonly in practice. The association between the two conditions is bidirectional, with each factor reinforcing the other. Additional factors, such as hypogonadism or cardiovascular disease, could contribute to the vicious cycle. Medical antidepressant therapy can exacerbate ED. The various classes of antidepressants vary in their sexual side effect profile, with the conventional SSRIs (paroxetine, fluoxetine, sertraline) being the worst offenders. Management of concomitant ED and depression involves careful titration of antidepressant dosage, switching antidepressants, or the use of additional agents. Of these, phosphodiesterase inhibitors have shown high efficacy in men who have concomitant ED and depression. Prospective trials of sildenafil and vardenafil showed that PDE5i monotherapy also could improve mild depression symptoms.

Understanding the interaction between these two conditions certainly will assist the urologist in managing the not-so-rare patient who presents with ED and depression. We recommend that urologists be proactive in eliciting symptoms of depression. A simple questionnaire, such as the CES-D, can be useful as a screening tool [21]. More elaborate questionnaires, such as the HAM-D or the male-specific Gotland Male Depression scale, also could be used [99,100]. The presence of depression symptoms should alert the clinician to the possibility of hypogonadism and consideration of supplementation [33]. A psychiatric referral is warranted in cases of positive questionnaire screening. For the patient who already is taking an antidepressant, coordination with the treating psychiatrist to adjust the medication and the addition of a phosphodiesterase inhibitor are recommended.

References

[1] Araujo AB, Durante R, Feldman HA, et al. The relationship between depressive symptoms and male erectile dysfunction: cross-sectional results from the Massachusetts Male Aging Study. Psychosom Med 1998;60(4):458–65.

[2] Seftel AD, Sun P, Swindle R. The prevalence of hypertension, hyperlipidemia, diabetes mellitus and depression in men with erectile dysfunction. J Urol 2004;171(6 Pt 1):2341–5.

[3] Shabsigh R, Klein LT, Seidman S, et al. Increased incidence of depressive symptoms in men with erectile dysfunction. Urology 1998;52(5):848–52.

[4] Ferguson JM. The effects of antidepressants on sexual functioning in depressed patients: a review. J Clin Psychiatry 2001;(62 Suppl 3):22–34.

[5] Rothschild AN. Sexual dysfunction associated with depression. J Clin Psychiatry 2001;(62 Suppl 3):3–4.

[6] Moore DP, Jefferson JW. Handbook of medical psychiatry. 2nd edition. Philadelphia: Mosby, Inc; 2004.

[7] Kessler RC, Berglund P, Demler O, et al. The epidemiology of major depressive disorder: results from the National Comorbidity Survey Replication (NCS-R). JAMA 2003;289(23):3095–105.

[8] Kessler RC, Berglund P, Demler O, et al. Lifetime prevalence and age-of-onset distributions of DSM-IV disorders in the National Comorbidity Survey Replication. Arch Gen Psychiatry 2005;62(6):593–602.

[9] Kennedy SH, Eisfeld BS, Dickens SE, et al. Antidepressant-induced sexual dysfunction during treatment with moclobemide, paroxetine, sertraline, and venlafaxine. J Clin Psychiatry 2000;61(4):276–81.

[10] Derogatis LR, Melisaratos N. The DSFI: a multidimensional measure of sexual functioning. J Sex Marital Ther 1979;5(3):244–81.

[11] Howell JR, Reynolds CF 3rd, Thase ME, et al. Assessment of sexual function, interest and activity in depressed men. J Affect Disord 1987;13(1):61–6.

[12] Nofzinger EA, Thase ME, Reynolds CF 3rd, et al. Sexual function in depressed men. Assessment by self-report, behavioral, and nocturnal penile tumescence measures before and after treatment with cognitive behavior therapy. Arch Gen Psychiatry 1993;50(1):24–30.

[13] Reynolds CF 3rd, Frank E, Thase ME, et al. Assessment of sexual function in depressed, impotent, and healthy men: factor analysis of a brief sexual function questionnaire for men. Psychiatry Res 1988;24(3):231–50.

[14] Mathew RJ, Largen J, Claghorn JL. Biological symptoms of depression. Psychosom Med 1979; 41(6):439–43.

[15] Mathew RJ, Weinman ML. Sexual dysfunctions in depression. Arch Sex Behav 1982;11(4):323–8.

[16] Derogatis LR, Meyer JK, King KM. Psychopathology in individuals with sexual dysfunction. Am J Psychiatry 1981;138(6):757–63.

[17] Thase ME, Reynolds CF 3rd, Jennings JR, et al. Nocturnal penile tumescence is diminished in depressed men. Biol Psychiatry 1988;24(1):33–46.

[18] Roose SP, Glassman AH, Walsh BT, et al. Reversible loss of nocturnal penile tumescence during depression: a preliminary report. Neuropsychobiology 1982;8(6):284–8.

[19] Steiger A, Holsboer F, Benkert O. Studies of nocturnal penile tumescence and sleep electroencephalogram in patients with major depression and in normal controls. Acta Psychiatr Scand 1993; 87(5):358–63.

[20] Feldman HA, Goldstein I, Hatzichristou DG, et al. Impotence and its medical and psychosocial correlates: results of the Massachusetts Male Aging Study. J Urol 1994;151(1):54–61.

[21] Radloff LS. The CES-D scale: a self-report depression scale for research in the general population. Applied Psychological Measurement 1977;1(3):385.

[22] Haringsma R, Engels GI, Beekman AT, et al. The criterion validity of the Center for Epidemiological Studies Depression Scale (CES-D) in a sample of self-referred elders with depressive symptomatology. Int J Geriatr Psychiatry 2004;19(6):558–63.

[23] Rosen RC, Fisher WA, Eardley I, et al. Men's Attitudes to Life Events and Sexuality (MALES) Study. The multinational Men's Attitudes to Life Events and Sexuality (MALES) study: I. Prevalence of erectile dysfunction and related health concerns in the general population. Curr Med Res Opin 2004;20(5):607–17.

[24] Kantor J, Bilker WB, Glasser DB, et al. Prevalence of erectile dysfunction and active depression: an analytic cross-sectional study of general medical patients. Am J Epidemiol 2002;156(11):1035–42.

[25] Meisler AW, Carey MP. Depressed affect and male sexual arousal. Arch Sex Behav 1991;20(6):541–54.

[26] Koukounas E, McCabe MP. Sexual and emotional variables influencing sexual response to erotica: a psychophysiological investigation. Arch Sex Behav 2001;30(4):393–408.

[27] Stoleru S, Gregoire MC, Gerard D, et al. Neuroanatomical correlates of visually evoked sexual arousal in human males. Archives of Sexual Behavior 1999;28(1):1–21.

[28] Goldstein I. The mutually reinforcing triad of depressive symptoms, cardiovascular disease, and erectile dysfunction. Am J Cardiol 2000;86(2A): 41F–5F.

[29] Musselman DL, Evans DL, Nemeroff CB. The relationship of depression to cardiovascular disease: epidemiology, biology, and treatment. Arch Gen Psychiatry 1998;55(7):580–92.

[30] Wald M, Meacham RB, Ross LS, et al. Testosterone replacement therapy for older men. J Androl 2006;27(2):126–32.

[31] Barrett-Connor E, Von Muhlen DG, Kritz-Silverstein D. Bioavailable testosterone and depressed mood in older men: the Rancho Bernardo Study. J Clin Endocrinol Metab 1999;84(2):573–7.

[32] Shores MM, Sloan KL, Matsumoto AM, et al. Increased incidence of diagnosed depressive illness in hypogonadal older men. Arch Gen Psychiatry 2004;61(2):162–7.

[33] Makhlouf AA, Mohamed MA, Seftel AD, et al. Hypogonadism is associated with overt depression symptoms in men with erectile dysfunction. Int J Impot Res 2007 Aug 16; [Epub ahead of print].

[34] Seidman SN, Araujo AB, Roose SP, et al. Low testosterone levels in elderly men with dysthymic disorder. Am J Psychiatry 2002;159(3):456–9.

[35] Traish AM, Munarriz R, O'Connell L, et al. Effects of medical or surgical castration on erectile function in an animal model. J Androl 2003;24(3): 381–7.

[36] Baba K, Yajima M, Carrier S, et al. Delayed testosterone replacement restores nitric oxide synthase-containing nerve fibres and the erectile response in rat penis. BJU Int 2000;85(7):953–8.

[37] Wang C, Swerdloff RS, Iranmanesh A, et al. Transdermal testosterone gel improves sexual function, mood, muscle strength, and body composition parameters in hypogonadal men. J Clin Endocrinol Metab 2000;85(8):2839–53.

[38] Seftel AD, Mack RJ, Secrest AR, et al. Restorative increases in serum testosterone levels are significantly correlated to improvements in sexual functioning. J Androl 2004;25(6):963–72.

[39] Shabsigh R, Kaufman JM, Steidle C, et al. Randomized study of testosterone gel as adjunctive therapy to sildenafil in hypogonadal men with erectile dysfunction who do not respond to sildenafil alone. J Urol 2004;172(2):658–63.

[40] Schiavi RC, White D, Mandeli J, et al. Effect of testosterone administration on sexual behavior and mood in men with erectile dysfunction. Arch Sex Behav 1997;26(3):231–41.

[41] Wang C, Alexander G, Berman N, et al. Testosterone replacement therapy improves mood in hypogonadal men–a clinical research center study. J Clin Endocrinol Metab 1996;81(10):3578–83.

[42] Seidman SN, Rabkin JG. Testosterone replacement therapy for hypogonadal men with SSRI-refractory depression. J Affect Disord 1998;48(2–3): 157–61.

[43] Seidman SN, Spatz E, Rizzo C, et al. Testosterone replacement therapy for hypogonadal men with major depressive disorder: a randomized, placebo-controlled clinical trial. J Clin Psychiatry 2001;62(6):406–12.

[44] Pope HG, Cohane GH, Kanayama G, et al. Testosterone gel supplementation for men with refractory depression: a randomized, placebo-controlled trial. Am J Psychiatry 2003;160(1):105–11.

[45] Bhasin S, Cunningham GR, Hayes FJ, et al. Testosterone therapy in adult men with androgen deficiency syndromes: an Endocrine Society clinical practice guideline. J Clin Endocrinol Metab 2006; 91(6):1995–2010, Epub 2006, May 23.

[46] Smith DM, Levitte SS. Association of fluoxetine and return of sexual potency in three elderly men. J Clin Psychiatry 1993;54(8):317–9.

[47] Power-Smith P. Beneficial sexual side-effects from fluoxetine. Br J Psychiatry 1994;164(2):249–50.

[48] Herman JB, Brotman AW, Pollack MH, et al. Fluoxetine-induced sexual dysfunction. J Clin Psychiatry 1990;51(1):25–7.

[49] Kennedy SH, Dickens SE, Eisfeld BS, et al. Sexual dysfunction before antidepressant therapy in major depression. J Affect Disord 1999;56(2–3):201–8.

[50] Montejo AL, Llorca G, Izquierdo JA, et al. Incidence of sexual dysfunction associated with antidepressant agents: a prospective multicenter study of 1022 outpatients. Spanish Working Group for the Study of Psychotropic-Related Sexual Dysfunction. J Clin Psychiatry 2001;(62 Suppl 3):10–21.

[51] Zajecka J, Mitchell S, Fawcett J. Treatment-emergent changes in sexual function with selective serotonin reuptake inhibitors as measured with the Rush Sexual Inventory. Psychopharmacol Bull 1997;33(4):755–60.

[52] Clayton AH, Pradko JF, Croft HA, et al. Prevalence of sexual dysfunction among newer antidepressants. J Clin Psychiatry 2002;63(4):357–66.

[53] Stahl SM. The psychopharmacology of sex, Part 1: neurotransmitters and the 3 phases of the human sexual response. J Clin Psychiatry 2001; 62(2):80–1.

[54] Meston CM. A randomized, placebo-controlled, crossover study of ephedrine for SSRI-induced female sexual dysfunction. J Sex Marital Ther 2004;30(2):57–68.

[55] Waldinger MD, Schweitzer DH, Olivier B. On-demand SSRI treatment of premature ejaculation: pharmacodynamic limitations for relevant ejaculation delay and consequent solutions. J Sex Med 2005;2(1):121–31.

[56] Hull EM, Muschamp JW, Sato S. Dopamine and serotonin: influences on male sexual behavior. Physiol Behav 2004;83(2):291–307.

[57] Millan MJ, Peglion JL, Lavielle G, et al. 5-HT2C receptors mediate penile erections in rats: actions of novel and selective agonists and antagonists. Eur J Pharmacol 1997;325(1):9–12.

[58] Finkel MS, Laghrissi-Thode F, Pollock BG, et al. Paroxetine is a novel nitric oxide synthase inhibitor. Psychopharmacol Bull 1996;32(4):653–8.

[59] Angulo J, Peiro C, Sanchez-Ferrer CF, et al. Differential effects of serotonin reuptake inhibitors on erectile responses, NO-production, and neuronal NO synthase expression in rat corpus cavernosum tissue. Br J Pharmacol 2001;134(6):1190–4.

[60] Ahn GJ, Kang KK, Kim DS, et al. DA-8159 reverses selective serotonin reuptake inhibitor-induced erectile dysfunction in rats. Urology 2005;65(1):202–7.

[61] Mendels J, Kiev A, Fabre LF. Double-blind comparison of citalopram and placebo in depressed outpatients with melancholia. Depress Anxiety 1999;9(2):54–60.

[62] Angulo J, Bischoff E, Gabancho S, et al. Vardenafil reverses erectile dysfunction induced by paroxetine in rats. Int J Impot Res 2003;15(2):90–3.

[63] Clayton AH, McGarvey EL, Clavet GJ. The Changes in Sexual Functioning Questionnaire (CSFQ): development, reliability, and validity. Psychopharmacol Bull 1997;33(4):731–45.

[64] Ackerman DL, Unutzer J, Greenland S, et al. Inpatient treatment of depression and associated hospital charges. Pharmacoepidemiol Drug Saf 2002; 11(3):219–27.

[65] Ashton AK, Rosen RC. Accommodation to serotonin reuptake inhibitor-induced sexual dysfunction. J Sex Marital Ther 1998;24(3):191–2.

[66] Mullins CD, Shaya FT, Meng F, et al. Persistence, switching, and discontinuation rates among patients receiving sertraline, paroxetine, and citalopram. Pharmacotherapy 2005;25(5):660–7.

[67] Pryor JL, Althof SE, Steidle C, et al. Efficacy and tolerability of dapoxetine in treatment of premature ejaculation: an integrated analysis of two double-blind, randomised controlled trials. Lancet 2006;368(9539):929–37.

[68] Labbate LA, Croft HA, Oleshansky MA. Antidepressant-related erectile dysfunction: management via avoidance, switching antidepressants, antidotes, and adaptation. J Clin Psychiatry 2003; (64 Suppl 10):11–9.

[69] Zajecka J. Strategies for the treatment of antidepressant-related sexual dysfunction. J Clin Psychiatry 2001;(62 Suppl 3):35–43.

[70] Taylor MJ, Rudkin L, Hawton K. Strategies for managing antidepressant-induced sexual dysfunction: systematic review of randomised controlled trials. J Affect Disord 2005;88(3):241–54, Epub 2005, Sep 12.

[71] Haddad PM. Antidepressant discontinuation syndromes. Drug Saf 2001;24(3):183–97.

[72] Rothschild AJ. Selective serotonin reuptake inhibitor-induced sexual dysfunction: efficacy of a drug holiday. Am J Psychiatry 1995;152(10):1514–6.

[73] Kavoussi RJ, Segraves RT, Hughes AR, et al. Double-blind comparison of bupropion sustained release and sertraline in depressed outpatients. J Clin Psychiatry 1997;58(12):532–7.

[74] Walker PW, Cole JO, Gardner EA, et al. Improvement in fluoxetine-associated sexual dysfunction in patients switched to bupropion. J Clin Psychiatry 1993;54(12):459–65.

[75] Ferguson JM, Shrivastava RK, Stahl SM, et al. Reemergence of sexual dysfunction in patients with major depressive disorder: double-blind comparison of nefazodone and sertraline. J Clin Psychiatry 2001;62(1):24–9.

[76] Edwards IR. Withdrawing drugs: nefazodone, the start of the latest saga. Lancet 2003;361(9365):1240.

[77] Ramasubbu R. Switching to moclobemide to reverse fluoxetine-induced sexual dysfunction in patients with depression. J Psychiatry Neurosci 1999;24(1):45–50.

[78] Koutouvidis N, Pratikakis M, Fotiadou A. The use of mirtazapine in a group of 11 patients following poor compliance to selective serotonin reuptake inhibitor treatment due to sexual dysfunction. Int Clin Psychopharmacol 1999;14(4):253–5.

[79] Boyarsky BK, Haque W, Rouleau MR, et al. Sexual functioning in depressed outpatients taking mirtazapine. Depress Anxiety 1999;9(4):175–9.

[80] Ashton AK, Mahmood A, Iqbal F. Improvements in SSRI/SNRI-induced sexual dysfunction by switching to escitalopram. J Sex Marital Ther 2005;31(3):257–62.

[81] Landen M, Eriksson E, Agren H, et al. Effect of buspirone on sexual dysfunction in depressed patients treated with selective serotonin reuptake inhibitors. J Clin Psychopharmacol 1999;19(3):268–71.

[82] Foley KF, DeSanty KP, Kast RE. Bupropion: pharmacology and therapeutic applications. Expert Rev Neurother 2006;6(9):1249–65.

[83] Ashton AK, Rosen RC. Bupropion as an antidote for serotonin reuptake inhibitor-induced sexual dysfunction. J Clin Psychiatry 1998;59(3):112–5.

[84] Masand PS, Ashton AK, Gupta S, et al. Sustained-release bupropion for selective serotonin reuptake inhibitor-induced sexual dysfunction: a randomized, double-blind, placebo-controlled, parallel-group study. Am J Psychiatry 2001;158(5):805–7.

[85] Clayton AH, Warnock JK, Kornstein SG, et al. A placebo-controlled trial of bupropion SR as an antidote for selective serotonin reuptake inhibitor-induced sexual dysfunction. J Clin Psychiatry 2004;65(1):62–7.

[86] Kang BJ, Lee SJ, Kim MD, et al. A placebo-controlled, double-blind trial of Ginkgo biloba for antidepressant-induced sexual dysfunction. Hum Psychopharmacol 2002;17(6):279–84.

[87] Goldstein I, Lue TF, Padma-Nathan H, et al. Oral sildenafil in the treatment of erectile dysfunction. Sildenafil Study Group. N Engl J Med 1998; 338(20):1397–404.

[88] Ashton AK, Bennett RG. Sildenafil treatment of serotonin reuptake inhibitor-induced sexual dysfunction. J Clin Psychiatry 1999;60(3):194–5.

[89] Nurnberg HG, Gelenberg A, Hargreave TB, et al. Efficacy of sildenafil citrate for the treatment of erectile dysfunction in men taking serotonin reuptake inhibitors. Am J Psychiatry 2001;158(11): 1926–8.

[90] Nurnberg HG, Hensley PL, Gelenberg AJ, et al. Treatment of antidepressant-associated sexual dysfunction with sildenafil: a randomized controlled trial. JAMA 2003;289(1):56–64.

[91] Fava M, Nurnberg HG, Seidman SN, et al. Efficacy and safety of sildenafil in men with serotonergic antidepressant-associated erectile dysfunction: results from a randomized, double-blind, placebo-controlled trial. J Clin Psychiatry 2006;67(2):240–6.

[92] Carson CC, Lue TF. Phosphodiesterase type 5 inhibitors for erectile dysfunction. BJU Int 2005; 96(3):257–80.

[93] Seidman SN. Exploring the relationship between depression and erectile dysfunction in aging men. J Clin Psychiatry 2002;(63 Suppl 5):5–12.

[94] Seidman SN, Roose SP, Menza MA, et al. Treatment of erectile dysfunction in men with depressive symptoms: results of a placebo-controlled trial with sildenafil citrate. Am J Psychiatry 2001;158(10): 1623–30.

[95] Rosen R, Shabsigh R, Berber M, et al, Vardenafil Study Site Investigators. Efficacy and tolerability of vardenafil in men with mild depression and erectile dysfunction: the depression-related improvement with vardenafil for erectile response study. Am J Psychiatry 2006;163(1):79–87.

[96] Segraves RT, Lee J, Stevenson R, et al. Tadalafil for treatment of erectile dysfunction in men on antidepressants. J Clin Psychopharmacol 2007;27(1): 62–6.

[97] Kell PD, Hvidsten K, Morant SV, et al. Factors that predict changing the type of phosphodiesterase type 5 inhibitor medication among men in the UK. BJU Int 2007;99(4):860–3.

[98] Nurnberg HG, Duttagupta S. Economic analysis of sildenafil citrate (Viagra) add-on to treat erectile dysfunction associated with selective serotonin reuptake inhibitor use. Am J Ther 2004;11(1):9–12.

[99] Zierau F, Bille A, Rutz W, et al. The Gotland Male Depression Scale: a validity study in patients with alcohol use disorder. Nord J Psychiatry 2002; 56(4):265–71.

[100] Hamilton M. A rating scale for depression. J Neurol Neurosurg Psychiatr 1960;23:56–62.

ELSEVIER
SAUNDERS

Urol Clin N Am 34 (2007) 575–579

UROLOGIC
CLINICS
of North America

Sexual Dysfunction Associated with Antidepressant Therapy

Robert Taylor Segraves, MD, PhD[a,b]

[a]Department of Psychiatry, MetroHealth Medical Center, Cleveland, OH, USA
[b]Case School of Medicine, Cleveland, OH, USA

Most of the commonly prescribed antidepressant drugs are associated with sexual side effects. Comparably little attention was paid to these side effects until the advent of the selective serotonin reuptake inhibitors (SSRIs), however. The tricyclic antidepressants (eg, amitriptyline) were associated with sedation, weight gain, dizziness, and anticholinergic side effects. When these were the predominantly prescribed antidepressants, more attention was devoted to these side effects than to drug-induced sexual dysfunction [1]. Monoamine oxidase inhibitors were associated with the potentially lethal side effect of hypertensive crisis precipitated by the coadministration of sympathomimetic drugs or the ingestion of foods containing tyramine. Most clinicians paid little attention to sexual side effects induced by monoamine oxidase inhibitors [2]. When the SSRIs were introduced, the clinician suddenly had available a class of drugs devoid of the side effect burden of the tricyclic antidepressants and monoamine oxidase inhibitors. Initially, the extent of sexual dysfunction with these compounds was grossly underestimated. With continued experience with these agents, more and more clinicians became aware of their sexual side effect burden [3]. Increased recognition of sexual side effects can partially be attributed to the pharmacologic industry, which used the lower frequency of sexual side effects with certain agents in major marketing initiatives.

The purpose of this article is to review the incidence and type of sexual side effects associated with modern psychopharmacologic therapies of depression and ways to minimize these side effects.

Methodologic issues

Several methodologic issues have to be appreciated in interpreting data concerning the incidence of sexual side effects with antidepressant drugs. First, studies relying on patient self-report have consistently underestimated the frequency of sexual side effects when compared with studies with direct inquiry [4]. Thus, prerelease data and postmarketing surveillance studies, which rely on spontaneous patient reporting, usually found low rates of sexual dysfunction associated with the SSRIs. Because of the high incidence of underreporting in studies not using direct inquiry, estimates of the incidence of antidepressant-induced sexual dysfunction should be based on studies employing direct inquiry. Second, there is a high prevalence of sexual dysfunction in the general population, and sexual dysfunction is associated with untreated major depressive disorder. For example, several studies have found the incidence of sexual dysfunction in untreated major depression to be approximately 35% to 50%. Major depressive disorder is especially associated with low sexual desire [5]. Interestingly, one study found low sexual desire to be an indicator of depression in all cohorts of elderly Finish patients, except for women older than 70 years of age [6]. Erectile dysfunction has also been associated with depressive disorders [7]. Anorgasmia, a common side effect of SSRIs, is rarely associated with untreated depression.

E-mail address: rsegraves@metrohealth.org

Thus, one encounters a potentially difficult situation when trying to tease apart effects of preexisting depressive disorder from the effects of treatment on libido and erectile disorders. Although most SSRIs cause sexual dysfunction, sexual function has been reported to improve with the successful alleviation of depression by antidepressant drugs [8]. This illustrates the complex relation between sexual dysfunction associated with depression, its possible alleviation by successful treatment, and its exacerbation or precipitation by SSRI therapy. Similarly, the presence of sexual dysfunction could result from ineffectively treated depressive disorder or could be a drug side effect. Attempts to tease apart sexual dysfunction as a drug side effect from the underlying depressive disorder require random assignment to placebo-controlled trials and concurrent measurement of depression.

Tricyclic antidepressants and monoamine oxidase inhibitors

There were numerous case reports about sexual dysfunction, especially anorgasmia, associated with tricyclic antidepressants and monoamine oxidase inhibitors. In fact, some clinicians used the increased latency to orgasm induced by monoamine oxidase inhibitors to treat premature ejaculation [8]. One double-blind study found that orgasmic delay was experienced by 20% to 30% of men and women taking imipramine and by 30% to 37% of those taking phenelzine [9]. Another controlled double-blind study found that more than 90% of patients taking clomipramine, a tricyclic antidepressant with serotonergic activity, experienced anorgasmia or marked delay in achieving orgasm [10]. Newer monoamine oxidase inhibitors, such as moclobemide (not available in the United States) and selegiline (available as a transdermal patch), seem to have a low rate of sexual dysfunction [5].

Selective serotonin reuptake inhibitors and multiple receptor inhibitors

Controlled clinical trials and large prospective clinical series have established that the SSRIs (paroxetine, sertraline, fluvoxamine, citalopram, s-citalopram, and fluoxetine), as a class, are all are associated with sexual dysfunction [11]. There is some evidence that paroxetine has a higher rate of sexual dysfunction than the other SSRIs and

that fluvoxamine may have a lower rate of sexual dysfunction [12]. The major side effect is anorgasmia or delayed orgasm, which seems to occur in 30% to 40% of patients depending on the threshold set for the diagnosis. Clinicians have used this side effect to treat premature ejaculation [13]. These problems usually occur within 1 to 2 weeks of starting the agent and well before the antidepressant effect is evident. The sexual side effects usually remit within days of drug discontinuation, although there have been rare reports of sexual dysfunction persisting after drug discontinuation [14]. Problems with decreased libido and erectile impairment occur less frequently, perhaps in approximately 20% and 10% of patients, respectively [15,16].

Several large clinical trials have specifically addressed the issue of the relative incidence of sexual dysfunction on different antidepressants. A multicenter study conducted in Spain [11] used a standardized questionnaire administered at baseline and after being on medication for several months. In this study, fluoxetine, fluvoxamine, and sertraline had similar rates of sexual dysfunction, but all these drugs had lower rates of sexual dysfunction than paroxetine. A large multicenter study in the United States examined the frequency of sexual dysfunction in 6297 men and women receiving antidepressant monotherapy [4]. From this large group, investigators identified a subgroup devoid of probable comorbid illness or concomitant medications that might independently be associated with sexual dysfunction. Within this subgroup, citalopram, sertraline, paroxetine, and fluoxetine all had higher rates of sexual dysfunction than bupropion, an antidepressant affecting norepinephrine and dopamine reuptake. Venlafaxine, an antidepressant affecting serotonin and norepinephrine reuptake, had a similar rate of sexual dysfunction as the SSRIs studied. This finding of venlafaxine having a similar rate of sexual dysfunction as the SSRIs is in contrast to a study by Kennedy and colleagues [5], who found that venlafaxine had a slightly lower rate of sexual dysfunction than the SSRIs.

Double-blind placebo-controlled studies have found that bupropion has a lower incidence of sexual dysfunction than sertraline [17], fluoxetine [18], and citalopram [19]. Several double-blind studies have demonstrated that duloxetine, a drug with norepinephrine and serotonin reuptake inhibition, has a lower rate of sexual dysfunction than paroxetine [20,21]. Serzone, a drug with norepinephrine and serotonin reuptake inhibition as well as 5HT-2 blockade, has been found to have a lower rate of sexual dysfunction than the SSRIs [22]. Evidence concerning the sexual side effect profile of mirtazapine, a drug with α_2-antagonism combining with blockade of serotonin 5HT-2 and 5HT-3 receptors, is inconsistent but generally supports the conclusion that this drug has a low incidence of sexual dysfunction [3]. Antidepressants with a low incidence of sexual side effects are as follows:

Bupropion
Nefazodone
Mirtazapine
Duloxetine

Medical management of antidepressant-induced sexual dysfunction

A variety of techniques have been described to reduce the sexual side effect burden of SSRIs while maintaining their therapeutic usefulness. These include waiting for tolerance to develop [23], dose reduction [24], scheduling sexual activity around drug dosing [25], drug holidays [26], the use of antidotes [27], and drug substitution [7]. These strategies are summarized as follows:

Waiting for tolerance to develop
Dose reduction
Scheduling sexual activity around drug dosing
Drug holidays
Drug substitution
Antidotes

Waiting for tolerance to develop is seldom used, because tolerance to sexual side effects develops in few patients on SSRIs. Dose reduction is rarely used, because it is difficult to achieve a dose reduction that relieves sexual side effects without also allowing the return of depressive symptoms. Drug holidays are rarely used because of the possibility of withdrawal symptoms and the concern that one may be encouraging treatment noncompliance. There is considerable evidence that switching from an SSRI to nefazodone, mirtazapine, or bupropion may alleviate SSRI-induced sexual dysfunction [3]. Drug substitution may not be feasible, however, because of other issues. For example, nefazodone has been associated with fatal liver toxicity, rendering its use problematic. Mirtazapine has been associated with significant sedation and weight gain. Bupropion may not be effective in patients who have comorbid obsessive-compulsive features and is contraindicated in patients who have a history of seizures. There is reason to believe that switching to duloxetine might be a preferred strategy in patients who have depression and comorbid anxiety. The most commonly used strategy for managing drug-induced sexual dysfunction in the United States is probably the use of antidotes. A large number of agents, including amantadine [27], dextroamphetamine, methylphenidate [28], gingko biloba [29] granisetron [30], cyproheptadine [31], yohimbine [32], atomoxetine [33], and others, have been reported to reverse SSRI-induced sexual dysfunction. Only bupropion, buspirone, and PDE-5 inhibitors have been shown to reverse SSRI-induced sexual dysfunction in double-blind trials, however [34]. The PDE-5 inhibitors clearly reverse SSRI-induced erectile dysfunction. This has been shown in double-blind trials [35] and large clinical series [36]. Whether PDE-5 inhibitors reverse SSRI-induced female sexual disorders is less well established. Whereas low-dose buspirone seems to be ineffective in reversing SSRI-anorgasmia and decreased libido, high-dose buspirone (60 mg/d) seems to be effective after 2 weeks of therapy [37]. Bupropion at doses of 300 to 450 mg/d has been shown to be effective in reversing SSRI-induced sexual dysfunction [38]. Interestingly, one double-blind placebo-controlled study found that bupropion increased various measures of sexual responsiveness in women with hypoactive sexual desire disorder [39]. SSRI-induced sexual dysfunction often seems to remain untreated, however. A recent study of SSRI-induced sexual dysfunction in 4557 French patients found that 42% of the patients waited for spontaneous remission, which rarely occurs [40]. Evidence-based antidotes are listed in Table 1.

Rare sexual side effects of antidepressants

There have been isolated case reports of priapism with paroxetine, sertraline, fluoxetine, citalopram, and trazodone [1]. Interestingly, isolated cases of increased sexual desire and spontaneous orgasm associated with clomipramine and SSRIs have also been reported [40–43].

Table 1
Evidence-based antidotes

Bupropion	300–450 mg/d
Buspirone	60 mg/d
Sildenafil	50–100 mg
Tadalafil	10–20 mg

Mechanisms

The mechanisms by which SSRIs cause sexual dysfunction is unknown, and various mechanisms have been proposed. The mechanism is probably multifactorial. It seems clear that SSRI-induced sexual dysfunction involves stimulation of the 5HT-2C receptor, because drugs that inhibit serotonin reuptake and also block the 5HT-2C receptor, such as nefazodone and mirtazapine, are minimally associated with sexual dysfunction [1]. Similarly, antidepressants with minimal or no effects on serotonin, such as bupropion, are not associated with sexual dysfunction.

SSRIs could cause serotonergically mediated inhibition of dopaminergic neurotransmission, however. Dopaminergic neurotransmission has been shown to have a facilitating effect on sexual behavior. Consistent with this hypothesis is the observation that bupropion has a positive effect on sexual function and the anecdotal reports that dopaminergic agents, such as amphetamines, reverse SSRI-induced sexual dysfunction [44]. Elevation of prolactin has been suggested as another mechanism by which SSRIs could cause sexual dysfunction. There is minimal evidence of a relation between prolactin elevation and SSRI-induced sexual dysfunction, however. Another proposed mechanism concerns anticholinergic mechanism and inhibition of nitric oxide synthase [7]. The evidence supporting these hypotheses is minimal, however.

Sexual dysfunction and other psychiatric drugs

It is important for clinicians also to appreciate that benzodiazepines are often used to treat anxiety and agitation associated with depression and may independently cause anorgasmia [1]. Antipsychotic agents are increasingly being used in the treatment of depression and may also cause sexual dysfunction. Risperidone, traditional antipsychotics, and clozapine seem to have a much higher rate of sexual dysfunction than such drugs as aripiprazole, olanzapine, and quetiapine [45–47].

Summary

Increasing numbers of patients are on psychiatric drugs, especially antidepressants. When patients complain of sexual dysfunction, it is important that the clinician take a careful history concerning psychopharmacologic agents. It is possible that simple interventions may maintain the desired effect of the psychiatric drugs while also eliminating sexual side effects caused by these agents.

References

[1] Segraves RT, Balon R. Sexual pharmacology: fast facts. New York: WW Norton; 2003.
[2] Segraves RT. Female sexual dysfunction: psychiatric aspects. Can J Psychiatry 2002;47:419–25.
[3] Balon R. Depression, antidepressants, and human sexuality. Prim Psychiatry 2007;14:42–50.
[4] Clayton A, Montejo A. Major depressive disorder, antidepressants, and sexual dysfunction. J Clin Psychiatry 2006;67(Suppl 6):33–7.
[5] Kennedy S, Eisfeld B, Dickens S, et al. Antidepressant-induced sexual dysfunction during treatment with paroxetine, sertraline and venlafaxine. J Clin Psychiatry 2000;61:276–81.
[6] Kivela S, Pahkala K. Symptoms of depression in old people in Finland. Z Gerontol 1988;21:257–63.
[7] Rosen R, Lane R, Menza M. Effects of SSRIs on sexual function: a critical review. J Clin Psychopharmacol 1999;19:67–84.
[8] Segraves RT. Antidepressant-induced sexual dysfunction. J Clin Psychiatry 1998;59(Suppl 4):48–54.
[9] Harrison W, Rabkin J, Erhardt A. Effects of antidepressant medication on sexual function: a controlled study. J Clin Psychopharmacol 1986;6:144–9.
[10] Monteiro W, Noshirvani H, Marks I. Anorgasmia from clomipramine in obsessive compulsive disorder: a controlled trial. Br J Psychiatry 1987;151:107–12.
[11] Montejo-Gonzalez A, Liorca G, Izquierdo J, et al. SSRI-induced sexual dysfunction: fluvoxamine, paroxetine, sertraline, fluvoxamine in a prospective, multicenter and descriptive clinical study of 344 patients. J Sex Marital Ther 1997;23:176–94.
[12] Waldinger M. Male ejaculation and orgasmic disorders. In: Balon R, Segraves R, editors. Handbook of sexual dysfunction. Boca Raton (FL): Taylor & Francis; 2005. p. 215–58.
[13] Waldinger M. Rapid ejaculation. In: Levine S, Risen C, Althof S, editors. Handbook of clinical sexuality for mental health professionals. New York: Brunner-Routledge; 2003. p. 257–74.
[14] Csoka A, Shipko S. Persistent sexual side effects after SSRI discontinuation. Psychother Psychosom 2006;75:187–8.
[15] Segraves RT. Recognizing and reversing sexual side effects of medications. In: Levine S, Risen C, Althof S, editors. Handbook of clinical sexuality for mental health professionals. New York: Brunner-Routledge; 2003. p. 377–92.
[16] Segraves RT, Kavoussi R, Hughes A, et al. Evaluation of sexual functioning in depressed outpatients: a double-blind comparison of sustained-release bupropion and sertraline treatment. J Clin Psychopharmacol 2000;20:122–8.

[17] Colemann C, Cunningham L, Foster V. Sexual dysfunction associated with the treatment of depression: a placebo-controlled comparison of bupropion sustained release and sertraline treatment. Ann Clin Psychiatry 2006;67:736–46.

[18] Colemann C, King B, Bolden-Watson C. A placebo-controlled comparison of the effects on sexual functioning of bupropion sustained release and fluoxetine. Clin Ther 2001;23:1040–58.

[19] Clayton AH, Croft H, Horrigan J. Bupropion sustained release compared with escitalopram; effects on sexual functioning in 2 randomized double-blind placebo-controlled studies. J Clin Psychiatry 2006; 67:736–46.

[20] Delgado P, Brannan S, Mallinckrodt C. Sexual functioning assessed in 4 double-blind placebo and paroxetine-controlled trials of duloxetine in major depressive disorder. J Clin Psychiatry 2005;66: 686–92.

[21] Fieger A, Kiev A, Shrivastava R, et al. Nefazodone versus sertraline in outpatients with major depressive disorder; focus on efficacy, tolerability, and effects on sexual function and satisfaction. J Clin Psychiatry 1996;57(Suppl 2):53–61.

[22] Herman J, Brotman A, Pollack M, et al. Fluoxetine-induced sexual dysfunction. J Clin Psychiatry 1990; 51:25–7.

[23] Patterson M. Fluoxetine-induced sexual dysfunction. J Clin Psychiatry 1993;54:71.

[24] Bennazi F, Mazzoli M. Fluoxetine-induced sexual dysfunction: a dose-dependent effect. Pharmacopsychiatry 1994;27:246.

[25] Olivera A. Sexual dysfunction due to clomipramine and sertraline; a nonpharmacological solution. J Sex Educ Ther 1994;20:119–22.

[26] Rothschild A. Sexual side effects of antidepressants. J Clin Psychiatry 2000;61(Suppl 11):28–36.

[27] Balon R. Intermittent amantadine for fluoxetine-induced sexual dysfunction. J Sex Marital Ther 1996; 22:290–2.

[28] Bartlick B, Kaplan P, Kaplan H. Psychostimulants apparently reverse sexual dysfunction secondary to selective serotonin reuptake inhibitors. J Sex Marital Ther 1995;21:264–71.

[29] Cohen A, Bartlick B. Gingko biloba for antidepressant-induced sexual dysfunction. J Sex Marital Ther 1998;24:139–43.

[30] Nelson E, Keck P, McElroy S. Resolution of fluoxetine-induced sexual dysfunction with the 5HT3 antagonist granisetron. J Clin Psychiatry 1997;58: 496–7.

[31] Goldbloom D. Adverse interaction of fluoxetine and cyproheptadine in two patients with anorexia nervosa. J Clin Psychiatry 1991;52:261–2.

[32] Segraves R. Treatment of drug-induced anorgasmia with yohimbine. Br J Psychiatry 1994;165:554.

[33] Carpenter L, Milosauljevic N, Schecter T, et al. Augmentation with open-label atomoxetine for partial or nonresponse to antidepressants. J Clin Psychiatry 2005;66:1234–8.

[34] Taylor M, Rudkin L, Hawton K. Strategies for managing antidepressant-induced sexual dysfunction: systematic review of randomized controlled studies. J Affect Disord 2005;88:241–54.

[35] Nurnberg HG, Hensley P, Gelenberg A, et al. Treatment of antidepressant-associated sexual dysfunction with sildenafil: a randomized controlled trial. JAMA 2003;289:56–64.

[36] Segraves RT, Lee J, Stevenson R, et al. Tadalafil for treatment of erectile dysfunction in men on antidepressants. J Clin Psychopharamcol 2007; 27:62–6.

[37] Landen M, Eriksson E, Agren H, et al. Effect of buspirone on sexual dysfunction in depressed patients treated with selective serotonin reuptake inhibitors. J Clin Psychopharmacol 1999;19:268–71.

[38] Clayton A, Warnock J, Kornstein S. A placebo controlled study of bupropion SR as an antidote for SSRI-induced sexual dysfunction. J Clin Psychiatry 2004;65:62–7.

[39] Segraves R, Clayton A, Croft H, et al. Bupropion sustained release for the treatment of hypoactive sexual desire disorder in premenopausal women. J Clin Psychopharmacol 2004;24:339–42.

[40] Bonierbale M, Lancon C, Tignol J. The ELIXIR study: evaluation of sexual dysfunction in 4557 depressed patients in France. Curr Med Res Opin 2003;19:114–24.

[41] Elmore J, Quattlebaum J. Female sexual stimulation during antidepressant treatment. Pharamcol Ther 1997;17:612–6.

[42] Berk M, Acton M. Citalopram associated with clitoral priapism: a case series. Int Clin Psychopharmacol 1997;12:121–3.

[43] Modell J. Repeated observation of yawning, clitoral engorgement and orgasm associated with fluoxetine administration. J Clin Psychopharmacol 1989;9: 63–5.

[44] McLean J, Forsythe R, Kaplin L. Unusual side effects of clomipramine associated with yawning. Can J Psychiatry 1983;28:569–70.

[45] Caerk D. SSRI and sexual functioning. J Am Acad Child Adolesc Pyschiatry 1996;35:110–6.

[46] Halaris A. Neurochemical aspects of the sexual response cycle. CNS Spectr 2003;8:211–6.

[47] Knegtering H, Bruggeman R. What are the effects of antipsychotics on sexual dysfunction. Prim Psychiatry 2007;14:51–6.

ELSEVIER
SAUNDERS

Urol Clin N Am 34 (2007) 581–589

UROLOGIC
CLINICS
of North America

Patient Reported Outcomes Used in the Assessment of Premature Ejaculation

Stanley E. Althof, PhD[a,b,c,]*, Tara Symonds, PhD[d]

[a]*Case Western Reserve University School of Medicine, Cleveland, OH, USA*
[b]*University of Miami Miller School of Medicine, Miami, FL, USA*
[c]*Center for Marital and Sexual Health of South Florida, West Palm Beach, FL, USA*
[d]*Global Outcomes Research, Pfizer Ltd., Kent, UK*

Sexuality questionnaires play an integral role in the diagnosis and treatment of male and female sexual dysfunctions. They are used to (1) identify/diagnose individuals with a particular dysfunction, (2) assess the severity of the dysfunction, (3) measure improvement or satisfaction with treatment, (4) examine the impact of the dysfunction on the individual's quality of life (eg, relationship satisfaction, mood, sexual confidence), and (5) study the impact of the dysfunction on the partner and his or her quality of life.

The development of new sexuality questionnaires and diaries, known as patient-reported outcomes (PROs), has been stimulated by the burgeoning sexual health pharmaceutical programs and guidance from regulatory agencies, such as the US Food and Drug Administration (FDA). The latter requires objective and PRO methods to document improvements in sexual function. For instance, the three phosphodiesterase Type 5 inhibitors (PDE5i) (sildenafil, tadalafil, and vardenafil) were approved, in part, because each compound demonstrated significant improvement on the International Index of Erectile Function (IIEF) [1], a 15-item validated PRO.

PROs for premature ejaculation (PE) have lagged behind the development of questionnaires for erectile dysfunction (ED). More recently, with the advent of pharmaceutical trials for PE [2], there has been renewed interest in creating and validating PROs that identify/diagnose the condition and measure improvement with treatment.

This article reviews the PE-related PROs that have appeared in the published literature. Each questionnaire's psychometric properties and its benefits and limitations are examined and discussed. The authors hope this helps clinicians and researchers to identify brief, reliable, and valid measures that document treatment effects or identify men with PE.

Definitions of premature ejaculation and problems with the current definitions

A universally accepted definition of PE remains to be established. To date, there are at least eight definitions of PE offered by different professional organizations or researchers (Table 1) [3–10]. All but one were derived from the consensus opinion of experts or from clinical wisdom; only the definition by Waldinger and colleagues [10] is the by-product of scientific data collection from a large observational study from the general population. All but two definitions (Waldinger and colleagues [10] and Masters and Johnson [9]) suffer from excessive vagueness, lack of precision, and undue subjectivity on the part of the diagnostician.

For example, examining the *Diagnostic and Statistic Manual of Mental Disorders, Fourth Edition, Text Revision* (DSM-IV-TR) [3], PE is defined as follows:

- Persistent or recurrent ejaculation with minimal sexual stimulation before, on, or shortly after penetration and before the person wishes it

* Corresponding author.
E-mail address: stanley.althof@case.edu (S.E. Althof).

Table 1
Definitions of premature ejaculation

Definition offered by	Definition
Diagnostic and Statistic Manual of Mental Disorders, Fourth Edition, Text Revision [3]	Persistent or recurrent ejaculation with minimal sexual stimulation before, on, or shortly after penetration and before the person wishes it. The condition must also cause marked distress or interpersonal difficulty and cannot be attributable exclusively to the direct effects of a substance.
International Statistical Classification of Disease, 10th Edition [4]	For individuals who meet the general criteria for sexual dysfunction, the inability to control ejaculation sufficiently for both partners to enjoy sexual interaction, which manifests as the occurrence of ejaculation before or soon after the beginning of intercourse (if a time limit is required, before or within 15 seconds) or the occurrence of ejaculation in the absence of sufficient erection to make intercourse possible. The problem is not the result of prolonged absence from sexual activity.
European Association of Urology, guidelines on disorders of ejaculation [5]	The inability to control ejaculation for a "sufficient" length of time before vaginal penetration. It does not involve any impairment of fertility when intravaginal ejaculation occurs.
International consultation on urological diseases [6]	Persistent or recurrent ejaculation with minimal stimulation before, on, or shortly after penetration, and before the person wishes it, over which the sufferer has little or no voluntary control, which causes the sufferer or his partner bother or distress.
American Urological Association guideline on the pharmacologic management of premature ejaculation [7]	Ejaculation that occurs sooner than desired, before or shortly after penetration, causing distress to one or both partners.
Metz and McCarthy [8]	The man does not have voluntary conscious control or the ability to choose in most encounters when to ejaculate.
Masters and Johnson [9]	The foundation considers a man to be a premature ejaculator if he cannot control his ejaculatory process for a sufficient length of time during intravaginal containment to satisfy his partner in at least 50% of their coital connections.
Waldinger et al [10]	Men with an IELT of less than 1 minute (belonging to the 0.5 percentile) have "definite" PE, whereas men with an IELT between 1 and 1.5 minutes (between 0.5 and 2.5 percentiles) have "probable" PE. An additional grading of severity of PE should be defined in terms of associated psychologic problems. Thus, definite and probable PE needs further psychologic subclassification in nonsymptomatic, mild, moderate, and severe PE.

- The disturbance causes marked distress or interpersonal difficulty
- The PE is not attributable exclusively to the direct effects of a substance

How would a clinician objectively define "minimal sexual stimulation" or "shortly after penetration" or "before the person wishes" or "marked distress or interpersonal difficulty"? One clinician's interpretation of the DSM-IV-TR criteria is likely to differ from another clinician's interpretation.

Failure to have an agreed-on definition of what constitutes PE has also hampered research efforts.

The validity of a PRO depends on the definition of the condition. PROs for PE need to discriminate between a group with the condition (PE) or those without the condition (non-PE) or to accurately assess treatment effects within a group of men with PE. Obviously, definitions without clearly defined objective criteria make development of PE PROs difficult.

Despite the convincing criticisms leveled at the eight definitions of PE (excessive vagueness, imprecision, and subjectivity), there is significant overlap among them. Four common factors emerge from the proposed definitions: intravaginal ejaculatory latency time (IELT), perceived control, distress, and interpersonal difficulty (related to the ejaculatory dysfunction).

Given these common factors, the issue becomes whether a diagnosis of PE should be unidimensional [11–13], based primarily on a defined IELT threshold, or multidimensional, using a defined IELT threshold and the variables of perceived lack of control, poor sexual satisfaction, and distress [14,15]. Recent publications of observational data in men with and without PE have clarified the answer to this controversy [16–18].

An observational study of men diagnosed by clinicians as having or not having PE by Patrick and colleagues [16] suggests that IELT alone is not sufficient to categorize the two groups accurately. There was significant overlap between the IELTs of men with and without PE. Further analysis of the data studied [18] the interrelation between IELT, perceived control over ejaculation, decreased satisfaction with sexual intercourse, personal distress, and interpersonal difficulty related to ejaculation. These investigators found that control over ejaculation was central to understanding how PE is associated with satisfaction with sexual intercourse and ejaculation-related distress. Furthermore, the association of IELT with satisfaction with intercourse and distress related to ejaculation was mediated by perceived control over ejaculation. The results were robust; how IELT was scaled did not have an impact on the model; neither did restricting the sample to men with an IELT of 2 minutes or less.

Given the evidence indicating the importance of assessing control, sexual satisfaction, and distress in relation to a man's PE, there needs to be a method to measure these subjective elements accurately. One way of doing this is by using a validated questionnaire (PRO) measure. Questionnaires have the advantage of allowing for a systematic/standardized approach to diagnosis.

Provided the measure is brief and accurate, it should facilitate the diagnosis of PE. Furthermore, in clinical research, such an approach of screening on control/sexual satisfaction/distress would allow a more comprehensive assessment of the impact of any novel treatment on PE.

In summary, the data suggest that the diagnosis of PE should be multidimensional and include IELT, the man's perceived control, sexual satisfaction, and distress. There remains some controversy as to the IELT threshold necessary to diagnose PE; further data analysis is likely to resolve this debate.

Psychometric properties of patient-reported outcomes

PRO development consists of multiple stepwise statistical procedures to ensure the measure meets or exceeds established psychometric principles. These psychometric requirements are listed and defined in Table 2. It is essential that PROs demonstrate reliability, validity (known groups, convergent and divergent), and sensitivity to detect changes in a specified population. Moreover, if the PRO contains scales or domains, the items within these scales and the relation between the scales and total score must also meet established psychometric standards. Developing a PRO in this manner ensures that the clinician or investigator has a reliable tool for diagnosis or detection of change.

Regulatory requirements for newly developed patient-reported outcomes

New measures being developed for use in a clinical trial program, which may lead to US labeling claims, need to satisfy the requirements of the FDA draft guidance for industry, PRO measures: use in medical product development to support labeling claims [19]. This document clearly sets forth the psychometric tests and properties that need to be demonstrated for a new PRO to be considered validated. The FDA draft guidance also stipulates that the content of the tool be developed by interviewing patients and that the language used in the PRO reflect the experience of patients. Additionally, the guidance suggests that an end point model be developed (research and model of Patrick and colleagues [18] are a good starting point for any new PE measure) to support why particular end points under

Table 2
Validation and reliability tests for development of a questionnaire

Questionnaire structure	Definition	Acceptability level
Principal components factor analysis	Principal components factor analysis can be conducted to determine the item-scale structure of a questionnaire	<ul><li>All items included in a scale should load on a single unrotated factor >0.40 to support unidimensionality</li><li>No item redundancy (inter-item correlations <0.80)</li><li>Variance explained by the second factor $>20\%$ after varimax rotation to be considered a second dimension of the questionnaire</li><li>No items should load >0.40 on more than one factor</li></ul>
Test-retest reliability	The stability of a measuring instrument, which is assessed by administering the instrument to respondents on two different occasions and examining the correlation between test and retest scores	Intraclass correlation coefficient ≥ 0.70 is considered satisfactory
Internal consistency reliability	To evaluate the extent to which individual items of the instrument are consistent with each other and reflect an underlying scheme or construct	Cronbach's α coefficient ≥ 0.70 is considered acceptable
Known groups validity	Known groups validity: ability of a measure to distinguish between groups known to differ, such as between different disease severity groups	Statistically significant differences are expected between these groups
Convergent and divergent validity	Convergent validity: dimensions measuring similar or overlapping concepts are expected to be substantially correlated ($r \geq 0.40$) Divergent validity: dimensions measuring dissimilar concepts are expected to correlate less strongly or not at all	Once the hypothesized domains have been determined, similar and dissimilar measures should be incorporated into the validation study to test for convergent and divergent validity
Responsiveness	Definition/test	Criteria for acceptability
Ability to detect change	To be useful for clinical trials, a measure must reflect changes in scores when change has occurred in health condition under study	Statistically significant change in scores
Interpretation of magnitude of change	Definition/test	Criteria for acceptability

(*continued on next page*)

Table 2 (*continued*)

Responsiveness	Definition/test	Criteria for acceptability
Anchor-based method	A clinical anchor or patient-reported anchor can be used to establish whether or not a patient has improved. Those improving at least "slightly" inform the MID in score at end of treatment expected to be shown to indicate a meaningful change [31]	This varies from measure to measure
Distribution-based method	Effect size [31]	≥ 0.5
Questionnaire as diagnostic	Definition	Acceptability level
Sensitivity and specificity	Sensitivity is defined as the proportion of subjects with the disease that are diagnosed as having the disease (true-positive rate), and specificity is defined as the proportion of subjects without a disease that are diagnosed as not having the disease (true-negative rate)	Point at which the sensitivity/specificity ratio is closest to unity (this maximizes sensitivity and specificity)
Positive and negative predictive value	Positive predictive value is the precision rate of patients being diagnosed with a condition and they do actually have the condition. Negative predictive value is the precision rate of patients not being diagnosed with condition when they do not have the condition.	Predictive values greater than 70% are considered acceptable

investigation have been chosen. Any changes to a measure, inclusive of medium of administration, or change in population would require revalidation.

Assessment techniques

Methods used to assess treatment outcome for PE include (1) patient self-report, (2) clinician judgment, (3) structured interview, (4) omnibus measures of sexual function, (5) focused self-report inventories designed specifically to evaluate outcome of treatments for rapid ejaculation, and (6) timing of ejaculatory latency by stopwatch.

Self-report

Investigators have been notoriously skeptical of the value of patient self-report when conducting outcome studies. A recent study by Rosen and colleagues [20] reported that self-estimated and stopwatch-measured IELT were interchangeable, however, correctly assigning PE status with 80% specificity and 80% sensitivity. Previously, Althof [21] correlated 13 patients' self-report of IELT during a telephone interview, a face-to-face

clinical interview, and stopwatch-assessed IELT. Correlation coefficients between telephone interview and actual time and structured interview and actual time were 0.619 and 0.627, respectively. These data would suggest that self-report of IELT might suffice in a clinical situation. Clinical research demands a higher standard of objectivity requiring IELT measurements, however.

Clinician judgment

There are no reported studies on clinician concordance in diagnosing PE. Clinician subjectivity in interpreting the current diagnostic criterion sets would likely hamper agreement. Subjectivity in interpretation would also interfere with reliability in gauging improvement with treatment or impact on the psychosocial parameters. Patient self-report and clinician judgment, however, remain unobtrusive means of obtaining data and are the least burdensome for patients.

Inventories of sexual function

The Derogatis Sexual Function Inventory (DSFI) [22] and the Golumbok Russ Inventory of Sexual Satisfaction (GRISS) [23] are omnibus sexual inventories, neither of which is specifically designed to assess any one particular sexual dysfunction. The DSFI is composed of 254 items comprising 10 subscales. This instrument offers investigators a reliable and valid means of measuring psychologic distress; however, it has few questions devoted to ejaculatory latency or voluntary control.

Similarly, the GRISS is a 28-item questionnaire designed to assess the existence and severity of sexual problems. It consists of 12 subscales, one of which is rapid ejaculation. The measure has good reliability and satisfactory validity but is more helpful with diagnosis than outcome.

Structured interviews

Designed by Metz and his colleagues, the Premature Ejaculation Severity Index (PESI) (Metz M, Pryor J, Nessvacil R, personal communication, 1997) is a 10-item interview scale that offers a severity of distress score. It may be most helpful to clinicians interested in pre- and post-therapy changes. It has limited utility as a research instrument, however, because the validity and reliability of this measure have never been established.

Timing of ejaculatory latency by stopwatch

Use of a stopwatch to time ejaculatory latency from vaginal penetration until ejaculation is a simple, objective, and reproducible outcome measure. The intrusiveness of stopwatch assessment may seem more severe to those unfamiliar with this approach than to subjects who participate in IELT studies. Surprisingly, most couples do not object to being asked to time their lovemaking. In fact, some men report that they enjoy competing with themselves to see if they can improve their ejaculatory latency. What remains unknown is what influence, if any, that asking couples to time lovemaking has on the outcome. Specifically, does timing, increase, decrease, or have no effect on ejaculatory latency? Is it possible that timing oneself serves as an occult treatment intervention?

It is, however, unlikely that physicians would be able to routinely require patients to time intercourse episodes before making a diagnosis of PE. It is too burdensome on the physician and patient. A simpler and less intrusive diagnostic assessment device must be developed.

Patient-reported outcomes for premature ejaculation

Table 3 lists the PROs available to identify/diagnose men with PE and PROs for detecting change when treating men with PE. Each measure's psychometric properties are described as well. Table 3 was compiled by reviewing the literature; only those measures in which the reliability and validity are documented have been included.

Patient-reported outcomes to identify/diagnose men with premature ejaculation

There are two measures available to diagnose PE. The first, the Chinese Index of Premature Ejaculation (CIPE) [24], has five items that assess perceived time to ejaculation from intromission, ability to prolong intercourse time, sexual satisfaction, partner satisfaction, and anxiety/depression related to sexual activity. This measure does not seem to have had any psychometric analyses conducted before determining the scoring system to diagnosis absence or presence of PE (only known groups validity). Although further validation seems to be necessary the CIPE may be used to identify men with PE but is not recommended as an outcome measure.

The second PRO, the Premature Ejaculation Diagnostic Tool (PEDT) [25,26], is a five-item measure that evaluates difficulty in delaying ejaculation, ejaculating before the person wishes, ejaculating with little stimulation, frustration related to ejaculating prematurely, and concerns about the partner being sexually unfulfilled. It has excellent sensitivity and specificity and makes an ideal diagnostic tool.

Psychometric analyses were conducted to ensure the items were valid and reliable. Testing was then conducted to determine the most appropriate scoring system to assess PE status. Although positive and negative predictive values were not calculated, a further study was conducted to test the PEDT concordance in diagnosis against expert clinician diagnosis. The level of agreement between the PEDT and clinical expert was high (κ statistic = 0.80; 95% confidence interval [CI]: 0.68–0.92).

The limitation to using questionnaires in busy clinical practices is the time required to have the patient complete the measure and the time necessary to score the PRO and make the diagnosis. The PEDT and CIPE are brief and are quickly completed and scored, however. They are less

Table 3
Psychometric properties of premature ejaculation measures

Instrument	Population	Reliability			Validity				Diagnostic tests	
		Factor analysis	Internal consistency	Test-retest	Convergent-divergent	Known groups	Responsiveness	MID	Sensitivity/specificity	Positive and negative predictive value
CIPE	n = 169 IELT: mean = 1.6 (SD = 1.2) minutes 61% lifelong 39% acquired	x	x	x	x	✓	x	x	✓	✓
Single-item PROs	n = 1587; n = 166 DSM-IV clinician diagnosis; DSM-IV clinician diagnosis plus IELT, 2 minutes > 50% intercourse episodes	n/a	n/a	✓	x	✓	✓	x	x	x
IPE	Study 1: 147 lifelong PE; DSM-IV clinician diagnosis Mean IELT = 1.92 (SD = 2.98) minutes Study 2: 939 acquired or lifelong PE; DSM-IV clinician diagnosis Mean IELT = 3.9 (SD = 37.4) seconds	✓	✓	✓	✓	✓	x	x	x	x
MSHQ-EjD	N = 1245 US men; n = 179 homosexual or bisexual men 6909 US men with LUTS/BPH No details on PE status within these samples	✓	✓	✓	✓	✓	x	x	x	x
PEDT	n = 292; IELT = 66 (SE = 1.78) seconds n = 309 self-reported PE; IELT = 279.4 (SE = 19.22)	✓	✓	✓	✓	✓	x	x	✓	x

Abbreviations: BPH, benign prostatic hyperplasia; CIPE, Chinese Index of Premature Ejaculation; IPE, Index of Premature Ejaculation; LUTS, lower urinary tract symptoms; MSHQ-EjD, Male Sexual Health Questionnaire–Ejaculatory Dysfunction; n/a, not applicable; PEDT, Premature Ejaculation Diagnostic Tool; Single-item PROs: control, sexual satisfaction, personal distress, and interpersonal difficulty.

✓, feature demonstrated; x, feature not demonstrated; ✓/x, feature not clearly demonstrated.

intrusive and burdensome than asking patients to time lovemaking and provide an immediate decision regarding diagnosis.

Patient-reported outcomes for determining treatment effects

There are five measures developed to assess the impact of treatment on men with PE. A summary of the development and validation of each PRO is given in Table 3.

The Premature Ejaculation Profile (PEP) [18] contains four questions assessing perceived control over ejaculation, satisfaction with sexual intercourse, personal distress related to ejaculation, and interpersonal difficulty related to ejaculation. Each item has been validated and has shown robust psychometrics. An assessment of the items' convergent and divergent validity needs to be considered, as does a criterion for showing a meaningful change, such as minimum important difference (MID) or responder definition.

The advantage of the PEP is its brevity. This may also be a limitation, however, because each domain (control, satisfaction, distress, and interpersonal difficulty) consists of only one question, which may have an impact on the reliability of the items and may limit the sensitivity of each domain.

The Index of Premature Ejaculation [27], with three domains covering control, sexual satisfaction, and distress, also showed strong psychometric properties. Responsiveness has yet to be shown, and an MID or responder definition needs to be defined.

The newly developed Male Sexual Health Questionnaire-Ejaculation [28] has four items: three to assess function (force, volume, and frequency of ejaculation) and one to assess bother. Validity and reliability analyses were conducted, but it is unclear what proportion of those who completed the measure had PE. How relevant the concepts of volume and force of ejaculation are in determining the impact on men's lives is unclear. The psychometric data did not provide any information on its diagnostic capability or its responsiveness or definition of MID or responder.

There were other measures mentioned in the literature; however, validation data were sparse or nonexistent. The PEQuest [29] was developed to investigate cognitive and partner-related factors in PE. Apart from information about how it was developed, however, there was limited information given as to its validation. The Yonsei-Sexual Function Inventory-II [30] similarly was developed to assess various factors related to PE (performance anxiety, patient and partner satisfaction, sexual desire, and overall sexual function); however, again, there was no validation information found in the literature to defend the measures used to assess outcome in PE clinical trials.

Summary

This article has reviewed the state of the art as it relates to PROs for PE. Controversy remains regarding the precise definition of PE, although recent publications have demonstrated the need for a multidimensional definition that includes a threshold for IELT and perceived controlled, distress, satisfaction, and interpersonal difficulty. The validity of any PE PRO depends on the operational definition of the condition. Use of the listed measures is limited to the populations on which they have been validated. The various populations used are a clear sign of lack of consensus in defining PE. The DSM-TR-IV is in the process of being revised; it is hoped that the definition for PE becomes more specific and easily operationalized.

Table 2 offers an in-depth review of the psychometric challenges that PROs must meet or exceed. Combined with the requirements of the regulatory agencies, such as the FDA, PROs have become increasingly sophisticated and reliable instruments for identifying men with PE and measuring treatment effects.

Table 3 reviews the available tools for clinicians and researchers and provides guidance concerning the benefits and limitations of these measures. It is important for the field to have brief but reliable instruments to make important judgments concerning diagnosis and treatment effects. The more a particular PRO is used, the more we learn about its reliability, validity, and diagnostic capability. Also, we begin to build a picture as to what an important change in score might look like. Rather than developing yet more measures for the diagnosis of PE and assessment of treatment effects, the authors encourage researchers to use and build on the existing measures. The PEDT and IPE publications state that use is available for any interested researchers, which is a positive move to consolidating and moving to one or two measures that all researchers can become familiar with and be more confident that diagnosis and treatment effects are reliable and valid.

References

[1] Rosen RC, Riley A, Wagner G, et al. The International Index of Erectile Function (IIEF): a multidimensional scale for assessment of erectile dysfunction. Urology 1997;49:822–30.

[2] Pryor J, Althof S, Steidle C, et al. Efficacy and tolerability of Dapoxetine in the treatment of premature ejaculation: integrated analysis of two randomized, double-blind, placebo-controlled trials. Lancet 2006;368:939–47.

[3] Diagnostic and statistical manual of mental disorders. 4th edition. Text revision: DSM-IV-TR. Washington, DC: American Psychiatric Association; 2000. p. 554.

[4] International statistical classification of diseases and related health problems. 10th edition. Geneva (IL): World Health Organization; 1994.

[5] Colpi GM, Hargreave TB, Papp GK, et al. European Association of Urology. Guidelines on disorders of ejaculation. 2001. Available at: http://www.uroweb.org/files/uploaded_files/guidelines/ejaculationdisor.pdf. Accessed July 3, 2007.

[6] McMahon CG, Abdo C, Incrocci L, et al. Disorders of orgasm and ejaculation in men. J Sex Med 2004;1:58–65.

[7] Montague DK, Jarow J, Broderick GA, et al. AUA guideline on the pharmacologic management of premature ejaculation. J Urol 2004;172:290–4.

[8] Metz M, McCarthy B. Coping with premature ejaculation: how to overcome PE, please your partner and have great sex. Oakland (CA): New Harbinber Publications; 2003.

[9] Masters W, Johnson V. Human sexual inadequacy. Boston: Little Brown Company; 1970.

[10] Waldinger MD, Zwinderman AH, Berend O, et al. Proposal for a definition of lifelong premature ejaculation based on epidemiological stopwatch data. J Sex Med 2005;2(4):498–507.

[11] Waldinger MD, Hengeveld MW, Zwinderman AH, et al. An empirical operational study of DSM-IV diagnostic criteria for PE. International Journal of Psychiatry in Clinical Practice 1998;2:287–93.

[12] Waldinger M, Schweitzer DH. Changing paradigms from a historical DSM-III and DSM IV view toward an evidenced-based definition of premature ejaculation. Part I—validity of DSM-IV-TR. J Sex Med 2006;3(4):682–92.

[13] Waldinger M, Schweitzer DH. Changing paradigms from a historical DSM-III and DSM-IV view toward an evidenced-based definition of premature ejaculation. Part II—proposals for DSM-V and ICD-11. J Sex Med 2006;3(4):693–705.

[14] Rowland DL. Treatment of premature ejaculation: selecting outcomes to determine efficacy. Bulletin of the International Society of Sexual Impotence Research 2003;10:26–7.

[15] Broderick GA. Premature ejaculation: on defining and quantifying a common male sexual dysfunction. J Sex Med 2006;4:S295–302.

[16] Patrick DL, Althof SE, Barada JH, et al. Premature ejaculation: an observational study of men and their partners. J Sex Med 2005;2:358–67.

[17] Waldinger MD, Quinn P, Dilleen M, et al. A multinational population survey of intravaginal ejaculation latency time. J Sex Med 2005;2(4):292–7.

[18] Patrick DL, Rowland D, Rothman M. Interrelationships among measures of premature ejaculation: the central role of perceived control. J Sex Med 2007; 4(3):780–8.

[19] US FDA draft guidance for industry, patient reported outcome measures: use in medical product development to support labeling claims, February, 2006. Available at: www.fda.gov/cder/guidance/5460dft.pdf.

[20] Rosen RC, McMahon CG, Niederberger C, et al. Correlates to the clinical diagnosis of premature ejaculation: results from a large observational study of men and their partners. J Urol 2007;177(3):1059–64.

[21] Althof S. Evidence based assessment of rapid ejaculation. Int J Impot Res 1998;10(2):74–6.

[22] Derogatis LR, Melisaratos N. The DSFI—a multidimensional measure of sexual functioning. J Sex Marital Ther 1979;5:244–81.

[23] Rust J, Golombok S. The GRISS: a psychometric instrument for the assessment of sexual dysfunction. Archives of Sexual Behavior 1986;13(2):157–65.

[24] Yuan JM, Xin ZC, Jiang H, et al. Sexual function of premature ejaculation patients assessed with the Chinese Index of Premature Ejaculation. Asian J Androl 2004;6:121–6.

[25] Symonds T, Perelman M, Althof S, et al. Development and validation of a premature ejaculation diagnostic tool. Eur Urol 2007;52:565–73.

[26] Symonds T, Perelman M, Althof S, et al. Further evidence of the reliability and validity of premature ejaculation diagnostic tool (PEDT). Int J Impot Res 2007;19:521–5.

[27] Althof S, Rosen R, Symonds T, et al. Development and validation of a new questionnaire to assess sexual satisfaction, control and distress associated with premature ejaculation. J Sex Med 2006;3(3):465–575.

[28] Rosen RC, Catania JA, Althof SE, et al. Development and validation of four-item version of the Male Sexual Health Questionnaire to assess ejaculatory dysfunction. Urology 2007;69(5):805–9.

[29] Hartmann U, Schedlowski M, Kruger TH. Cognitive and partner-related factors in rapid ejaculation: differences between dysfunctional and functional men. World J Urol 2005;23(2):93–101.

[30] Lee HS, Song DS, Kim CY, et al. An open clinical trial of fluoxetine in the treatment of premature ejaculation. J Clin Pharmacol 1996;16:379–82.

[31] Guyatt GH, Osoba D, Wu D, et al. Methods to explain clinical significance of health status measures. Mayo Clin Proc 2002;77:371–83.

ELSEVIER
SAUNDERS

Urol Clin N Am 34 (2007) 591–599

UROLOGIC
CLINICS
of North America

Premature Ejaculation: State of the Art

Marcel D. Waldinger, MD, PhD[a,b,*]

[a]*Department of Psychiatry and Neurosexology, HagaHospital Leyenburg, The Hague, The Netherlands*
[b]*Section of Psychopharmacology, Department of Pharmaceutical Sciences, Utrecht University,*
Utrecht, The Netherlands

It has become customary to start an article on premature ejaculation (PE) with the following introduction: "PE is the most prevalent male sexual *disorder* affecting some 20% to 30% of men." This sentence mirrors a general belief that PE always represents a male sexual "disorder." However, if one distinguishes PE as a "complaint" versus PE as a "disorder," it appears more appropriate to state "PE is the most prevalent male sexual *complaint* affecting some 20% to 30% of men. The prevalence of PE as a sexual *disorder* has not yet been investigated in the general male population, but is assumed to be much lower." The omission of the distinction complaint versus disorder has been blurring the debate on definition, classification, epidemiology, and treatment of PE.

Diagnostic and Statistical Manual of Mental Disorders and International Classification of Diseases definition of premature ejaculation

Currently, there are two official definitions of PE. In the *Diagnostic and Statistical Manual of Mental Disorders* (*DSM-IV-TR*), which is issued by the American Psychiatric Association, premature ejaculation is defined as a "persistent or recurrent ejaculation with minimal sexual stimulation before, on, or shortly after penetration and before the person wishes it. The clinician must take into account factors that affect duration of the excitement phase, such as age, novelty of the sexual partner or situation, and recent frequency of sexual activity" [1]. According to this

definition, PE can only be diagnosed when "the disturbance causes marked distress or interpersonal difficulty" [1]. According to the International Classification of Diseases (ICD-10), issued by the World Health Organization, PE is defined as "the inability to delay ejaculation sufficiently to enjoy lovemaking, which is manifested by either an occurrence of ejaculation before or very soon after the beginning of intercourse (if a time limit is required: before or within 15 seconds of the beginning of intercourse) or ejaculation occurs in the absence of sufficient erection to make intercourse possible" [2].

Interestingly, in contrast to the *DSM* definition, the ICD-10 uses a cutoff point for the ejaculation time of 15 seconds, but does not provide literature on which this quantification is based. In reverse, and in contrast to the ICD-10, according to the *DSM-IV-TR*, PE needs to cause marked distress and/or interpersonal difficulty before it can be classified as the sexual disorder PE.

However, the distress and/or interpersonal difficulty requirement for the diagnosis of PE is not based on evidence-based studies but on the subjective idea of the *DSM-IV* Task Force that any mental disorder in the *DSM* should cause distress and/or interpersonal difficulty [3].

It should be noted that both the *DSM* and ICD definition of PE are based on authority-based opinions and not on well-controlled clinical and epidemiologic studies [3]. Recently, it has been shown that the *DSM-IV-TR* definition of PE has a low positive predictive value when the required criterium "short ejaculation latency time" is not applied [3]. This low positive predictive value is therefore related to the absence in the *DSM* definition of a quantified cutoff point of the intravaginal ejaculation latency time (IELT), which is the time between vaginal intromission and intravaginal ejaculation.

* Department of Psychiatry and Neurosexology, HagaHospital Leyenburg, Leyweg 275, 2545 CH The Hague, The Netherlands.
E-mail address: md@waldinger.demon.nl

This means that erroneously men with long IELT values of, for example 10 to 20 minutes, may be diagnosed as having PE in case they perceive themselves as suffering from PE [4]. The existence of men who complain of PE, while at the same time having normal and even long durations of the IELT, became evident in the study of Patrick and colleagues [5], in which experienced clinicians diagnosed PE according to the *DSM-IV-TR* criteria of PE thereby ignoring the required criterium "short ejaculation latency time". Obviously, due to the low positive predictive value of the *DSM-IV-TR* definition, there is a high chance of false-positive diagnoses of PE, which hampers clinical practice and epidemiologic and drug treatment research [3].

Proposal for new definition of premature ejaculation

Recently, a new proposal for the pending *DSM-V* and ICD-11 definition of PE has been put forward [6,7]. According to this proposal, PE should be classified according to a "syndromal" approach, incorporating well-controlled clinical and epidemiologic stopwatch studies [6]. PE as a clinical entity or a syndrome has for the first time been described by Schapiro in 1943 [8]. He distinguished Types A and B that were later termed "lifelong" and "acquired" PE by Godpodinoff [9]. Both types have been mentioned but not further operationalized in the *DSM-IV-TR* definition of PE.

Recently, the existence of two other PE syndromes have been proposed: "natural variable PE" [3] and "premature-like ejaculatory dysfunction" [7]. In natural variable PE, men only occasionally suffer from early ejaculations. This should be regarded as part of the normal variability of ejaculatory performance and not a symptom of pathology. As such, natural variable PE is not a real syndrome [3]. In premature-like ejaculatory dysfunction men experience and/or utter complaints of PE, while having objectively normal and even long durations of the IELT of 5 to 20 minutes [6]. In the new proposal, the four PE syndromes are defined according to the following symptomatology.

Lifelong premature ejaculation

Lifelong PE is a syndrome characterized by the cluster of the following core symptoms:

1) ejaculation occurs too early at nearly every intercourse,

2) with (nearly) every woman,
3) from about the first sexual encounters onward,
4) in the majority of cases (80%) within 30 to 60 seconds, or between 1 and 2 minute (20%) and
5) remains rapid during life (70%) or can even aggravate during aging (30%)
6) the ability to control ejaculation (ie, to withhold ejaculation at the moment of imminent ejaculation) may be diminished or lacking, but is not obligatory for the diagnosis.

Some men already get an ejaculation during foreplay, before penetration, or soon as their penis touches the vagina (ejaculatio ante portas). It should be noted that there are no hard indications that lifelong premature ejaculation can be cured, either by drug treatment or psychotherapy. In other words, lifelong PE is a chronic ejaculatory dysfunction.

Acquired premature ejaculation

The complaints of acquired premature ejaculation differ in relation to the underlying somatic or psychologic problem.

1) early ejaculation occurs at some point in a man's life,
2) the man has usually had normal ejaculation experiences before the start of complaints
3) there is either a sudden or gradual onset
4) the dysfunction may be due to:
   • urologic dysfunctions, for example, erectile dysfunction or prostatitis [10].
   • thyroid dysfunction [11].
   • psychologic or relationship problems [12,13].
5) the ability to control ejaculation (ie, to withhold ejaculation at the moment of imminent ejaculation) may be diminished or lacking, but is not obligatory for the diagnosis.

In contrast to lifelong PE the acquired form of PE can be cured by treatment of the underlying cause.

Natural variable premature ejaculation

In natural variable PE men only coincidentally and situationally experience early ejaculations. This type of PE should not be regarded as a symptom or manifestation of true pathology but of normal variation in sexual performance [3]. The syndrome is characterized by the following symptoms

1) early ejaculations are inconsistently and occur irregularly

2) the ability to control ejaculation, that is, to withhold ejaculation at the moment of imminent ejaculation may be diminished or lacking, but is not obligatory for the diagnosis
3) experiences of diminished control of ejaculation go along with either a short or normal ejaculation time, that is, an ejaculation of less or more than 1.5 minutes.

Premature-like ejaculatory dysfunction

Men with premature-like ejaculatory dysfunction experience or complain of PE while the ejaculation time is in the normal range, that is, around 3 to 6 minutes, and may even be of very long duration, that is, between 5 and 25 minutes [7]. This type of PE should not be regarded as a symptom or manifestation of true medical pathology. Psychologic and/or relationship problems may underlie the complaints [7]. The syndrome is characterized by the following symptoms.

1) Subjective perception of consistent or inconsistent rapid ejaculation during intercourse.
2) Preoccupation with an imagined early ejaculation or lack of control of ejaculation.
3) The actual intravaginal ejaculation latency time is in the normal range or may even be of longer duration (ie, an ejaculation that occurs between 5 and 25 minutes).
4) Ability to control ejaculation (ie, to withhold ejaculation at the moment of imminent ejaculation) may be diminished or lacking, but is not obligatory for the diagnosis.
5) The preoccupation is not better accounted for by another mental disorder.

Continuum of neurobiology and psychology

The distinction of the four PE syndromes shows a continuum of PE along a line from mainly neurobiologically to mainly psychologically determined forms (Fig. 1). For example, from both human and animal research it may be derived that lifelong PE is presumably highly neurobiologically and perhaps also genetically determined. However, as yet, one cannot rule out that certain forms of lifelong PE are psychologically determined. As is the case in major depression, a biologic marker of lifelong PE has not yet been found. However, the positive response on daily selective serotonin reuptake inhibitor (SSRI) drug treatment indicates that both major depression and PE are neurobiologically, that is, serotonergically, mediated, and may have a neurobiologic etiology. Acquired PE may be medically (prostatitis, thyroid dysfunction) or psychologically (relationship problems) determined. The sporadic early ejaculations in natural variable PE have been postulated to represent the normal variation of ejaculatory performance in men, and are presumably not an expression of underlying pathology. The complaints of early ejaculations in men with premature-like ejaculatory dysfunction that occurs at normal and even long durations of the IELT, have been postulated to be due to mainly psychologic factors [7].

Prevalences

Epidemiologic research has repeatedly shown a prevalence of PE of 20% to 30% [14]. Erroneously, by not distinguishing PE as a complaint and as a syndrome, it has been concluded that

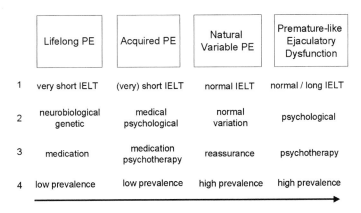

Fig. 1. Continuum of the four PE syndromes; Lifelong PE is more neurobiologically determined while Premature-like Ejaculatory Dysfunction is more psychologically determined. 1. Duration IELT, 2. Etiology, 3. Treatment, 4. Prevalence.

the "disorder" PE has a high prevalence. However, these studies have only shown that the "complaint" of PE in the general male population has a high prevalence of 20% to 30%. Studies into the prevalence of lifelong PE and acquired PE have never been conducted. However, it is of note that the prevalence of lifelong PE, defined in terms of lifelong consistent IELTs of <1 to 1.5 minutes along feelings of diminished control, has been suggested to be rather low (2%–5%). Further epidemiologic research to confirm this hypothesis is warranted. It is suggested that in case the prevalence of lifelong PE appears to be rather low, it should be argued that only a small percentage of men with "complaints" of PE suffer from PE that is mainly neurobiologically and genetically determined. This is of major importance for genetic studies on PE. New epidemiologic research may also contribute to confirm the hypothesis that the high percentage of "complaints" of PE (20%–30%) is due to the large number of males in the general population that either have natural variable PE or premature-like ejaculatory dysfunction.

Pathophysiology

The distinction of the four PE syndromes illustrates that there is not one particular pathophysiology of PE, but that there a different pathophysiologies dependent on the type of PE. For example, the serotonin hypothesis of PE, that is, a disturbance of serotonin neurotransmission and/or serotonin receptor functioning [15], pertains only to lifelong PE and partly to acquired PE. In other words, the serotonin hypothesis explains probably only a small percentage (2%–5%) of complaints of PE in the general population. The pathophysiology of acquired PE is related to disturbances of peripheral neuronal functioning, whereas the pathophysiology of premature-like ejaculatory dysfunction is speculated to be related to cognitive and unconscious mental processes.

Diagnosis of premature ejaculation syndromes

Lifelong, acquired, natural variable PE, and premature-like ejaculatory dysfunction are recognizable by taking a brief medical and sexual history with special attention to the duration of the ejaculation time, the frequency of occurrences, and the course since the first sexual encounters. In daily clinical practice, diagnosis of the four PE syndromes is not difficult, and therefore,

evaluation with questionnaires or the use of a stopwatch is not required [4]. However, for drug treatment trials and epidemiologic research, stopwatch assessment and questionnaires of satisfaction and quality of (sexual) life are a prerequisite.

Treatment

The distinction of the four PE syndromes has consequences for treatment. Lifelong PE should be treated with drugs that strongly delay ejaculation. It is a matter of debate whether additional counseling is always needed for these men. A lot of these men will manage without additional counseling. However, clinicians should take time to talk with these men, to inform them about the current knowledge of lifelong PE, and to regularly check their well-being, particularly when using SSRIs on a daily basis.

Acquired PE needs to be treated with either drugs to treat underlying medical pathology, or psychotherapy to treat underlying psychologic pathology, or both with or without additional other drug treatment options like SSRIs or topical anesthetics.

Men with natural variable PE usually cope well with their coincidental early ejaculations, but in case of seeking treatment, it is advised to inform them that the occurrence of sporadic early ejaculation is part of normal ejaculatory performance. Presumably, psychoeducation will probably be sufficient for these men to regain confidence. Due to the incidental nature of early ejaculations, one should not a priori treat these men with ejaculation delaying drugs with potential side effects. Men with premature-like ejaculatory dysfunction should better not be treated with ejaculation delaying drugs but with counselling, psychoeducation, psychotherapy, or couple therapy. One should inform these men that the actual ejaculation time is in the normal range, but that psychologic or relationship factors are likely to contribute to their complaint.

Evidence-based drug treatment

Apart from randomized, double-blind controlled study designs, drug treatment studies of PE should include a baseline and a drug treatment period in which the IELT is measured prospectively at each coitus using a stopwatch handled by the female partner. The IELT is expressed in seconds or minutes, and in case an ejaculation occurs outside the vagina (ejaculatio ante portas), the IELT is by definition equal to zero. As the IELT distribution is positively skewed, IELT values should be logarithmically transformed and results should be reported as geometric mean IELT or median IELT [4]. In addition, ejaculation delay should be expressed as percentage or fold increase from baseline with 95% confidence intervals (CIs) [4]. Adverse effects should be assessed with a validated questionnaire. Moreover, side effects of on-demand treatment should be assessed at the day of drug intake and the next day [4].

Daily selective serotonin reuptake inhibitor treatment

During the last decade, daily use of SSRIs, on-demand use of the tricyclic antidepressant clomipramine, and topical use of anesthetics has become most popular to treat PE [16]. Although none of these treatment options have been approved by the Food and Drug Administration, their use has been recognized and is supported by evidence-based studies [16]. The serotonergic antidepressants modify the course of PE by modulating the central serotonergic system, and the anesthetics suppress the sensitivity of the glans penis. A number of studies further reported efficacy of the on-demand use of phosphodiesterase type 5 (PDE-5) inhibitors, but their role in the treatment of PE without erectile dysfunction is disputable. Recently, two studies reported ejaculation-delaying effects of the on-demand use of tramadol. Actually, one can distinguish two major strategies to treat PE by medication: daily and on-demand treatment.

Daily treatment with clomipramine

In 1973, Eaton [17] published the first publication on the efficacy of clomipramine, the most serotonergic tricyclic antidepressant, to treat premature ejaculation. Particularly, in the 1970 to 1980s, but also in the 1990s, various studies demonstrated its efficacy in delaying ejaculation in daily rather low dosages of 10 to 30 mg [18].

Daily treatment with selective serotonin reuptake inhibitors

The introduction of the SSRIs in psychiatry, however, would lead to a revolutionary change in the understanding of and treatment of PE. After the first publication in 1994 [19] on the efficacy of daily treatment with paroxetine hemihydrate, various studies confirmed its strong ejaculation-delaying effects at dosages of 20 to 40 mg [16,20].

Moreover, it appeared that nearly all SSRIs, except fluvoxamine, exerted a clinically relevant ejaculation-delaying effect [16]. Currently, daily treatment with SSRIs or combined daily treatment with on-demand use of some SSRIs has become the first choice of treatment. In 2004, Waldinger and colleagues [16] published a systematic review and meta-analysis of all drug treatment studies that have been published between 1943 and 2003. Of all 79 studies, a meta-analysis was only feasible on 35 clomipramine and SSRI daily treatment studies that were conducted between 1973 and 2003 [16]. The outcome data of the few SSRI treatment studies published between 2003 and 2007 hardly distort the findings of the systematic review and meta-analysis, and therefore its conclusions are still valid today. The meta-analysis revealed a placebo effect of a geometric mean 1.4-fold IELT increase (95% CI: 1.2–1.7). Furthermore, it was demonstrated that the rank order of efficacy (geometric mean fold-increase of IELT) was (a) paroxetine (8.8; 95% CI: 5.9–13.2), (b) clomipramine (4.6; 3.0–7.4), (c) sertraline (4.1; 2.6–7.0), and (d) fluoxetine (3.9; 3.0–5.4). Thus, in general, daily SSRI treatment studies generate a 2.6-fold to 13.2-fold geometric mean IELT increase, dependent on the type of SSRI. Daily treatment can be performed with paroxetine 20 to 40 mg, clomipramine 10 to 50 mg, sertraline 50 to 100 mg, fluoxetine 20 to 40 mg, citalopram 20 to 40 mg, and 10 to 20 mg escitalopram [4]. Ejaculation delay usually starts a few days after drug intake, but becomes more manifest after 1 to 2 weeks. The delay continues to exist for years, but sometimes may diminish after 6 to 12 months. The cause of this tachyphylaxis of SSRIs has not yet been clarified [4].

Daily SSRI treatment is most often, but not always, effective in delaying ejaculation. The reason that SSRIs sometimes fail to delay ejaculation has not yet been clarified. Patients should be informed about the short-term and long-term side effects of SSRIs. On the short-term fatigue, yawning, mild nausea, loose stools, or perspiration may occur. These side effects are usually mild, start in the first 1 to 2 weeks of treatment, and most often gradually disappear within 2 to 3 weeks. Although a head-to-head comparative study has not yet been performed, drug treatment studies seem to indicate that in contrast to the side effects in depressed patients, diminished libido and erectile dysfunction are less frequently and also to a lesser extent reported by healthy nondepressed men with lifelong PE.

Waldinger has hypothesized that this may be related to the involvement of an increased oxytocin release in men with lifelong PE [4,21]. Obviously, further controlled research to confirm and elucidate this phenomenon is needed.

A rather rare side effects of SSRIs is the risk of bleeding. Clinicians should caution patients about combining SSRIs with aspirin or nonsteroidal anti-inflammatory drugs, as this may further increase the risk of bleeding. A very rare side effect is priapism [22]. Although very rare, it is advised to inform all patients using SSRIs about the risk of priapism and its need for immediate medical treatment. One should not prescribe these drugs to young men < 18 years, and to men known with depressive disorder, particularly when associated with suicidal thoughts. In those cases, referral to a psychiatrist is indicated. On the long term, weight gain might occur with an associated risk for diabetes mellitus type II.

Patients should be advised not to stop taking the medication acutely to prevent the occurrence of an SSRI discontinuation syndrome, which is characterized by symptoms like tremor, shock-like sensations when turning the head, nausea, and dizziness [23].

Generic versus brand-name selective serotonin reuptake inhibitors

A special note should be made to the use of generic SSRIs. The most relevant studies on SSRI treatment of PE have been conducted in the early and mid-1990s using the brand name SSRIs, simply because at that time generic SSRIs where not yet on the market. In contrast, today, generic SSRIs are frequently prescribed. In a review of the few publications comparing the bioequivalence and efficacy of brand name and generic psychoactive drugs, it was shown that there are differences between the generic drugs and the brand name drugs that had not been noted in the original bioequivalence studies [24]. This issue has consequences for drug treatment of PE [4].

Paroxetine hemihydrate

Daily treatment studies of PE with paroxetine, has been investigated with paroxetine hydrochloride hemihydrate and not with the generic drug paroxetine hemihydrate and/or paroxetine mesylate. The ejaculation delaying efficacy and relative mild side effect profile of paroxetine hemihydrate has been repeatedly demonstrated in well-controlled studies [16]. Based on these studies, there are no real objective contraindications to use the generic paroxetine hemihydrate to treat PE [4].

Paroxetine mesylate

Drug treatment studies on PE have not been performed with paroxetine *mesylate*. There are some indications that particularly the side-effect profile of the generic paroxetine mesylate is different from paroxetine hemihydrate [24,25]. Therefore, and due to the lack of placebo-controlled comparative studies investigating the efficacy and side effect profile of both paroxetine hemihydrate and paroxetine mesylate in the treatment of PE, it is advised to prescribe only paroxetine hydrochloride hemihydrate to men with lifelong PE and not paroxetine mesylate [4].

Daily treatment with α_1 adrenoceptor antagonists

Ejaculation is peripherally controlled by the sympathetic nervous system. Blocking the sympathetic system by α_1 adrenoceptor antagonists (α_1-blockers) may theoretically delay ejaculation. Terazosin and alfuzosin are two selective α_1-blockers whose ejaculation delaying effects have been investigated in men with PE. In a placebo-controlled study in 91 men with PE both terazosin 5 mg/d and alfuzosin 6 mg/d proved effective in approximately 50% of the cases [26]. In another placebo-controlled study in 90 men with PE and urinary tract symptoms without chronic prostatitis and benign prostatic hyperplasia, daily use of terazosin 5 to 10 mg showed a clinically significant improvement [27]. However, the methodology of both studies has been rather weak. Efficacy was measured by merely qualitative measures like satisfaction and subjective feelings of improvement. Prolongation of the IELT was not assessed by a stopwatch. Although α_1-blockers may affect ejaculatory performance, they do not always delay ejaculation [28]. Despite the aforementioned limitations in methodology and the rather low rate of clinically relevant ejaculation delaying effects, α_1-blockers, and particularly terazosin 5 to 10 mg, may be a good alternative to treat men with PE who also have urinary tract dysfunction. However, further well-designed studies are pivotal to evaluate the place of α_1-blockers in the armentarium of drugs in the treatment of PE.

On-demand drug treatment

Despite any study investigating patient preferences, it has recently become rather fashionable to state that on-demand treatment of PE would be more favorable than daily treatment. This is rather peculiar, as contrary to daily treatment, on-demand strategies may quite negatively interfere with the spontaneity of having sex, particularly as one usually decides to have sex at the spur of the moment. This is particularly so in young adults with children when the couple often take the opportunity to have sex at a sudden moment when the chance to be disturbed is very low. Also, the argument that daily treatment is not preferable because one has to wait 1 to 2 weeks before ejaculation delay occurs is not based on evidence. Most men with lifelong PE will report that after many years of having had PE, it is no problem to wait another 1 to 2 weeks before medication becomes effective. Moreover, a clear advantage of daily treatment is that ejaculation is delayed at every moment of the day that one wished to have intercourse. Recently, Waldinger and colleagues [29] conducted the first study investigating the preferences of men with lifelong PE for the currently existing PE treatment options. In this study in 88 men with lifelong PE, it was shown that 81% preferred *daily* drug treatment mainly because patients feared that on-demand treatment would negatively interfere with the spontaneity of having sex [29].

Nevertheless, on-demand drug treatment contributes to the armamentarium of drug treatment of PE. In recent years, on-demand treatment studies have been conducted with topical anesthetics, clomipramine, SSRIs, dapoxetine, tramadol, and PDE-5 inhibitors. Due to differences in methodology and design, a meta-analysis comparing the efficacy of these drugs has not yet been feasible.

On-demand treatment with topical anesthetics

The use of topical local anesthetics such as lidocaine and/or prilocaine in the form of a cream, gel, or spray is the oldest drug treatment strategy and is still practiced today [30]. The topical anesthetics delay ejaculation by reducing the sensitivity of the glans penis. However, only a few studies have been conducted to show their efficacy. The application is rather simple, but still may lead to side effects like complete anesthesia of the penis, which may lead to erectile difficulties. Patients should be informed that its use may also lead to vaginal numbness. This may be prevented by the use of a condom.

On-demand treatment with clomipramine

On-demand use of 20 to 40 mg clomipramine can effectively delay ejaculation after 3 to 5 hours [31,32]. However, it might also give rise to nausea at the day of intercourse and the next day.

On-demand treatment with selective serotonin reuptake inhibitors

In the systematic review of 2003 only eight studies on on-demand treatment with SSRIs and clomipramine were reported [16]. These eight on-demand studies greatly differed in methodology. A meta-analysis on the published on-demand SSRI studies could not be performed as the studies were unbalanced for the antidepressants used, baseline IELT values, design (double-blind versus open) and assessment techniques (questionnaire versus stopwatch) [16]. Despite the absence of a meta-analysis on on-demand SSRI treatment studies, there are indications that on-demand use of SSRIs, like 20 mg paroxetine, do not strongly delay ejaculation after 3 to 5 hours of intake [33].

On-demand treatment with dapoxetine

Recently, a multicenter study with dapoxetine, an SSRI with a short half-life, has shown that despite minimal ejaculation delay, objectivated with stopwatch assessment, feelings of satisfaction and control were improved [34]. However, the study did not use the appropriate statistics to measure ejaculation delay and did not use the appropriate method to investigate the dapoxetine-induced side effects [35]. In 2005, the Food and Drug Administration did not approve dapoxetine for the treatment of PE.

On-demand treatment with tramadol

Recently, two studies in men with PE have shown the ejaculation delaying effects of on-demand use of 50 mg tramadol [36]. Tramadol is registered as a centrally acting analgesic agent combining µ-opioid receptor activation and reuptake inhibition of serotonin and noradrenaline. The most common adverse of tramadol were nausea (15.6%), vomiting (6.2%), and dizziness (6.2%), but they were reported to be mild. However, it should be noted that despite that tramadol has a weak µ-opioid agonistic effect, long-term follow-up studies are also needed to investigate the risk of opioid addiction.

On-demand treatment with phosphodiesterase type 5 inhibitors

In recent years, a number of authors have suggested that on-demand use of PDE-5 inhibitors is effective to treat PE. However, most of these studies lack a good methodology, which makes the results difficult to interpret. Recently, McMahon and colleagues [37] published a well-designed systematic review of all publications on the use of PDE-5 inhibitors against PE that have been published between 2001 until 2006. The review analyzed 14 studies, which reported the use of sildenafil, vardenafil, and tadalafil [37]. The majority of these studies did not fulfil the current criteria of evidence-based medicine. Of the 14 studies, only one fulfilled these criteria. It was concluded that there is no convincing evidence of any direct effect of PDE-5 inhibitors on the central or peripheral control of ejaculation, or for any role in the treatment of PE, except for men with PE and comorbid erectile dysfunction [37].

On-demand treatment with intracavernous vasoactive drug injection

A special comment should be made regarding intracavernous self-injection treatment. This strategy to treat premature ejaculation is advocated by a few institutions. However, it should be noted that there is not any evidence-based support for the efficacy of this strategy. Actually, there has only been one single study investigating this treatment method [38]. In this open study of eight men, patients injected vasoactive drugs into the corpus cavernosum. From the eight men, three stated that they were cured and stopped the treatment, whereas the other five men continued using the medication after 14 months. However, the methodology of this study was very weak. There were no baseline assessments of the IELT, and a prolongation of the IELT was not measured with a stopwatch. Moreover, success of treatment was defined by prolongation of erectile function after ejaculation and not by the measure of a delayed ejaculation. As long as there are no well-controlled studies showing the efficacy of injection treatment to delay ejaculation time, one should not treat PE with intracavernosal injection of vasoactive drugs.

Summary

The *DSM-IV-TR* definition has a high risk for false-positive diagnoses of PE. Recently, a new classification of four PE syndromes has been proposed for the pending *DSM-V*. According to this classification PE can no longer be defined in one overall descriptive definition, but should be defined according to the symptomatology of the underlying PE syndrome.

The high prevalence rate of 20% to 30% is more likely to reflect the percentage of men that has "complaints" of PE, rather than the percentage of men that suffer from the "disorder" lifelong PE and acquired PE. The percentage of men that are in need for drug treatment is probably much lower than the high percentage of men than have "complaints" of PE without suffering from PE syndromes. Similarly, it is likely that only a small percentage of PE is neurobiologically and/or genetically determined. It has been suggested that a much higher percentage of men only occasionally experience early ejaculations, representing the normal variation of ejaculatory performance. Similarly it has been suggested that presumably a high percentage of men complain of early ejaculation while having normal and even long durations of the IELT. Treatment of PE is dependent of its etiology. Drug treatment is particularly indicated for men with lifelong PE and acquired PE. This may be combined with counselling or behavioral therapy. Psychotherapy is particularly indicated for men with premature-like ejaculatory dysfunction or secondary PE due to psychologic problems. Psychoeducation should be provided to men with natural variable PE. Of the various drug treatment options, daily drug treatment with SSRIs, particularly paroxetine, on-demand use of clomipramine, and/or topical anesthetics has become most popular, and their efficacy has been based on evidence-based research.

References

[1] American Psychiatric Association. Diagnostic and statistical manual of mental disorders. 4th edition, Text Revision DSM-IV-TR. Washington, DC: American Psychiatric Association; 2000.
[2] World Health Organization. The ICD-10 classification of mental and behavioural disorders: diagnostic criteria for research. Geneva (IL): World Health Organization; 1993.
[3] Waldinger MD, Schweitzer DH. Changing paradigms from an historical *DSM-III* and *DSM-IV* view towards an evidence based definition of premature ejaculation. Part I: validity of *DSM-IV-TR*. J Sex Med 2006;3:682–92.
[4] Waldinger MD. Premature ejaculation: definition and drug treatment. Drugs 2007;67:547–68.
[5] Patrick DL, Althof SE, Pryor JL, et al. Premature ejaculation: an observational study of men and their partners. J Sex Med 2005;2:358–67.

[6] Waldinger MD, Schweitzer DH. Changing paradigms from an historical *DSM-III* and *DSM-IV* view towards an evidence based definition of premature ejaculation. Part II: proposals for *DSM-V* and ICD-11. J Sex Med 2006;3:693–705.

[7] Waldinger MD. The need for a revival of psychoanalytic investigations into premature ejaculation. Journal Men's Health & Gender 2006;3:390–6.

[8] Schapiro B. Premature ejaculation: a review of 1130 cases. J Urol 1943;50:374–9.

[9] Godpodinoff ML. Premature ejaculation: clinical subgroups and etiology. J Sex Marital Ther 1989; 15:130–4.

[10] Screponi E, Carosa E, Stasi SM, et al. Prevalence of chronic prostatitis in men with premature ejaculation. Urology 2001;58:198–202.

[11] Carani C, Isidori AM, Granata A, et al. Multicenter study on the prevalence of sexual symptoms in male hypo- and hyperthyroid patients. J Clin Endocrinol Metab, in press.

[12] Althof SE. Psychological treatment strategies for rapid ejaculation: rationale, practical aspects, and outcome. World J Urol 2005;23:89–92.

[13] Hartmann U, Schedlowski M, Kruger THC. Cognitive and partner-related factors in rapid ejaculation: differences between dysfunctional and functional men. World J Urol 2005;23:93–101.

[14] St. Lawrence JS, Madakasira S. Evaluation and treatment of premature ejaculation: a critical review. Int J Psychiatry Med 1992;22:77–97.

[15] Waldinger MD. The neurobiological approach to premature ejaculation. J Urol 2002;168:2359–67.

[16] Waldinger MD, Zwinderman AH, Schweitzer DH, et al. Relevance of methodological design for the interpretation of efficacy of drug treatment of premature ejaculation: a systematic review and meta-analysis. Int J Impot Res 2004;16:369–81.

[17] Eaton H. Clomipramine in the treatment of premature ejaculation. J Int Med Res 1973;1:432–4.

[18] Assalian P. Clomipramine in the treatment of premature ejaculation. J Sex Res 1988;24:213–5.

[19] Waldinger MD, Hengeveld MW, Zwinderman AH. Paroxetine treatment of premature ejaculation: a double-blind, randomized, placebo-controlled study. Am J Psychiatry 1994;151:1377–9.

[20] McMahon CG, Touma K. Treatment of premature ejaculation with paroxetine hydrochloride. Int J Impot Res 1999;11:241–5.

[21] de Jong TR, Veening JG, Olivier B, et al. Oxytocin involvement in SSRI-induced delayed ejaculation: a review of animal studies. J Sex Med 2007;4: 14–28.

[22] Rand EH. Priapism in a patient taking sertraline. J Clin Psychiatry 1998;59:538.

[23] Black K, Shea C, Dursun S, et al. Selective serotonin reuptake inhibitor discontinuation syndrome; proposed diagnostic criteria. J Psychiatry Neurosci 2000;25:255–61.

[24] Borgherini G. The Bioequivalence and therapeutic efficacy of generic versus brand-name psychoactive drugs. Clin Ther 2003;25:1578–92.

[25] Vergouwen AC, Bakker A. Adverse effects after switching to a different generic form of paroxetine: paroxetine mesylate instead of paroxetine HCL hemihydrate. Ned Tijdschr Geneeskd 2002;146:811–2 [in dutch].

[26] Cavallini G. Alpha-1 blockade pharmacotherapy in primitive psychogenic premature ejaculation resistant to psychotherapy. Eur Urol 1995;28:126–30.

[27] Basar MM, Yilmaz E, Ferhat M, et al. Terazosin in the treatment of premature ejaculation: a short-term follow-up. Int Urol Nephrol 2005;37:773–7.

[28] Buzelin JM, Fonteyne E, Kontturi MJ, et al. Comparison of tamsulosin with alfuzosin in the treatment of patients with lower urinary tract symptoms suggestive of bladder outlet obstruction (symptomatic benign prostatic hyperplasia). Br J Urol 1997;80: 597–605.

[29] Waldinger MD, Zwinderman AH, Olivier B, et al. Majority of men with lifelong premature ejaculation prefer daily drug treatment: an observational study in a consecutive group of Dutch men. J Sex Med 2007;4:1028–37.

[30] Berkovitch M, Keresteci AG, Koren G. Efficacy of prilocaine-lidocaine cream in the treatment of premature ejaculation. J Urol 1995;154:1360–1.

[31] Segraves RT, Saran A, Segraves K, et al. Clomipramine vs placebo in the treament of premature ejaculation: a pilot study. J Sex Marital Ther 1993;19: 198–200.

[32] Haensel SM, Rowland DL, Kallan KTHK, et al. Clomipramine and sexual function in men with premature ejaculation and controls. J Urol 1996;156: 1310–5.

[33] Waldinger MD, Zwinderman AH, Olivier B. On-demand treatment of premature ejaculation with clomipramine and paroxetine: a randomized, double-blind fixed-dose study with stopwatch assessment. Eur Urol 2004;46:510–6.

[34] Pryor JL, Althof SE, Steidle C, et al. Efficacy and tolerability of dapoxetine in treatment of premature ejaculation: an integrated analysis of two double-blind, randomised controlled trials. Lancet 2006; 368:929–37.

[35] Waldinger MD, Schweitzer DH, Olivier B. Dapoxetine treatment of premature ejaculation [letter]. Lancet 2006;368:1869–70.

[36] Safarinejad MR, Hosseini SY. Safety and efficacy of tramadol in the treatment of premature ejaculation. J Clin Psychopharmacol 2006;26:27–31.

[37] McMahon CG, McMahon CN, Liang JL, et al. Efficacy of type-5 phophodiesterase inhibitors in the drug treatment of premature ejaculation: a systematic review. BJU Int 2006;98:259–72.

[38] Fein RL. Intracavernous medication for treatment of premature ejaculation. Urology 1990;35:301–3.

ELSEVIER
SAUNDERS

Urol Clin N Am 34 (2007) 601–618

UROLOGIC
CLINICS
of North America

Penile Rehabilitation Following Radical Prostatectomy: Role of Early Intervention and Chronic Therapy

Craig D. Zippe, MD*, Geetu Pahlajani, MD

*Cleveland Clinic Foundation, Glickman Urological and Kidney Institute,
Prostate Center, Cleveland, OH 44195, USA*

The concept of early penile rehabilitation following radical prostatectomy (RP) started in the 1990s, with the evolution of several dynamic themes regarding prostate cancer diagnosis and management. First, with the maturation of the prostate-specific antigen (PSA) era, the detection of lower-volume cancers changed the surgical margin rate, and the rate of biochemical cures rose substantially to the 80% to 90% range. Most of our newly diagnosed tumors were histologic Gleason score 6/7 cancers and were pathologically organ confined. Recent cancer statistics for the year 2006 report that 91% of new prostate cancer cases are expected to be diagnosed at local or regional stages with 5-year cancer-specific survivals approaching 100% [1]. A second major theme of the 1990s was the substantial drop in patient age at diagnosis due to earlier screening with serum PSA testing and improved office-based ultrasound-guided biopsy techniques. The Seattle-Puget Sound Surveillance, Epidemiology and End Results (SEER) cancer registry from 1995 to 1999 reported that 33% of all incident prostate cancer cases were diagnosed in men under age 65 [2–4] and this figure will invariably be higher in the subsequent 5-year report.

This diagnostic shift toward earlier age and lower tumor volumes suggests that prostate cancer survivors will have longer life expectancies after diagnosis, regardless of treatment, and higher expectations on health-related quality-of-life issues (foremost, urinary continence and erectile function). Another theme of the 1990s was a reexamination of our potency rates following various treatments for erectile dysfunction (ED) after prostate cancer treatment. Younger prostate cancer patients now want information on short- and long-term potency rates following prostate cancer treatments and the efficacy of the various treatment options in treating their ED. The demands of the younger patient for higher potency rates pushed many of us into using earlier intervention strategies to improve our potency rates following RP. During the 1990s, with many experienced retropubic surgeons focusing rigorously on improving their nerve-sparing surgical technique, it became evident that the volume of surgeries (ie, doing 1000 or more cases) was not the answer to improving potency rates following RP. It was the realization, or concession, that technical improvements in nerve-sparing retropubic surgery could not be advanced to any great extent that motivated the prostate cancer community to consider the role of early penile rehabilitation.

Approaches to radical prostatectomy: potency rates

Retropubic approach

When analyzing the reported potency rates following radical retropubic prostatectomy (RRP), we find the results from bilateral nerve-sparing procedures vary widely. Erectile function following retropubic prostatectomy in the hands of experienced surgeons (> 1000 cases) at centers of excellence ranges from 40% to 86% [5–9]. However, most urologists rarely report or experience potency rates higher than 40%, with the range being from 9% to 40% [10–12]. Table 1 lists

---

* Corresponding author.

E-mail address: zippec@ccf.org (C.D. Zippe).

Table 1
Potency rates following bilateral nerve-sparing radical retropubic prostatectomy

Investigator	Mean age (y)	n	Mean follow-up (mo)	Partial erections	Vaginal potency w/wo adjuvant 5-phosphodiesterase inhibitors
Quinlan et al (1991) [6]	> 50	29	18	n/a	90%
	50–59	141	18	14%	82%
	60–69	112	18	21%	69%
	> 70	9	18	22%	22%
Leandri et al (1992) [12]	68	106	6/12	38%/15%	30%/56%
Jonler et al (1994) [10]	64	93	22.5	38%	9%
Geary et al (1995) [11]	64	69	18	16%	32%
Talcott et al (1997) [9]	65	37	12	89%	11%
Walsh et al (2000) [7]	57	64	2/18	n/a	73%/86%
Kundu et al (2004) [76]	> 50	125	18	n/a	93%
	50–59	675	18	n/a	85%
	60–69	794	18	n/a	71%
	> 70	176	18	n/a	52%

Abbreviation: n/a, not applicable.

the selected potency rates of various investigators from major American hospitals. Table 2 summarizes the author's (C.D. Zippe) personal experience with patients' potency rates from the period of 2003 to 2005 from a consecutive series of bilateral nerve-sparing retropubic prostatectomies; all patients were younger than 65 years old, with a minimum follow-up of 18 months. At 18 months, only 38% had natural spontaneous erections sufficient for vaginal intercourse, and the use of sildenafil citrate increased this percentage to 56%. Also, in 2002, Schover and colleagues [13],

Table 2
Potency rates following bilateral nerve-sparing retropubic prostatectomy: personal and Cleveland Clinic Foundation series

Follow-up	Vaginal potency	Adjuvant 5-phosphodiesterase inhibitors
Personal series[a]		
3 mo	0%	0%
6 mo	18%	28%
12 mo	33%	44%
18 mo	38%	56%
Cleveland Clinic Foundation series[b]		
48 mo (CCF)	18%	33%

[a] 100 consecutive surgeries; 2003–2005; preoperative International Index of Erectile Function-5 score > 20; age < 65 years.

[b] Published review by Schover et al [13] in 2002 of open radical prostatectomies performed by multiple Cleveland Clinic Foundation surgeons between 1992 and 1999. This review includes the author's (C.D. Zippe) series of prostatectomies.

who analyzed 1207 patients from the Cleveland Clinic with a mean follow-up of 4.3 years following surgery, reported a natural potency rate of 18%, which improved to 33% with oral 5-phosphodiesterase (PDE-5) inhibitors.

Although several prominent retropubic surgeons have set the gold standard for emulating potency rates with percentages in the high 60%- to 90%-range, these numbers are probably achieved only with a large volume of surgeries (> 3000 cases) and a large volume of younger patients (< 60 years old) [14]. Unfortunately, in the years ahead, it will be very difficult for an individual surgeon to accrue this volume of cases, with the competing influences of prostate brachytherapy and the more integrated external beam radiation techniques.

Perineal approach

In one of the earliest reports, Frazier and colleagues [15] from Duke University reported in 1991 on 51 patients who underwent radical perineal prostatectomy (RPP). In the radical perineal group who underwent bilateral nerve sparing, 77.3% were reported to be potent 1 year after surgery. This study from 1991 did not define potency as vaginal intercourse and lacked a validated questionnaire.

In 1988, Weldon and Tavel [16] first described the technique of nerve-sparing RPP. However, it was not until 1997 that Weldon and associates published potency rates in a subset of only 50 patients (mean age 67) who had excellent preoperative potency and underwent nerve-sparing procedures (22 bilateral, 28 unilateral). Weldon and Tavel [17] reported potency returning to 24% of patients by 6 months, 50% by 12 months, 64% by 18 months, and 70% by 24 months. Unilateral nerve sparing preserved potency in 68%. However, this study used physician-reported, rather than patient-reported, outcomes, and did not use a validated questionnaire.

In 2001, Ruiz-Deya and associates [18] reported the outcome of 250 consecutive patients who underwent outpatient RPP. Bilateral or unilateral nerve-sparing surgery was performed in only 54 of the 250 patients. Follow-up results at 18 months revealed that 56% of these patients had unassisted potency and satisfactory sexual function, although eight were not satisfied with the quality of erection and sought erectaids.

In 2003, Harris [19] reported outcome data on 508 RPPs performed by a single surgeon over the past 8.5 years. Unfortunately, until recently, the technique of performing bilateral nerve sparing in the perineal approach was not well understood. In Harris' series, only 12 bilateral nerve- sparing procedures had been performed since July 2001, with 83% recovering spontaneous erections (no reports of vaginal potency) within 6 months. In the unilateral nerve-sparing group, 74% reported spontaneous erections in a follow-up period ranging from 2 months to 2 years. The limitations of this study were the short follow-up period in the bilateral nerve-sparing group; the lack of standardized questionnaires; and that the definition of potency was not defined as vaginal intercourse.

Table 3 summarizes most of the literature reports on erectile function following RPP [20]. Reports are few, with no current, contemporary series in younger patients, where bilateral nerve-sparing procedures are principally performed.

Laparoscopic approach

Laparoscopic radical prostatectomy (LRP) emerged as a minimally invasive surgical technique in 2000, as an alternative to open retropubic prostatectomy [21–23]. A major impetus for the development of minimally invasive techniques for prostate cancer was to minimize patient morbidity, length of stay, and postoperative pain. Initially, because of the lengthy learning curve, the development of nerve-sparing techniques was not a priority, and the percentage of patients receiving bilateral nerve-sparing procedures was less than expected.

In 2000, Guillonneau and Vallancien [24] were the first to report potency outcomes following LRP. Of the 120 laparoscopic procedures performed, only 20 were bilateral nerve sparing. Of these 20, 45% reported spontaneous erections, including 1 with rigidity sufficient for sexual intercourse 12 months following surgery. In a recent updated study with 550 LRPs, Guillonneau and colleagues [25] report that only 47 patients underwent bilateral nerve-sparing procedures. Of these 47, 66% of patients experienced intercourse with or without adjuvant sildenafil, and 85% recovered spontaneous erections. The period of time for the recovery of vaginal intercourse ranged from 3 weeks to 4 months. These figures at 3 weeks to 4 months are just too good to go unconfirmed, and suggest that the laparoscopic approach may significantly shorten the period of neurapraxia. Table 4 reviews potency rates following bilateral nerve-sparing LRP, with reports ranging from 14% to 81% [25–31].

In 2003, Anastasiadis and associates [26] prospectively evaluated 300 patients who underwent RP (70 retropubic, 230 laparoscopic). At the 1-year follow-up, this group reported an overall potency rate of 30% by way of the retropubic approach and 41% by way of the laparoscopic approach ($P > .05$). With preservation of one neurovascular bundle, the potency rates were 27% (retropubic) and 46% (laparoscopic). After bilateral nerve-sparing procedures, the potency rate increased to 44% (retropubic) and 53%

Table 3
Potency rates following bilateral nerve-sparing perineal radical prostatectomy

Investigator	Mean age (y)	n	Mean follow-up (mo)	Partial erections	Vaginal potency w/wo adjuvant PDE-5 inhibitors
Frazier et al (1992) [15]	65.0	22	12	n/a	78%
Lerner et al (1994) [20]	63.0	27	23	30%	22%
Weldon et al (1997) [17]	67.0	22	12/24	n/a	50%/70%
Ruiz-Deya et al (2001) [18]	62.9	54	18	n/a	41%
Harris (2003) [19]	65.8	12	6	83%	25%

Abbreviation: n/a, not applicable.

(laparoscopic) $(P > .05)$. For patients younger than 60 with bilateral neurovascular bundle preservation, the potency rates were 72% (retropubic) and 81% (laparoscopic) 1 year after surgery $(P > .05)$ [26].

In 2003, Roumeguere and colleagues [27] reported no significant difference in potency rates following RRP and LRP. They followed 77 patients after RRP and 85 patients after LRP prospectively at 1, 3, 6, and 12 months. At the 1-year follow-up, 54.5% from the bilateral nerve-sparing retropubic group had erections sufficient for vaginal potency versus 65.3% from the bilateral nerve-sparing laparoscopic group. In 2005, Rozet and associates [28] reported potency rates following extraperitoneal LRP. Of the 599 extraperitoneal surgeries, 23.2% underwent bilateral nerve sparing. With a mean follow-up of 6 months in 89 bilateral nerve-sparing patients, the rate of partial erections and vaginal potency was 64% and 43% respectively.

In 2006, Curto and colleagues [31] described their nerve-sparing technique of using an intrafascial approach during laparoscopic nerve sparing. This approach was performed in 425 patients, with reported postoperative potency rates of 30% at 3 months, 43% at 6 months, and 58.5% at 12 months. Erections not sufficient for sexual intercourse were observed in 31% at 3 months, 44.5% at 6 months, and 35% at 1 year.

Table 4 lists the reported potency rates following LRP. The conclusion from the laparoscopic literature is that the potency rates are equivalent to, if not better than, those reported from open retropubic series [26,27,32]. Although this procedure is minimally invasive, it is still apparent that the laparoscopic nerve-sparing technique causes enough neurovascular injury and damage to produce the routine neuropraxia that we commonly see.

Robotic-assisted laparoscopic approach

Dr. Menon and associates [33] pioneered and popularized the da Vinci robot (Intuitive, Inc., Sunnyvale, CA), demonstrating that this technology could overcome the counterintuitive pitfalls of standard laparoscopic surgery. Robotic assistance provides three-dimensional (3D) visualization, 10- to 15-fold magnification, wristed instrumentation, intuitive finger-controlled movements, and a comfortable seated position for the surgeon, all of which makes for an advanced ergonomic operation. With the 3D magnification and nonexistent blood loss, it has never been easier to identify and fine-tune the neurovascular dissection (Fig. 1).

Early potency rates from robotic-assisted laparoscopic prostatectomy (RALP) are impressive (Table 5) [34–42]. In 2003, Bentas and colleagues [34] described their early outcomes at 1 year with RALP. Of 37 potent patients before surgery, 22% had regained sexual activity, all requiring adjuvant medical therapy. In the same year (2003), Menon and associates [35], from the Vattikuti Institute, reported their interim results with RALP in 200 patients. Patients were followed at baseline and at 1, 3, 6, 12, and 18 months after surgery with validated questionnaires referred to as Expanded Prostate Cancer Index Composite. They reported that at 6 months, 82% of the men younger than 60, and 75% of men older than 60, had return of partial erections and 64% and 38%, respectively, had erection sufficient for vaginal intercourse. In the same year, this group compared their outcomes using the Vattikuti Institute Prostatectomy (VIP) technique (RALP) and RRP in 300 patients (100 RRP, 200 VIP). It was reported that after VIP, patients had return of erections earlier than after RRP (180 versus 440 days, $P < .5$) and earlier median return to

Table 4
Potency rates following bilateral nerve-sparing laparoscopic radical prostatectomy

Investigator	Mean age (y)	n	Mean follow-up (mo)	Partial erections	Vaginal potency rate w/wo adjuvant PDE-5 inhibitors
Guillonneau (2002) [25]	<70.0	47	4	85%	66%
Hara (2002) [30]	<70.0	7	3	71%	14%
Roumegure (2003) [27]	62.5	26	12	n/a	65%
Anastasiadis (2003) [26]	<60.0	77	12	n/a	81%
Rozet (2005) [28]	62.0	89	6	64%	43%
Rassweiler (2006) [29]	<55.0	n/a	12	n/a	78%
Curto (2006) [31]	62.0	137	12	35%	59%

Abbreviation: n/a, not applicable.

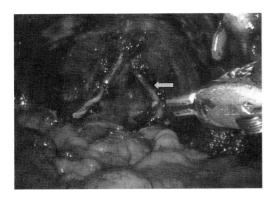

Fig. 1. Intraoperative photograph during robotic-assisted nerve-sparing RP. Three-dimensional and 10–15 times magnification allows unparalleled exposure of the neurovascular bundle. Arrow marks the right neurovascular bundle. (*Courtesy of* J. Kaouk, MD, Cleveland, OH.)

intercourse (340 versus 700 days, $P < .05$) [36]. This early return of sexual function was attributed to better visualization and a better anatomic dissection, which resulted from the 3D vision and reduced blood loss [43].

In 2005, Kaul and colleagues [44], from the Vattikuti Institute, described the feasibility and efficacy of preserving the prostatic fascia (veil of Aphrodite) during RALP. Anatomically, this fascia is composed of numerous smaller neurovascular components that theoretically can influence the return of potency postoperatively. Kaul and colleagues reported potency rates in patients who had undergone conventional bilateral nerve-sparing RALP versus those who had undergone the more skeletonized procedure with preservation of the prostatic fascia. At 12 months, 74% of the conventional nerve-sparing RALP and 97% of the "veil technique" achieved erections strong enough for intercourse. Seventeen percent of the conventional RALP and 51% of the "veil" patients achieved

normal erections (International Index of Erectile Function [IIEF] > 21) without medication [37].

In 2006, Kaul and associates [38] updated their results, using the "veil technique" of prostatic fascia sparing at 1 year in 154 patients. In this series, 102 men with normal sexual function before surgery (IIEF-5 > 21) were included in the analysis. At 1 year, 96% of the men reported having vaginal intercourse and 71% recovered normal erectile function. The mean IIEF-5 (Sexual Health Inventory for Men [SHIM]) scores before and after surgeries were reported as 24.3 and 20.6, respectively, with a median IIEF-5 score of 22 postsurgery.

In 2005, Chien and associates [39], from the University of Chicago, reported potency rates following RALP series using modified, clipless, antegrade nerve preservation. Fifty-six patients were prospectively followed after nerve-sparing procedures. The overall return to baseline sexual function was 47%, 54%, 66%, and 69% at 1, 3, 6, and 12 months postoperatively. No statistically significant difference was found between the unilateral or bilateral nerve-sparing groups. Also in 2005, Ahlering and colleagues [40] reported on short-term potency outcomes with a cautery-free technique to preserve the neurovascular bundles during RALP in 23 patients. At 3 months, 43% of the patients in the cautery-free group had erections sufficient for vaginal penetration versus 9% in the bipolar cautery group. This interval is very short for reporting potency outcomes, so long-term follow-up is necessary.

In 2006, Joseph and associates [41] evaluated their experience with 325 patients who had undergone da Vinci robot–assisted extraperitoneal LRP. Erectile function was assessed using the IIEF-5 (SHIM) validated questionnaire in 150 patients. All patients used oral PDE-5 inhibitors for at least 1 month postoperatively. Looking specifically at the bilateral nerve-sparing group, at

Table 5
Potency rates following bilateral nerve-sparing robotic-assisted radical prostatectomy

Investigator	Mean age (y)	n	Mean follow-up (mo)	Partial erections	Vaginal potency rate w/wo adjuvant PDE-5 inhibitors
Menon (2005) [37]	57.4	58	12	17/51%[a]	74%/97%[a]
Ahlering (2005) [40]	<66.0	23	3	n/a	43%
Tewari (2005) [42]	60.0	n/a	6	n/a	78%
Joseph (2006) [41]	60.0	129	6	n/a	80%
Kaul (2006) [38]	57.0	102	12	71%	96%[a]

Abbreviation: n/a, not applicable.
[a] Veil of Aphrodite nerve-sparing surgery (prostatic fascia sparing).

a mean follow-up of 6 months, 80% had an IIEF-5 score of greater than 16. These results and those from the Vattikuti Institute are landmark contributions to the literature on potency following RALP.

Table 5 lists the reported potency rates following RALP, which would appear to be generally much better than previously observed with open perineal or open RRP. The robotic approach appears to produce excellent potency rates, with a much shorter learning curve. RALP may truly be the first major surgical advancement in the last 10 to 15 years that can improve potency rates and be performed universally. Having stated that, even the most experienced practitioner using robotic hands still faces problems with at least 25% to 30% of ED cases. Consequently, even if 100% of patients with a mean age of 55 are having RALP in 2010, at least one quarter to one third are ultimately going to need some form of sexual rehabilitation for long-term potency.

Concept of early penile intervention

To understand the potential advantage of early intervention, the authors have summarized the literature on the reported efficacy of delayed treatments of ED following RP. Table 6 lists the efficacy and discontinuation rates of various pre-oral treatments for ED following RP [45]. What is apparent is that known treatments for ED do not have long-term durability, whether it is with intracavernosal injections (IC), vacuum constriction devices (VCDs), intraurethral alprostadil, or oral 5-phosphodiesterace inhibitors. Patients have very high noncompliance rates with these treatments at 1 year and little (if any) data exists on 5-year outcomes. Thus, with a younger male population with 10 to 15 years of sexual longevity, it is apparent that we do not have a durable and permanent solution for treating ED following RP.

Currently, the best treatment is to continue to perform and perfect a good bilateral nerve-sparing technique. The robotic nerve-sparing

technique with the aid of 3D vision may be the most significant advance in the last decade in improving the short- and long-term potency rates of younger patients. Nonetheless, even with the robotic technique, the sexual recovery of the patient is not perfect by any means. A significant period of neurapraxia is still observed in the first year and the 1-year IIEF-5 scores postsurgery are usually lower than the baseline IIEF-5 scores, indicating some degree of nerve damage from the procedure.

Pathophysiology of nerve injury: historical evidence

In 1982, Goldstein and colleagues [46] first reported the role of the cavernosal smooth muscle in the normal erection. Since then, several investigators have demonstrated that normal smooth muscle content and function are essential in initiation and maintenance of erection. The integrity and function of any smooth muscle depend on tissue oxygenation. This phenomenon has been well established in cardiac myocytes. Similarly, the cavernosal smooth muscle function has been reported to be dependent on tissue oxygenation. Historically, collagen accumulation (fibrosis) has been reported as the most probable cause of ED in patients who have penile arterial insufficiency [47–49]. However, the exact mechanism of collagen accumulation in patients who have penile hypoxia has not been established. In 1995, Moreland and colleagues [50] reported that penile hypoxia induces transforming growth factor-beta$_1$ (TGF-β_1) in the culture of cavernosal smooth muscle, which was implicated in the collagen deposition. They also reported that prostaglandin E 1 (PGE1) added to the cavernosal culture suppressed the TGF-β_1-induced collagen synthesis. Daley and colleagues [51,52] reported in 1996 that the production of PGE1 in the cavernosal muscle, which suppresses the TGF-β_1-induced collagen accumulation, was also oxygen dependent. These initial reports have shown that penile

Table 6
Efficacy and discontinuation rates of non-oral treatments for erectile dysfunction following radical prostatectomy (Cleveland Clinic Foundation data)

Options	n	Presurgery vaginal potency (%)	Postsurgery vaginal potency (%)	Vaginal potency with treatment (%)	Discontinuation rate after 1 y of use (%)
VCD	74	100	4.5	55	45
ICI	98	100	0	68	40
Intraurethral alprostadil	27	100	0	32	74

Abbreviations: ICI, intracavernosal penile injections; VCD, vacuum constriction device.

hypoxia is the key factor in collagen deposition in hypoxic cavernosal muscle, and that PGE1 reduced the expression of TGF-β_1 and opened a new era of interest in the field of pharmacologic prevention of ED following RP.

Nocturnal erections have been implicated in preserving normal erectile function by providing regular tissue oxygenation [53]. The lack of any erections during the period of neurapraxia has been implicated in the production of persistent penile hypoxia and fibrosis. Leungwattanakij and colleagues [54] reported that 3 months after cavernous nerve damage in the rat model, the penile tissue biopsy revealed significant overexpression of TGF-β_1 and collagen. Similarly, User and colleagues [55] in 2003 demonstrated significant apoptosis in the cavernosal smooth muscle, and high proportion of trabecular smooth muscle replaced by collagen. The consequence of cavernosal apoptosis and collagen deposition leads to veno-occlusive disease. It also causes penile shortening in both length and girth because of scar tissue.

Similarly, Iacono and colleagues [56] from Italy recently studied the changes in penile biopsy in human models before and after RP (2 months and 12 months). They reported a significant decrease in the elastic fibers and smooth muscle content and a significant increase in the collagen content in the postoperative biopsies compared with the biopsy before surgery, which is implicated in the reduction of penile length.

Progressive cavernosal fibrosis produced because of persistent penile hypoxia has been shown to produce veno-occlusive dysfunction. In 2002, Mulhall and colleagues [57] reported that the incidence of venous leak increases with the postoperative time interval. They showed that the incidence of postoperative venous leak was 14% at 4 months, which increased to 35% between 9 and 12 months. Similarly, Montorsi and colleagues [58] reported in 1997 that the incidence of venous leak was much higher in a control group (no treatment) compared with the treatment group (alprostadil injections three times/wk) (53% versus17%). These two studies revealed that postoperative venous leak was proportional to the time interval from the surgery, and that early treatment could result in a considerable decrease in venous leak. It is evident from the literature that ED after RP is multifactorial in cause. Penile hypoxia has been one of the most important precipitating factors in the formation of cavernosal fibrosis. The formation of cavernosal fibrosis, with the

subsequent venous leak, has been implicated as one of the most important causes of long-term ED after RP.

In any one patient who undergoes RP, the insult can be primarily neurogenic, vasculogenic, or mixed. It is a dynamic process from surgery to recovery. Either nerves or blood flow are compromised in every surgery, evident by that the fact it takes 9 to 12 months for resolution of the associated neurapraxia.

Clinical evidence for (studies of) early intervention

Unfortunately, the available clinical data come from a number of small studies with relatively few subjects, and which are often nonrandomized. Overall, the circumferential, or indirect, evidence from multiple studies is that early intervention strategies can improve sexual activity and the return of natural spontaneous erections, and may improve, at least marginally (10%–25%), the return of natural erections sufficient for vaginal penetration or vaginal potency. Larger, randomized studies are needed to prove the last potential advantage, that early intervention improves the return of natural erections sufficient for vaginal potency. The current potential clinical options for early intervention are listed in Box 1 and the current clinical data regarding these treatment options are summarized below.

Box 1. Potential early treatment options for erectile dysfunction following radical prostatectomy

1. Pharmacologic agents
   Oral (daily/14–20 d/mo)
   a. PDE-5 inhibitors (sildenafil, tadalafil, and vardenafil)
   IC injections (three times per week)
   a. PGE1 (alprostadil)
   b. Low-dose Trimix (alprostadil, papaverine, phentolamine)
   c. Bimix (papaverine, phentolamine)
   Intraurethral alprostadil (three times per week, 125 or 250 µg)
2. Nonpharmacologic agents
   VCD (daily for 5–10 minutes without ring)
3. Combination of above treatments

Early use of vacuum constriction devices

Considerable interest exists in early intervention protocols with the use of VCDs to encourage corporeal rehabilitation and prevention of post-RP veno-occlusive dysfunction. Early penile rehabilitation after RP may enhance earlier recovery of nocturnal erections by enhancing oxygenation of the corpora cavernosa and preventing formation of collagen and fibrosis, a cofactor in smooth muscle relaxation and erectile function. Clinically, this finding is evident in the preservation of penile length and girth that is seen with early use of the VCD following RP.

Several years ago, the authors' group completed a prospective, but nonrandomized, study of the use of early VCDs after retropubic prostatectomy at the Cleveland Clinic [59]. Of the 109 patients, 74 (group 1) patients used early VCDs daily for 9 months, and 35 patients were observed without any early maintenance erectogenic treatment (group 2). Patients in group 2 occasionally used oral PDE-5 inhibitors on an as-needed basis. With a minimum follow-up of 9 months, 80% in group 1 successfully used their VCDs with a constriction ring for vaginal intercourse at a frequency of twice a week, with an overall spousal satisfaction rate of 55% (Table 7). Thirty-two percent reported return of natural erections, with 17% having erections sufficient for sexual intercourse. The abridged IIEF-5 score significantly increased after VCD use in both the nerve sparing and non-nerve sparing groups (Table 8). After a mean use of 3 months, 18% discontinued treatment. In group 2, 37% of the patients regained spontaneous erections and 11% had erections sufficient for successful vaginal intercourse, with the remaining 26% of patients seeking adjuvant treatment.

RP has a significant effect on penile length and girth. In 2001, Munding and colleagues [60] reported that 71% of men had a decrease in penile stretched length after RRP and 48% had a significant decrease in length of 1 cm or more.

Similarly, Savoie and colleagues [61] in 2003 reported a decrease in penile length in 68% of their patients after RRP, with 19% having a decrease of 15% or greater. In the authors' study, in the observation group (no VCD), 63% reported a decrease in penile length and girth; in contrast, only 23% reported this in the VCD group. Recently, the authors' study has been confirmed; early use of VCDs preserves penile length and girth. In 2007, Dalkin and colleagues [62] at the Society of Urologic Oncology presented an abstract demonstrating that early use of VCDs for 10 minutes per day reduced the likelihood of penile shortening from 48% in historical control to 3.5% in this study.

A multicenter study at Ohio State University, Duke University, the Prostate Center in Austin, and the Cleveland Clinic is investigating the role of the VCD pump immediately following robotic RP. This study currently includes 500 patients with a 9-month follow-up. Preliminary results show patient compliance at 90%, maintenance of length and girth in 80% of patients, and a faster return of erections sufficient for intercourse.

Evolving data suggest that VCDs following RP facilitates early sexual intercourse, early patient/spousal sexual satisfaction, potentially an earlier return of natural erections sufficient for vaginal potency, and preservation of penile length and girth. The other advantages of the VCD include a high patient compliance and the fact that it is medically affordable, because the VCD is covered by most insurance.

Early use of intraurethral alprostadil

The authors' group completed a prospective, nonrandomized study of 91 patients on the use of early intraurethral alprostadil after RRP at the Cleveland Clinic [63]. Of the 91 patients, 56 received early intraurethral alprostadil, and 35 (the control group) did not receive any early erectogenic treatment. The control group occasionally used oral PDE-5 inhibitors on an as-needed basis. Patients

Table 7
Early use of vacuum constriction device following radical prostatectomy: results at 9 months

Variables	Early use of vacuum constriction device (n = 60)	Observation (PDE-5 inhibitors prn) (n = 35)
Total IIEF-5 score	16 + 7.3	12.06
Sexually active w/wo VCD	60/60 (100%)	13/35 (37%)
Return of natural (partial) erections	19/60 (32%)	13/35 (37%)
Natural erection sufficient for vaginal potency (no VCD)	10/60 (17%)	4/35 (11%)
Decrease in penile length/girth	14/60 (23%)	22/35 (63%)

Table 8
Response to early vacuum constriction device in relation to nerve-sparing status: results at 9 months

	Bilateral nerve sparing (n = 31)	Unilateral nerve sparing (n = 22)	Non–nerve sparing (n = 21)
Using VCD for sexual intercourse	25/31 (80.6%)	19/22 (86%)	16/21 (76%)
Spousal satisfaction	13/25 (52%)	11/19 (57%)	9/16 (57%)
Return of natural (partial) erections with VCD	9/31 (29%)	7/22 (32%)	3/21 (14%)
Natural erection sufficient for vaginal intercourse	5/31 (16%)	4/22 (18%)	1/21 (5%)

in the early intraurethral alprostadil group received 125 μg three times per week for the first 6 weeks. At 6 weeks the intraurethral alprostadil dose was titrated to 250 μg three times per week for 4 months. Patients who could not tolerate 250 μg doses remained at 125 μg for 4 months. In the intraurethral alprostadil group, 68% continued intraurethral alprostadil treatment. At 9 months, 74% of the patients resumed sexual activity, 40% had natural erections sufficient for vaginal potency without intraurethral alprostadil, and 34% continued to use intraurethral alprostadil as an adjuvant treatment for successful vaginal potency. In the control group, 37% regained spontaneous natural erections, but only 11% had natural erections sufficient for vaginal potency (Table 9).

The authors concluded that early intraurethral alprostadil therapy (at low doses of 125/250 μg) increased the frequency of sexual activity, shortened the period of neurapraxia, increased the incidence of spontaneous erections, and increased the incidence of erections sufficient for vaginal potency. The disadvantages of early intraurethral alprostadil therapy included the high incidence of urethral irritation, the cost of the intraurethral alprostadil, and lack of insurance coverage.

Early use of oral therapy with 5-phosphodiesterase inhibitors

Interest is growing among urologists regarding the early use of daily oral PDE-5 inhibitors. In 2004, Schwartz and colleagues [64] analyzed cavernosal smooth muscle content in a postprostatectomy population. A total of 40 patients were included in the study and a first cavernosal biopsy was performed at the time of surgery. Patients were stratified to receive two different doses of sildenafil: group 1 (n = 20) received 50 mg/day and group 2 (n = 20) received 100 mg every other day. At 6 months, group 2 had significantly more smooth muscle content in the second biopsy (56.85%) compared with the first biopsy (42.82%; $P<.05$). In group 1 (50 mg daily dose), no significant difference was observed in the smooth muscle content in second biopsy (51.67%), compared with the first biopsy (51.52%; $P>.05$). The study concluded that early use of sildenafil (50 mg daily) following RP preserves smooth muscle content, and at higher doses (100 mg every other day), it increases the smooth muscle content.

The benefit of early sildenafil has been reported by Padma-Nathan and colleagues [65], who conducted a randomized, controlled study in 76 men given oral sildenafil daily (50 mg [n = 23]; 100 mg [n = 28]; placebo [n = 25]) who underwent nerve-sparing RP with normal preoperative erectile function. Sildenafil was given for 36 weeks in the study group. Two months later, at 48 weeks (11 months), 27% patients receiving sildenafil had natural erections sufficient for intercourse, compared with one patient (4%) in the placebo group (Table 10). This study revealed that oral daily sildenafil increased the return of erections sevenfold, compared with the placebo group, and was well tolerated. In a subset of 54 patients from this study (35 sildenafil group, 19 control group), measurement of nocturnal penile tumescence and evaluation of penile rigidity revealed that 29%

Table 9
Early use of intraurethral alprostadil following radical prostatectomy: results at 9 months

Variables	Early use of intraurethral alprostadil (n = 38)	Observation (PDE-5 inhibitors prn) (n = 35)
Total IIEF-5 score	18.92	12.06
Sexually active w/wo intraurethral alprostadil	28/38 (74%)	13/35 (37%)
Return of natural (partial) erections	21/38 (56%)	13/35 (37%)
Natural erections sufficient for vaginal intercourse (no erectaids)	15/38 (39%)	4/35 (11%)

Table 10
Early use of sildenafil following radical prostatectomy:
International Index of Erectile Function-5 results at 9
months

Variables	Group 1 (sildenafil 50/100 mg for 36 wk)	Observation (no sildenafil)
N	51	25
Vaginal potency (%)	14 (27%)	1 (4%)
Positive NPT (%)[a]	10/35 (29%)	1/19 (5%)

[a] Patient is having spontaneous nocturnal penile erections.

of the sildenafil group demonstrated return of spontaneous erectile function, compared with 5% in the control group [65]. This study also demonstrated that tip rigidity of more than 55% appears to be the most important parameter to discriminate between responders and nonresponders. However, the study has been criticized because the rate of vaginal potency in the placebo group was only 4%, which is low compared with the other reported series in the literature. Although the study was randomized, the low rate of vaginal potency in the control group at 11 months softened the study's impact.

In 2005, Gallo and colleagues [66] from Italy evaluated the role of vardenafil in the recovery of erectile function following pelvic urologic surgeries (RRP and cystectomy). After 6 months of daily therapy, vardenafil therapy increased the mean IIEF-5 score to 12.9 points in the bilateral nerve-sparing group, to 8.0 points in the unilateral nerve-sparing group, and to 11.3 points in the bilateral nerve- sparing radical cystectomy group. This study showed that vardenafil was well tolerated and potentially effective for recovery of erectile function following major pelvic urologic surgery. However, the lack of a contemporary control group may be a limiting factor in the study.

The role of early use of PDE-5 inhibitors appears to give minimal to moderate benefit in early ED. This benefit appears to be a 20% increase at 1 year in erectile function, defined by vaginal penetration.

Early use of intracavernosal penile injections

In 1997, Montorsi and colleagues [58] first demonstrated the advantage of penile injection therapy as an early intervention strategy in a randomized, controlled study of patients after

bilateral nerve-sparing RP. Patients were randomized to treatment (receiving IC alprostadil 2–3 times/wk for 12 weeks, n = 15) and a control group (no treatment, n = 15). The mean IC PGE1 dose was 8 µg (range: 4–12). After a minimum follow-up of 6 months, 67% in the treatment group were reported to have spontaneous erections sufficient for satisfactory vaginal potency, compared with 20% in the control group. Penile Doppler studies revealed veno-occlusive dysfunction in only 17% of the treatment group, compared with 53% of the control group. This paper was published in 1997, but the data were never confirmed. The concept of early PGE1 injections has been used anecdotally by various groups but has not become a mainstream option because of the lack of patient compliance secondary to penile pain. Patients rarely forgive even a single episode of throbbing penile discomfort secondary to long-lasting prostaglandin effects.

The authors' group reexamined the role of IC injections immediately following RP. Their objective was to adjust the PGE1 dose to achieve 100% compliance. They felt injection therapy may be the strongest pharmacologic stimulus to facilitating an earlier response to PDE-5 inhibitors. In this report, they identified 49 patients using IC injections for more than 1 year. Of these 49 patients, 36 agreed to use sildenafil orally (50–100 mg) for a minimum of 4 weeks, or eight attempts. Of the 36 patients, 41% successfully switched to sildenafil and discontinued IC injection; 38% found sildenafil ineffective and remained on IC injection; 19% found sildenafil alone to be suboptimal but continued to use it, enhancing the efficacy of IC injections alone [67]. Because of the potential of injection therapy to potentate the response of PDE-5 inhibitors, the authors' group initiated an early injection program in combination with sildenafil. Patients were asked to use IC injection two to three times per week and to take 50 mg sildenafil on the remaining days.

This prospective study included 22 patients who underwent bilateral nerve-sparing RRP after October 2004 (Tables 11 and 12) [68,69]. A sildenafil dose of 50 mg/day was started at the time of hospital discharge. Of the 22 patients, 18 were started on IC alprostadil PGE1 (1–8 µg) and 4 were started on low-dose Trimix (20–30 units) two to three times per week. These patients were followed at regular intervals (3, 6, 9, 12, and 18 months) with IIEF-5 questionnaires. The authors optimized the dose to achieve 95% compliance. This compliance rate was sustained for almost 6 months; then, 10 of

Table 11
Early use of combination therapy following radical prostatectomy

Group	Total (n)	Initial injection dose (µg)	9-Mo follow-up(Sexually active[a] [n = 21/22, 96%])			
			Injection alone	PDE-5 + VCD	Partial erections (no erectaids)	Vaginal potency w/wo PDE-5 inhibitors
PGE1[b] (mean-4 µg)	4	8	1	0	4	3
	6	4	3	2	6	1
	6	2	3	2	2	1
	2	1	2	0	1	0
Total	18	—	9	4	13	5
Trimix[c] (low dose)	4	30 U	2	1	2	1
Total (%)	22	—	11 (52)	5 (23)	15 (71)	6 (28)

[a] One patient on injections alone was not sexually active because of spousal ill health.

[b] PGE1 = intracavernosal alprostadil.

[c] Low-dose Trimix = PGE1 (5.88 ug/mL), papaverine (17.65 mg/mL), and phentolamine (0.59 mg/mL).

the 22 patients refused to do further injections. These 10 patients were amenable to switching to VCD/PDE-5 inhibitors. With a mean follow-up of 9 months, 71% had return of spontaneous partial erections. Of the 22 patients, 96% were sexually active, 52% of these with injections and sildenafil, and 46% with VCDs/sildenafil. Overall, 28% of patients achieved vaginal potency with sildenafil alone. At 6 months, penile Doppler studies revealed arterial insufficiency in 17 out of the 22 patients and venous insufficiency in only 1 out of the 22 patients. Baseline and 9-month IIEF-5 scores for the patients continuing injections or VCDs were comparable (22.3 ± 1.6 at baseline and 22.1 ± 0.3 at 9 months). In the six patients using sildenafil alone to achieve vaginal potency, the mean IIEF score was 11.5 ± 1.8.

The authors' early conclusion in this pilot study was that combination therapy using IC injections and sildenafil facilitated early sexual intercourse, patient satisfaction, earlier return of spontaneous erections, and potentially an earlier

Table 12
Sexual activity (vaginal potency) of patients following early combination therapy: results at 9 months (summary)

Sexual activity (vaginal potency)	21/22 (96%)[a]
Injections alone	10/21 (46%)
VCD and PDE-5 (sildenafil)[b]	5/21 (23%)
PDE-5 (sildenafil) alone	6/21 (28%)

[a] One patient was not sexually active because of spousal ill health.

[b] After 6 months, 10 patients declined further injections; 5 switched to VCD/PDE-5 inhibitors (sildenafil), and another 5 were able to achieve vaginal potency with PDE-5 inhibitors alone.

return of natural erections sufficient for vaginal potency. However, with 9-month follow-up, results were still marginal in terms of vaginal potency. What is apparent in conducting this study is that patient compliance, even in well-motivated patients with pain-free injections, is difficult to maintain after 6 months, with 50% of the patients refusing to continue injections.

A summary of early intervention therapies

The authors' work on early intervention therapies still leaves them uncertain as to the best form of early therapy (Table 13). They feel that the use of oral PDE-5 inhibitors alone is not strong enough in the first 9 to 12 months to produce erections sufficient for vaginal penetration. This delay will affect penile physiology and anatomy (length and girth) and changes in marital sexual relations and partner satisfaction. For this reason, they are committed to using adjunctive combination therapy, using oral PDE-5 inhibitors along with VCD, intraurethral alprostadil, or IC penile injections. Currently, the logistics of administering an early injection program in a normal office practice is sometimes prohibitive. Multiple visits are sometimes required to regulate the dose, and the cost of the injections and needles can be an issue. These patients often need to be followed every 1 to 2 weeks to make sure the injections are technically done correctly and the proper dose is used, and to ensure there is no pain. The chronic patient demands of an early injection program can overwhelm the office resources and may not be the right answer.

Thus, in the present office urologic environment, an early VCD/PDE-5 inhibitor program

Table 13
Summary of early intervention therapies following radical prostatectomy

Treatment	Follow-up (mo)	Natural erections (partial)	Vaginal potency w/wo PDE-5 inhibitors
Oral drugs (USA) [62]	11	n/a	27%
VCD (CCF) [59]	9	37%	17%
Intraurethral alprostadil (CCF) [60]	9	35%	39%
Injections (CCF) [66]	8	71%	28%
Injections (Italy) [58]	6	n/a	69%
Control (CCF) [60]	9	39%	11%

Abbreviations; n/a, not applicable; CCF, Cleveland Clinic Foundation.

may be the most effective, time-efficient, and cost-effective option. Most patients are compliant on a daily basis with a VCD. The authors' current early intervention program following RP includes a regimen of daily VCD therapy 5 minutes twice a day and maximum use of oral PDE-5 inhibitors. Because of a lack of insurance coverage for PDE-5 inhibitors, VCD therapy has emerged as the dominant therapy in their intervention strategies.

Does early penile rehabilitation following robotic-assisted laparoscopic prostatectomy have a role?

Although potency results following RALP are impressive at remarkably shorter intervals than previously reported in the retropubic literature, the ultimate quality of the erection as defined by IIEF-5 (SHIM) scores still remains less than baseline in most series. Despite technically excellent nerve-sparing surgery done by robotic surgeons, a temporary period of neurapraxia continues to be observed [35,43]. Although the robotic surgical system, with its 3D-dimensional vision and 10- to 15-fold magnification (see Fig. 1), provides a significant technical advantage over conventional open surgery, reports still show that erections sufficient for vaginal intercourse do not return for 3 to 12 months following surgery [39,40,42–44]. In 2003, Menon and associates reported that only 50% of patients achieved return of partial erections at a mean follow-up of 180 days and a return to vaginal intercourse at a mean of 340 days [36]. Similarly, Chien and associates [39] reported a return to baseline sexual function in 66% and 69% of patients under 60 years old at 6 and 12 months following RALP, respectively. These reports illustrate that, even with robotic technology performing nerve-sparing surgery, a significant period of neurapraxia occurs.

The ultimate outcome measure regarding potency and the approach will be the long-term follow-up. Thus far, the longest reported follow-up on a robotic series is 12 months, and it is becoming apparent that this end point may be premature. A recent study from the authors' group indicates that the attrition in potency or sexual activity (50%) in the first 5 years is significant [70]. The exact reasons for the attrition appear to be lack of interest, diminished potency, and comorbidities, with only 11% of these patients remaining naturally potent. This finding raises the ultimate question of whether early intervention strategies should extend into chronic intervention treatments. Would chronic therapy or chronic dosing ultimately mitigate this decline or attrition in sexual activity seen in the surgical prostate patient following definitive treatment? Whether patients are treated with prostate brachytherapy, external beam therapy, or RP, the most potent patients fail to ever recover their baseline status. This reality should help stimulate and drive the concept of chronic dosing for high-risk groups for ED. High-risk groups include patients who have significant hypertension, hyperlipidemia, diabetes mellitus, obesity, and patients who receive definitive local treatment for localized prostate cancer.

Concept of chronic therapy

ED is reported in 70% to 80% of patients 5 years after RP [71,72]. Penson and colleagues [73] assessed temporal changes in sexual function in a cohort of 1288 men who underwent RP. They reported that at 60 months, 46% of patients reported no sexual activity, 77% of patients had little or no interest in sexual activity, and only 28% had erections firm enough for vaginal intercourse. It is unclear if the lack of spontaneous vaginal potency with or without oral therapy adversely affects the interest level.

Unfortunately, a significant attrition in potency is observed after 5 years in patients who have recovered natural potency following RP. At the annual American Urological Association in 2005, Zippe and colleagues presented an abstract on the natural history of sexual activity of patients who have recovered potency following RRP (Table 14) [70]. In this study of 141 sexually active patients (mean age 65.08 ± 6.68), it was noted that at 1 year, 80% of patients were sexually active. Of these, 3% were active naturally, 49% with PDE-5 inhibitors, 8% with intraurethral alprostadil, 23% with IC penile injections, and 17% with a VCD. However, the 5-year analysis showed that only 50% of patients were sexually active; 11% of patients were having intercourse without erectaids, 40% with PDE-5 inhibitors, 14% with IC injections, 7% with a VCD, and none with intraurethral alprostadil. Most of the patients who were still sexually active at 5 years were using PDE-5 inhibitors. The two main reasons for sexual discontinuation were loss of interest and diminished potency, and medical comorbidities. If more sophisticated clinical inquiries are done, the loss of interest and medical comorbidities are probably related to the loss of obtaining a natural erection easily, with or without oral therapy. What becomes evident is that these patients are not being followed closely enough, and opportunities for intervention, whether pharmacologic or psychologic, are not being pursued. This subject of loss of long-term desire and interest resulting from the loss of natural vaginal potency has not been appropriately studied in the urologic literature and illustrates the long-term marriage that exists between the prostate cancer specialist and the problems of erectile function.

In 2005, Stephenson and colleagues [74] reported their outcomes from two major population-based studies: SEER and Prostate Cancer Outcomes Study. In this review, 1977 men with localized prostate cancer who received either external beam radiation therapy or RP were surveyed 6, 12, 24, and 60 months after the initial prostate cancer diagnosis. It was observed that 50.5% of the men used multiple types of erectaids for their ED during the 60 months following the prostate cancer diagnosis. Most of these patients (38%) were compliant with oral therapy, but only 5.7% and 2% continued to use VCDs and IC penile injections, respectively. The most satisfied group was the penile prosthetic group, but it only comprised 1.6% of the patients. Men who used no treatment (49.2%) reported low sexual success, 50% of what was predicted (Table 15). It was felt that this large "no treatment" group resulted not only from patient reluctance but also failure of the physicians to offer therapy. This report also concluded that the effectiveness of currently available ED treatments is, at best, modest. Similar to the findings of Schover and colleagues [13], their results indicate substantial room for improvement in the use, effectiveness, and acceptability of therapy for ED following treatment of localized prostate cancer.

Table 14
Natural history of sexual activity patients (Sexual Health Inventory for Men score > 21) following radical prostatectomy at 1 and 5 years

Vaginal potency	At 1 year, number of patients (%)	At 5 years, number of patients (%)
Total sexually active	113 (80.0)	70 (50.0)
Natural potency (no erectaids)	4 (2.8)	16 (11.3)
PDE-5 inhibitor	55 (48.7)	28 (40.0)
PDE-5 inhibitor plus (VCD, ICI, intraurethral alprostadil)	0 (0.0)	5 (7.0), 5 (7.0), 1 (1.4)
Intraurethral alprostadil	9 (8.0)	0 (0.0)
ICI	26 (23.0)	10 (14.3)
VCD	19 (16.8)	5 (7.1)
Discontinuation of sexual activity and reasons		
Total	28 (14.0)	71 (50.4)
Loss of interest	10 (46.0)	44 (31.0)
Medical comorbidities (CVS and CNS)	0 (0.0)	25 (18.0)
Urinary incontinence	15 (53.0)	0 (0.0)
Loss of partner	0 (0.0)	3 (2.1)
Others	0 (0.0)	2 (1.4)

In this study, n = 141; mean age was 65.08 ± 6.68 years; mean follow-up was 6.4 ± 1.5 years.
Abbreviations: CNS, central nervous system; CVS, cardiovascular system; ICI, intracavernosal penile injections.

Table 15
Treatment of erectile dysfunction at 12 and 60 months following radical prostatectomy and radiation therapy: outcomes from the Surveillance, Epidemiology and End Results cancer registry and the Prostate Cancer Outcomes Study

Variables	At 12 mo (% of patients[a])	At 60 mo (% of patients[b])
Any ED treatment	25.4 ± 1.19	50.8 ± 1.53
VCD	9.8 ± 0.82	5.7 ± 0.69
Penile injection	6.6 ± 0. 68	2.0 ± 0.43
Nonsildenafil medication	1.6 ± 0.32	0.8 ± 0.25
Psychosexual counseling	2.0 ± 0.44	0.8 ± 0.25
Penile prosthesis	1.1 ± 0.30	1.6 ± 0.35
Sildenafil only	—	16.7 ± 1.18
Sildenafil + others	—	20.9 ± 1.21
Other multiple treatments	4.3 ± 0.55	2.3 ± 0.47
No ED treatment	74.6 ± 1.19	49.2 ± 1.53

[a] 1753 patients.
[b] 1462 patients.

Definitive treatment of localized prostate cancer, whether it is surgery or radiation, is a significant comorbidity in the sexual longevity of our younger patients. It is not any different from having a diagnosis of diabetes mellitus, severe hypertension, or hyperlipidemia, requiring daily medication. In exploring the feasibility of a chronic therapy or dosing model, the authors chose to investigate a pharmacologic stimulus in a subset of patients who underwent prostate brachytherapy. They hypothesized that beginning a daily oral dose of a PDE-5 inhibitor (sildenafil) at the time of radioactive seed placement may mitigate the subsequent radiation damage and fibrosis. Between December 2002 and January 2004, data on 44 sexually active patients (mean age 68.6) was collected. Group 1 (24 patients) received a daily maintenance dose of sildenafil (50 mg/d for 12 months, then as needed). The PDE-5 inhibitor was started immediately following brachytherapy (mean: 3 days, range: 1–5). Group 2 (20 patients) did not receive any early treatment. All patients were assessed after a minimum follow-up of 12 months using IIEF-5. In group 1, IIEF-5 scores were totally preserved at 12 months follow-up (pre-brachytherapy IIEF score was 24 ± 3.0 versus post-brachytherapy IIEF-5 score of 21± 3.6). Group 2 showed a significant decline in IIEF-5 scores (pre-brachytherapy IIEF-5 of 22.4 ±2.67 versus post-brachytherapy IIEF-5 of 10.6 ± 6.86) (Table 16) [75]. This pilot study is one of the first models in the radiation literature to demonstrate that early intervention, and perhaps chronic therapy, may impact subsequent potency rates.

Applying a chronic therapy model to prevent ED in the current medical environment is probably unrealistic if we are asking patients to use a daily medicine for years and insurance payers to reimburse this request. However, it may be possible to convince patients to use a daily medicine for the period of neurapraxia (0–12 months) following definitive prostate cancer treatments, and then use oral therapy as adjuvant treatment on an as-needed basis to augment erectile performance. A model of chronic maintenance therapy for ED in high-risk subsets needs to be explored further to help preserve sexual activity in younger patients.

Summary

Dynamic themes that emerged in the 1990s regarding prostate cancer diagnosis and management were largely due to the mainstream use of PSA testing and office-based ultrasound-guided biopsy techniques. PSA screening contributed to the detection of lower-volume cancers, which increased biochemical cure rates to upwards of 80% to 90%. A second important consequence of

Table 16
Response to International Index of Erectile Function-5 questionnaire by patients on chronic sildenafil dosing following prostate brachytherapy

IIEF-5 (SHIM)	Early sildenafil group (n = 24) mean ± SD		Control group (n = 20) mean ± SD	
Follow-up (mo)	14.4 ± 3.9		17.1 ± 4.0	
Status	Prebrachytherapy	Postbrachytherapy	Prebrachytherapy	Postbrachytherapy
Confidence	4	4	4.3 ± 0.48	2.8 ± 1.03
Erection firmness	4.5 ± 1.0	3.75 ± 0.96	4.7 ± 0.67	1.7 ± 1.25
Maintenance ability	4.1 ± 1.01	3.65 ± 0.87	4.8 ± 0.63	1.75 ±1.3
Maintenance frequency	4.5 ± 1.03	3.79 ± 1.9	4.27 ±1.08	2.3 ± 1.57
Intercourse satisfaction	4.5 ± 1.04	4.0 ± 1.1	4.8 ± 0.63	2.1 ±1.05
Total	24 ± 3.0	21 ± 3.6	22.4 ± 2.67	10.6 ± 6.85*

* $p < 0.05$.

rigorous prostate cancer screening was that the patient age of diagnosis dropped substantially. Younger cancer patients have higher expectations regarding quality-of-life issues (foremost, urinary incontinence and erectile function). It is the demand of the younger patients that pushed many of us to consider early penile rehabilitation strategies to improve potency rates following RP.

When analyzing the reported potency rates following various RP approaches, one finds that the results from various procedures vary widely. The vaginal potency rate following RRP in the hands of experienced surgeons at centers of excellence ranges from 40% to 86%. Perineal RP, which did not gain universal popularity, suffered because of the paucity of literature on potency rates in younger patients following bilateral nerve-sparing surgery. The reported potency rates following bilateral nerve-sparing LRP range from 14% to 81%. But very few surgeons can climb the steep learning curve necessary to perform bilateral nerve-sparing laparoscopic surgery well. Although the short-term vaginal potency rates following RALP are unprecedented (43%–97%), erections sufficient for vaginal intercourse still require 3 to 12 months of recovery, which suggests that, despite robotic technology and technically superior vision and magnification, the neurovascular bundle still has some degree of injury.

The available clinical data on the early use of PDE-5 inhibitors, VCDs, IC penile injections, and combinations of the above would suggest a short-term benefit of 20% to 40% in the rate of vaginal potency and a 30% to 70% improvement in the rate of partial (spontaneous) erections. Thus, the authors conclude that an early program with one of the erectaids, with or without a PDE-5 inhibitor, improves erectile physiology and performance following RP. Logistically, the combination of a PDE-5 inhibitor and a VCD may prove to be the most user-friendly, cost-effective, and patient-compliant. Ultimately, even with the superior potency results reported from robotic-assisted laparoscopic surgery, early intervention or penile rehabilitation therapies will always have a role.

The sexual longevity of the prostate cancer patient, however, greatly exceeds the interval of current reporting. A number of recent studies illustrate the fact that nearly 50% of baseline sexually active patients are no longer active at 5-year follow-up. Several dominant issues have been identified in these databases. Patients exponentially lose their natural erectile ability to achieve vaginal penetration, requiring the frequent use of erectaids.

The most compliant erectaids for the long-term are PDE-5 inhibitors, which usually require some degree of partial erections for success. The other issues that occur with longer follow-up include a loss of interest and fear of, or reluctance to undertake, sexual activity because of other comorbidities. These issues illustrate the need and urgency of long-term care and follow-up by the prostate cancer specialist. Our prostate cancer patients will be best served by a prostate cancer specialist who understands this long-term commitment.

References

[1] Jemal A, Siegel R, Ward E, et al. Cancer statistics, 2006. CA Cancer J Clin 2006;56(2):106–30.

[2] Stanford JL, Stephenson RA, Coyle LM, et al. Prostate cancer trends 1973–1994, NIH publication no. 99-4543. Bethesda (MD): SEER Program. National Cancer Institute; National Institute of Health; 1999.

[3] Stephenson RA. Prostate cancer trends in the era of prostate-specific antigen. An update of incidence, mortality, and clinical factors from the SEER data base. Urol Clin N Am 2002;29:173–81.

[4] Greene KL, Cowan JE, Cooperberg MR, et al. Who is the average patient presenting with prostate cancer? Urology 2005;66(Suppl 5A):76–82.

[5] Catalona WP, Basler JW. Return of erections and urinary continence following nerve-sparing radical retropubic prostatectomy. J Urol 1993;150:905–7.

[6] Quinlan DM, Epstein JI, Carter BS, et al. Sexual function following radical prostatectomy: influence of preservation of neurovascular bundles. J Urol 1991;145:998–1002.

[7] Walsh PC, Marschke P, Ricker D, et al. Patient-reported urinary continence and sexual function after anatomic radical prostatectomy. Urology 2000; 55:58–61.

[8] Rabbani F, Stapleton AM, Khattan MW, et al. Factors predicting recovery of erections after radical prostatectomy. J Urol 2000;164:1929–34.

[9] Talcott JA, Rieker P, Propert KJ, et al. Patient reported impotence and incontinence after nerve-sparing radical prostatectomy. J Natl Cancer Inst 1997;89:1117–23.

[10] Jonler M, Messing EM, Rhodes PR, et al. Sequelae of radical prostatectomy. Br J Urol 1994;73:352–8.

[11] Geary ES, Dendinger TE, Freiha FS, et al. Nerve sparing radical prostatectomy: a different view. J Urol 1995;154:145–9.

[12] Leandri P, Rossignol G, Gautier JR, et al. Radical retropubic prostatectomy: morbidity and quality of life. Experience with 620 consecutive cases. J Urol 1992;147(3 Pt 2):883–7.

[13] Schover L, Fouladi R, Warneke C, et al. Defining sexual outcomes after treatment for localized prostate carcinoma. Cancer 2002;95:1773–85.

[14] Kundu SD, Roehl KA, Eggener SE, et al. Potency, continence, and complications in 3,477 consecutive radical retropubic prostatectomies. J Urol 2004; 172:2227–31.

[15] Frazier HA, Robertson JE, Paulsen DF. Radical prostatectomy: the pros and cons of the perineal versus the retropubic approach. J Urol 1992;147:888–90.

[16] Weldon VE, Tavel FR. Potency sparing radical perineal prostatectomy: anatomy, surgical technique, and initial results. J Urol 1988;140:559–62.

[17] Weldon VE, Tavel FR. Potency and morbidity after radical perineal prostatectomy. J Urol 1997;158: 1470–5.

[18] Ruiz-Deya G, Davis R, Srivstav SK, et al. Outpatient radical prostatectomy; impact of standard perineal approach on patient outcome. J Urol 2001;166:581–6.

[19] Harris M. Radical perineal prostatectomy: cost efficient, outcome, effective, minimally invasive prostate cancer management. Eur Urol 2003;44:303–8.

[20] Lerner SE, Fleischmann J, Taub HC, et al. Combined laparoscopic pelvic lymph node dissection and modified belt radical perineal prostatectomy for localized prostatic adenocarcinoma. Urol 1994; 43:493–8.

[21] Abbou CC, Salmon L, Hozek A, et al. Laparoscopic radical prostatectomy: preliminary results. Urology 2000;55:630–4.

[22] Guillonneau B, Vallancien G. Laparoscopic radical prostatectomy: the Montsouris technique. J Urol 2000;163:1643–9.

[23] Arai Y, Egawa S, Terachi T, et al. Morbidity of laparoscopic radical prostatectomy: summary of early multi-institutional experience in Japan. Int J Urol 2000;10:430–4.

[24] Guillonneau B, Vallancien G. Laparoscopic radical prostatectomy: the Montsouris experience. J Urol 2000;163:418–22.

[25] Guillonneau B, Cathelineau X, Doublet JD, et al. Laparoscopic radical prostatectomy: assessment after 550 procedures. Crit Rev Oncol Hematol 2002; 43:123–33.

[26] Anastasiadis A, Salomon L, Katz R, et al. Radical retropubic versus laparoscopic prostatectomy: a prospective comparison of functional outcome. Urology 2003;62:292–7.

[27] Roumeguere T, Bollens R, Bossche MV, et al. Radical prostatectomy: a prospective comparison of oncological and functional results between open and laparoscopic approaches. World J Urol 2003;20:360–6.

[28] Rozet F, Galiano M, Cathelineau X, et al. Extraperitoneal laparoscopic radical prostatectomy: a prospective evaluation of 600 cases. J Urol 2005;174:908–11.

[29] Rassweiler J, Hruza M, Teber D, et al. Laparoscopic and robotic assisted prostatectomy: critical analysis of the results. Eur Urol 2006;49:612–24.

[30] Hara I, Kawabata G, Miyake H, et al. Feasibility and usefulness of laparoscopic radical prostatectomy: Kobe University experience. Int J Urol 2002; 11:635–40.

[31] Curto F, Benijits AP, Barmoshe S, et al. Nerve sparing laparoscopic radical prostatectomy: our technique. Eur Urol 2006;49:344–52.

[32] Namiki S, Egawa S, Terachi T, et al. Changes in quality of life in first year after radical prostatectomy by retropubic, laparoscopic, and perineal approach: multi-institutional longitudinal study in Japan. Urology 2006;67:321–7.

[33] Menon M, Shrivastava A, Tewari A, et al. Laparoscopic and robot assisted radical prostatectomy: establishment of a structured program and preliminary analysis of outcomes. J Urol 2002;168:945–9.

[34] Bentas W, Wolfram M, Jones J, et al. Robotic technology and the translation of open radical prostatectomy to laparoscopy: the early Frankfurt experience with robotic radical prostatectomy and one year follow up. Eur Urol 2003;44:175–81.

[35] Menon M, Tewari A, Members of the Vattikuti Institute Prostatectomy team. Robotic radical prostatectomy and the Vattikuti Urology Institute technique: an interim analysis of results and technical points. Urology 2003;61:15–20.

[36] Tewari A, Srivasatava A, Menon M, members of the VIP team. A prospective comparison of radical retropubic and robot-assisted prostatectomy: experience in one institution. BJU Int 2003;92:205–10.

[37] Menon M, Kaul S, Bhandari A, et al. Potency following robotic radical prostatectomy: a questionnaire based analysis of outcome after conventional nerve sparing and prostatic fascia sparing techniques. J Urol 2005;174:2291–6.

[38] Kaul S, Savera A, Badani K, et al. Functional outcomes and oncological efficacy of Vattikuti Institute prostatectomy with veil of Aphrodite nerve sparing: an analysis of 154 consecutive patients. BJU Int 2006;97:467–72.

[39] Chien WG, Mikhail AA, Marcelo AO, et al. Modified clipless antegrade nerve preservation in robotic-assisted laparoscopic radical prostatectomy with validated sexual function evaluation. Urology 2005;66:419–23.

[40] Ahlering TE, Eichel L, Skarecky D. Rapid communication: early potency outcomes with cautery-free neurovascular bundle preservation with robotic laparoscopic radical prostatectomy. J Endourol 2005; 19:715–8.

[41] Joseph JV, Rosenbum RM, Erturk E, et al. Robotic extraperitoneal radical prostatectomy: an alternative approach. J Urol 2006;175:945–51.

[42] Tewari A, Kaul S, Menon M. Robotic radical prostatectomy: a minimally invasive therapy for prostate cancer. Curr Urol Rep 2005;6:45–8.

[43] Tewari A, Peabody JO, Fischer M, et al. An operative and anatomic study to help in nerve sparing during laparoscopic and robotic radical prostatectomy. Eur Urol 2003;299:1–12.

[44] Kaul S, Bhandari A, Hemal A, et al. Robotic radical prostatectomy with preservation of the prostatic fascia: a feasibility study. Urology 2005;66:1261–5.

[45] Zippe CD, Raina R, Thukral M, et al. Management of erectile dysfunction following radical prostatectomy. Curr Urol 2001;2:495–503.

[46] Goldstein AM, Meehan JP, Zakhary R, et al. New observation on micro architecture of corpora cavernosa in man and possible relationship to mechanism of erection. Urology 1982;20:259–66.

[47] Persson C, Diederichs W, Lue TF, et al. Correlation of altered penile ultrastructure with clinical arterial evaluation. J Urol 1989;142:1462–8.

[48] Jevtich MJ, Khawand NY, Vidic B. Clinical significance of ultrastructural findings in the corpora cavernosa of normal and impotent men. J Urol 1990; 143:289–93.

[49] Luangkhot R, Rutchik S, Agarwal V, et al. Collagen alterations in the corpus cavernosum of men with sexual dysfunction. J Urol 1992;148:467–71.

[50] Moreland RB, Traish A, McMillin MA, et al. PGE1 suppresses the induction of collagen synthesis by transforming growth factor-beta 1 in human corpus cavernosum smooth muscle. J Urol 1995;153:826–34.

[51] Daley JT, Brown ML, Watkins T, et al. Prostanoid production in rabbit corpus cavernosum: I. Regulation by oxygen tension. J Urol 1996;155(4):1482–7.

[52] Daley JT, Watkins MT, Brown ML, et al. Prostanoid production in rabbit corpus cavernosum. II. Inhibition by oxidative stress. J Urol 1996;156(3):1169–73.

[53] Moreland RB. Is there a role of hypoxemia in penile fibrosis: a viewpoint presented to the Society for the Study of Impotence. Int J Impot Res 1998;10:113–20.

[54] Leungwattanakij S, Bivalacqua TJ, Usta MF, et al. Cavernous neurotomy causes hypoxia and fibrosis in rat corpus cavernosum. J Androl 2003;24:239–45.

[55] User HM, Hairston JH, Zelner DJ, et al. Penile weight and cell subtype specific changes in a postradical prostatectomy model of erectile dysfunction. J Urol 2003;169:1175–9.

[56] Iacono F, Giannella R, Somma P, et al. Histological alterations in cavernous tissue after radical prostatectomy. J Urol 2005;173:1673–6.

[57] Mulhall JP, Slovick R, Hotaling J, et al. Erectile dysfunction after radical prostatectomy: hemodynamic profiles and their correlation with the recovery of erectile function. J Urol 2002;167:1371–5.

[58] Montorsi F, Guazzoni G, Strambi LF, et al. Recovery of spontaneous erectile function after nerve-sparing radical retropubic prostatectomy with and without early intracavernous injections of alprostadil: results of a prospective, randomized trial. J Urol 1997;158:1408–10.

[59] Raina R, Agarwal A, Ausmundson S, et al. Early use of vacuum constriction device (VCD) following radical prostatectomy (RP) facilitates early sexual activity and potential return of erection. Int J Impot Res 2006;18:77–81.

[60] Munding M, Wessels H, Dalkin B. Pilot study of changes in stretched penile length 3 months after radical retropubic prostatectomy. Urology 2001; 58(4):567–9.

[61] Savoie M, Kim S, Soloway M. A prospective study measuring penile length in men treated with radical prostatectomy for prostrate cancer. J Urol 2003; 169:1462–4.

[62] Dalkin B. Preservation of penile length after radical prostatectomy (RP): early intervention with a vacuum erection device (VED). Society of Urologic Oncology [Abstract] 2007.

[63] Raina R, Pahlajani G, Agarwal A, et al. The early use of transurethral alprostadil after radical prostatectomy potentially facilitates an earlier return of erectile function and successful sexual activity. BJU Int 2007; in press.

[64] Schwartz EJ, Wong P, Graydon RJ. Sildenafil preserves intracorporeal smooth muscle after radical retropubic prostatectomy. J Urol 2004;171:771–4.

[65] Padma-Nathan H, et al. Postoperative nightly administration of sildenafil citrate significantly improves the return of normal spontaneous erectile function after bilateral nerve-sparing radical prostatectomy [abstract 1402]. J Urol 2003;169:375.

[66] Gallo L, Perdona S, Autorino R, et al. Recovery of erection after pelvic urologic surgery: our experience. Int J Impot Res 2005;17:484.

[67] Raina R, Lakin MM, Agarwal A, et al. Long-term intracavernosal therapy responders can potentially switch to sildenafil citrate after radical prostatectomy. Urology 2004;63:532–7.

[68] Nandipati KC, Raina R, Bhatt A, et al. Early combination therapy following radical prostatectomy: intracorporeal alprostadil and sildenafil promotes early return of natural erections. Poster # 72 in 79th Annual Meeting of North Central Section AUA, Chicago, September 7–10, 2005.

[69] Nandipati K, Raina R, Agarwal A, et al. Early combination therapy: intracavernosal sildenafil following radical prostatectomy increases sexual activity and the return of natural erections. Int J Impot Res 2006;16:1–6.

[70] Nandipati K, Rupesh R, Agarwal A, et al. Five-year potency status after radical prostatectomy: role of oral therapy in erectaids. American Urological Association Annual Meeting [abstract #270] May 21–26, 2005.

[71] Potosky AL, Davis WW, Hoffman RM, et al. Five year outcomes after prostatectomy or radiotherapy for prostate cancer: the prostate cancer outcomes study. J Natl Cancer Inst 2004;96:1358–67.

[72] Korfage IJ, Essink-Bot ML, Borsboom GJJM, et al. Five-year follow-up of health related quality of life after primary treatment of localized prostate cancer. Int J Cancer 2005;116:291–6.

[73] Penson DF, McLerran D, Feng Z, et al. 5-Year urinary and sexual outcomes after radical prostatectomy: results from the prostate cancer outcomes study. J Urol 2005;173:1701–5.

[74] Stephenson RA, Mori M, Yi-Ching Hsieh, et al. Treatment of erectile dysfunction following therapy for clinically localized prostate cancer: patient

reported use and outcomes from the Surveillance, Epidemiology and End Results prostate cancer outcomes study. J Urol 2005;174:646–50.

[75] Nandipati K, Rupesh R, Agarwal A, et al. Role of early sildenafil in preservation of erectile function following prostate brachytherapy. North Central Section American Urology Association Annual Meeting [abstract]. May 21–26, 2005.

[76] Kundu SD, Roehl KA, Eggener SE, et al. Potency, continence and complications in 3,477 consecutive radical retropubic prostatectomies. J Urol 2004; 172:2227–31.

ELSEVIER
SAUNDERS

Urol Clin N Am 34 (2007) 619–630

UROLOGIC
CLINICS
of North America

Gene Therapy for Male Erectile Dysfunction

Arnold Melman, MD

Department of Urology, Albert Einstein College of Medicine,
Bronx, NY, USA

Human gene therapy has been described as a promising, but unfulfilled, approach to treat diseases—a virtual "roller coaster" of ups and downs since the first reported gene therapy clinical trial in 1990 [1,2]. The complexities of delivery systems and setbacks, in large part due to the use of viral vectors, have led to some initial successes but many failures. Providentially, smooth muscle disorders of the genitourinary system, including erectile dysfunction (ED), share important differences that make them attractive targets for gene therapy and, in particular, allow the use of naked DNA without requiring viral vectors to effect cell membrane penetration by the gene of interest. The therapeutic goal of therapy in these disorders is modulation of smooth muscle tone, rather than more radical alterations of structure, function, or induction of apoptosis. Additionally, major smooth muscle organs, including the penis, bladder, gut, and lungs, are easily accessible for local, targeted administration of the gene product. Therefore, the need for systemic delivery of gene product with its attendant generalized, nonspecific biodistribution is eliminated. The author's laboratory has taken advantage of these properties in an attempt to develop a safe, durable treatment for ED based on knowledge of the physiology, pharmacology, and electrical activity of corporal smooth muscle cells [1,3–5]. With publication of preclinical data and, more recently, results from the first human trial of *h*Maxi-K gene transfer in

men who have ED [6,7], we have begun to show that ion channel gene therapy is a viable option to treat smooth muscle cell disorders.

Although the current generation of oral phosphodiesterase-5 (PDE-5) inhibitors for the treatment of ED represents a significant advancement over earlier, more invasive treatments, there are unmet needs among men who have ED. That family of products is least effective in men who have more severe ED, including men who have diabetes, and is contraindicated in association with some families of drugs or medical conditions. The short duration of currently available members of the PDE-5 inhibitor class limits the spontaneity of the sexual act. Many men and their partners are unhappy with the concept of "planned sex." Current approved oral therapies also have a high incidence of untoward side effects, such as nasal stuffiness and headaches, and the recently described occurrence of nonarteritic ischemic optic neuropathy leading to blindness [8] is troubling to many potential users of the medications.

Several groups have taken diverse approaches to gene therapy for ED. A variety of vectors have been used to insert genes to enhance the production of vascular endothelial growth factor, nitric oxide synthase, preprocalcitonin gene-related peptide, and vasoactive intestinal peptide in the corporal bodies of rodents [9–15]. Although all of these studies demonstrated improved erections and cavernous pressures in response to stimuli in the rat, mostly they relied on viral vectors that insert genes into the host chromosomes. This approach introduces the potential for insertion into unintended targets or outcomes. It is of interest that the plasticity of the erectile apparatus is such that positive outcome has been the case in each of the published reports in animal models;

Portions of this text were published previously in Melman A, Bar-Chama N, McCullough A, et al. hMaxi-K gene transfer in males with erectile dysfunction: results of the first human trial. Hum Gene Ther 2006;18:1165–76; with permission.

E-mail address: amelman@aecom.yu.edu

however, for use in humans, the product must be proven safe and practical to pass the muster of the US Food and Drug Administration (FDA) as well as the target population. Detailed reviews of these varied gene therapy approaches for ED were published recently [3,5,16,17].

Our rationale for ion channel gene therapy that led to the first human trial of hMaxi-K for ED is based on the unique ultrastructural features of the smooth muscle of the genitourinary system and the role of ion channel function in the cavernous bodies.

Penis ultrastructural features and ion channels

The penis is an easily accessible external organ, and placement of a tourniquet at the base before administration limits potential biodistribution of the injected gene to other organs. Therefore, the issues related to intravenous injection of gene product are avoided. Smooth muscle cells form a functional synctium that lines the cavernous bodies of the penis along with endothelial cells, fibroblasts, and collagen [18]. These cells are joined by gap junctions that allow for intracellular communication and transfer of neurotransmitters and second messengers [19]. Flux of ions through these channels governs many of the physiologic properties and activities of muscles in the body. Ion channels for potassium, calcium, and chloride govern many of the contractile properties seen in smooth muscles, including cavernous smooth muscles. The intermittent opening of the Maxi-K channels in response to regional increases of intracellular calcium ion concentration controls the tone of the penile smooth muscle. Proper function of those potassium channels is necessary for the induction of smooth muscle cell relaxation and the induction of a penile erection. Normal erectile function is governed by the limitation of influx of calcium ions into the smooth muscle cells that results in smooth muscle relaxation. The initiating process occurs in response to a sexual stimulus causing production and release of nitric oxide (from nerves and endothelium) diffusing into the cells and causing the production and accumulation of cyclic GMP that facilitates some of the downstream events listed above that cause smooth muscle relaxation.

At least four types of potassium channels are present in the plasma membranes of human smooth muscle cells [20–24]. With respect to penile erection, these ion channels respond to endogenous intracellular events by opening and allowing K^+ to flow down its electrochemical gradient out of the smooth muscle cell. The resulting hyperpolarization (ie, increased negativity), in turn, limits calcium entry and promotes relaxation of the corporal and arterial smooth muscle cells (Fig. 1). The Maxi-K is a well-studied potassium channel subtype that is involved in smooth muscle relaxation [22,25,26]. It exhibits little activity in the normal corporal smooth muscle population. When these cells are stimulated, the open time or activity of the Maxi-K channel increases dramatically. This effect represents the convergence point for several upstream signaling pathways [27]. The central role of potassium channels in controlling membrane potentials and excitability makes them an attractive target for gene therapy [21]. Because potassium channels also control ion flux through other channel types, their augmentation modulates the flux of other ions (eg, calcium). The proposed increase in functional membrane potassium channels as a consequence of gene transfer should lead to normalization of smooth muscle cell hyperpolarization and subsequent smooth muscle cell relaxation in the presence of aging or disease (Fig. 2).

A possible mechanism by which Maxi-K gene transfer can improve erectile function

Davies and colleagues [28,29] recently reported from work in the author and colleagues' laboratory, that, in the rat model of aging, there are remarkable changes posttranscriptionally in the expression of Maxi-K protein in corporal smooth muscle cells. In older animals there is a significant decrease in the amount of Maxi-K protein expressed in the membranes and an increase in the amount of Maxi-K retained in the cytosol. The down-regulated expression of the Maxi-K channel in the membranes correlates with a significant increase in the levels of a dominant negative transcript of the Slo gene (SV1) in older animals. As depicted in Fig. 3, Davies and colleagues proposed that the increase in SV1 in older animals traps the Maxi-K protein in the cytoplasm. It was shown that dominant negative mutants trapping Maxi-K in the cytoplasm can lead to an overall decrease in the expression of the Maxi-K protein, probably through protein degradation pathways. Potentially, the physiologic effect of down-regulating the Maxi-K channel activity could lead to heightened tone of the corporal smooth muscle tissue through an increase in intracellular calcium, which

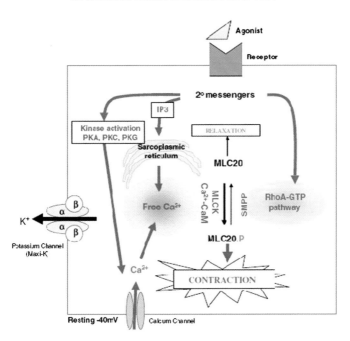

Fig. 1. Smooth muscle cell contraction. The relationship of the smooth muscle cell to the potassium ion channels, intracellular calcium ion, procontractile and relaxant second messengers, and contractile proteins. Because smooth muscle contractility is regulated primarily by intracellular Ca^{2+}, the moment-to-moment control of calcium ion entry by potassium channel activity regulates the tone of the smooth muscle cell. Furthermore, the change to the open state of the channel is in response to an event. Most of the time, the K^+ channels are in the closed state. With the opening of the channel, the membrane potential of the cell becomes more negative (ie, hyperpolarized), and the voltage-sensitive calcium channel closes and prevents influx of calcium ion into the cell. IP3, inositol triphosphate; MLC20, myosin light chain 20; MLCK, myosin light chain kinase; PKA, protein kinase A; PKC, protein kinase C; PKG, protein kinase G; SMPP, smooth muscle myosin phosphatase.

results in heightened contractility and ED. These results suggest that if Maxi-K gene transfer were applied to the treatment of ED in an aging patient, the mechanism of action would be to overcome posttranscriptional events that limit the expression of Maxi-K channel activity.

Although the precise mechanism by which the Maxi-K gene transfer works in diabetic animals is not known, it is likely to again involve a change in splicing of the Slo transcript. The author and colleagues recently demonstrated that, in diabetic animals, alternative splicing of the Slo transcript might represent an important compensatory mechanism to increase the ease with which relaxation of corporal tissue may be triggered as a result of a diabetes-related decline in erectile capacity [29]; however, there seems to be a transcriptional upper limit of the Slo gene expression, which when reached, can no longer compensate for the physiologic pressure resulting in ED. We proposed, at this point, that gene transfer of plasmids expressing a functional channel can supplement endogenous gene transcription, which leads to recovery of erectile function.

Thus, a gene transfer approach that provides the ability to locally overexpress a potassium channel gene in a target tissue theoretically could overcome the age- or disease-related changes in end organ contractility that contribute to ED. Therefore, thus far we have focused on recombinant hSlo, which encodes the α, or pore-forming, subunit of the human Ca^{2+}-activated K^+ potassium channel (Maxi-K).

Vector

Naked DNA was selected as the vector for hMaxi-K gene transfer. Naked DNA has been unpopular as a gene transfer vector because of its reported lack of efficacy and limited duration of effect in systemic trials; however, in an appropriate targeted, local, nonsystemic application, naked DNA is recognized for its lack of chromosomal integration and its lack of toxicity.

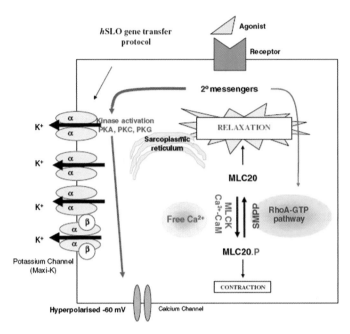

Fig. 2. Insertion of Maxi-K channels into smooth muscle cell. A representative cell into which the a-subunit of the MaxiK channel has been transferred. Three additional MaxiK channels are shown in the cell membrane. Because it is not know if the additional channels expressed by the hMaxi-K possess the β-subunit, that unit was not included. In the presence of an appropriate neural or ionic signal, the potassium channels open, hyperpolarize the cell to approximately −60 mV, and inhibit the influx of calcium ion, thus causing the cell to relax. MLC20, myosin light chain 20; MLCK, myosin light chain kinase; PKA, protein kinase A; PKC, protein kinase C; PKG, protein kinase G; SMPP, smooth muscle myosin phosphatase.

Most previous gene therapy protocols used retroviral vectors to integrate DNA into the target (Fig. 4). This results in integration of the DNA into the host nucleus. With naked plasmid DNA transfer, the plasmid is incorporated into the cell and then translocates into the nucleus, but is not integrated [22]. Theoretically, at least, plasmid DNA could integrate into the nuclear DNA; however, experimentally this has not been seen at a sensitivity of one copy per 1 μg of DNA, or three orders of magnitude below the spontaneous mutation frequency. The hSlo plasmid construct (hMaxi-K) illustrated in Fig. 5 has demonstrated excellent uptake into cavernosal smooth muscle cells in rats [4,30,31]. Experiments have demonstrated excellent uptake of the plasmid vector into cells and excellent functional results in terms of restoring intracavernosal pressures in response to stimuli (Fig. 6). Overall, the unique properties of the genitourinary smooth muscle cells seem to overcome the perceived disadvantages of limited efficacy and duration of the naked DNA plasmid.

The extensive preclinical evidence showing the safety, effectiveness, and long duration of action of hMaxi-K led to the design and approval to implement the first human trial of gene transfer therapy for ED.

Phase 1 human safety trial of hMaxi-K: initiating a human gene transfer trial for a nonfatal indication

All gene transfer trials are conducted under the auspices of the Center for Biologics Evaluation and Research of the FDA. Those trials must be reviewed first by the Recombinant DNA Advisory Committee (RAC) of the Office of Biotechnology of the National Institutes of Health (NIH). The output of the RAC is advisory to the FDA; however, by law, the FDA cannot act on an Investigational New Drug (IND) application unless that review is undertaken. The RAC must review and make recommendations for the proposed clinical trial before an Institutional Review Board and the Institutional Biosafety Committee of private and institutional based trials can allow a study to proceed. The RAC reviews the

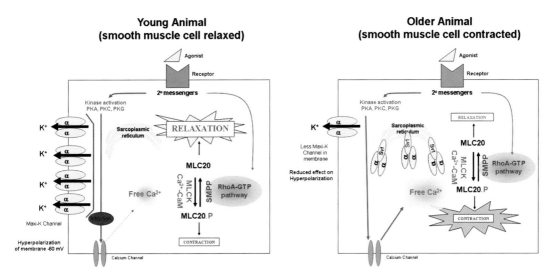

Fig. 3. Potential mechanism of Maxi-K gene transfer in old versus young animals. In young animals, most of the Maxi-K channel is expressed on the surface of the corporal smooth muscle cells. Upon activation, they hyperpolarize the membrane, an effect that inhibits the activity of the calcium channel. This results in a reduction in the intracellular free calcium levels and activity of the myosin light chain kinase (MLCK) through the action of the calcium-calmodulin complex. Less myosin light chain is in the phosphorylated (contracted) state, leaving the smooth muscle cell in a relaxed state. In older animals, increased expression of the dominant-negative Maxi-K channel (Sv1) reduces the amount of Maxi-K expressed on the cell surface. The reduction in the ability of the Maxi-K channels may cause hyperpolarization and, thereby, inhibit calcium channels, which leads to an increase in intracellular calcium that ultimately results in the smooth muscle cell being in a more contracted state. CaM, calmodulin; MLC20, myosin light chain 20; PKA, protein kinase A; PKC, protein kinase C; PKG, protein kinase G; SMPP, smooth muscle myosin phosphatase.

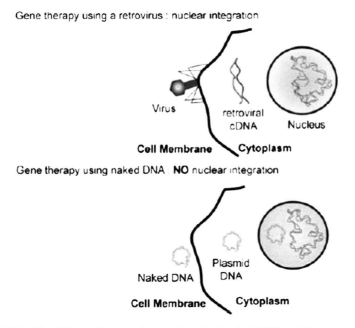

Fig. 4. Viral vector DNA. The difference between the use of viral and naked DNA to effect gene transfer. In the upper panel, in which a retrovirus is used as the vector, the DNA passes across the cell and nuclear membrane into the nucleoplasm, where it is integrated into the chromosomal apparatus. When naked DNA is used to effect the transfer, the DNA passes across both membranes but is not incorporated into the nuclear apparatus.

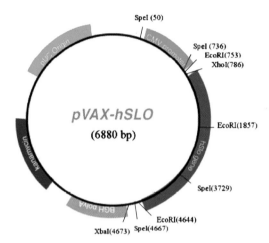

Fig. 5. hMaxi-K. Plasmid construct (hMaxi-K, 6880 base pairs): cytomegalovirus (CMV) promoter (positions 137–724), viral; hSlo gene (positions 888–4428), human; bovine growth hormone (BGH) polyadenylation [poly(A)] signal (positions 4710–4940), bovine; kanamycin gene (positions 5106–5901), bacterial; pUC origin of replication (positions 6200–6874), bacterial. Plasmid description: hMaxi-K is a double-stranded naked plasmid DNA molecule carrying the human hSlo gene, which encodes the α, or pore-forming, subunit of the human smooth muscle Maxi-K channel. hSlo is under the control of the CMV promoter positioned upstream of the transgene, and the construct also contains the BGH poly (A) site, kanamycin resistance gene, and pUC origin of replication. (From Melman A, Bar-Chama N, McCullough A, et al. The first human trial for gene transfer therapy for the treatment of erectile dysfunction: Preliminary results. Eur Urol 2005;48:314–8; with permission.)

submitted protocol and has the option of requiring a public, Web cast presentation by the principal investigator or the sponsor, at which time a recommendation for approval or additional data is made.

Most clinical trials that use gene transfer are for the indications of cancer, end-stage vascular disease, or genetic disorders. The NIH's Genetic Modification Clinical Trial Research Information System (www.gemcris.od.nih.gov) lists only one ongoing gene transfer trial for the indication of ED, and that is the one described below.

The ethics of using gene transfer as a therapy for ED, a nonfatal disease, was addressed recently by Dr. Arthur Caplan [32] as a prelude to the published results of the clinical trial. The text was as follows:

> The report by Melman and his team in this issue of Human Gene Therapy of a safety trial of gene therapy for men afflicted with erectile dysfunction is certain to raise more than a few ethical eyebrows. The history of clinical trials utilizing gene therapy is, to say the least, ethically contentious. Many would argue that the slow rate of progress and the established risks associated with various vectors should make it clear that gene therapy ought only be utilized in the pursuit of life and death disorders for which no current therapeutic modalities exist. Otherwise, many are likely to argue, the risks involved with gene therapy could not possibly be balanced by the potential for serious benefit.
>
> This line of reasoning is however in my view deeply flawed. It presumes that conditions such as erectile dysfunction are not 'serious' enough to merit attention by those working on the cutting edge of gene therapy research. Dismissing erectile dysfunction out of hand as a condition for which risks ought not be permitted in research undervalues the importance of medical efforts aimed at maintaining or restoring the quality of life of patients. And, disparaging safety trials involving subjects with erectile dysfunction also fails to address the question of what sorts of conditions and what organ systems are likely to be the most

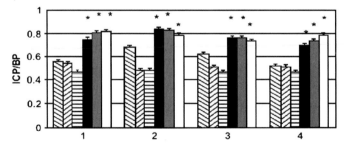

Fig. 6. Restoration of intracavernous pressure in impotent diabetic rats by hSlo gene therapy. Restoration of intracavernosal pressure (ICP) in impotent diabetic rats by hSlo gene therapy. Control treated and untreated groups demonstrate no improvement in ICPs compared with baseline pressure (BP), whereas all hSlo-treated rats demonstrated increases in ICPs that persisted up to 4 months after treatment: non-diabetic aged matched controls (▨), plasmid cDNA (▨), untreated (▤), 100 μg of hSlo (■), 300 μg of hSlo (▨), and 1000 μg of hSlo (☐) (* = significant difference from controls at the $p < 0.05$ level).

useful in understanding the utility and safety of various gene vectors and their potential for efficacy.

Erectile dysfunction is a serious medical problem. There are many men who decline life-saving surgery for prostate cancer when told that such surgery may leave them impotent. The degree to which this condition matters in relationships and to the individual self-esteem of persons is reflected in the surgical measures that men were willing to endure before the advent of pharmacological treatments for impotency. Sexual behavior is a key aspect of the quality of life that we all enjoy. If existing treatments cannot help all those in need then there is absolutely no reason not to pursue new and pioneering strategies to resolve dysfunction and disorder in this area of life.

As Melman and his co-authors note there are sound physiological reasons to think that gene transfer into smooth muscle in the penis might provide a safer and more useful model for understanding gene therapy than is afforded by targeting other tissues and organs. The generation of key safety data from subjects suffering from a serious and sometimes devastating medical condition is an ethical course for gene therapy researchers to follow as long as their science is sound, their consent of subjects thorough and their reports of results modest, balanced and fair.

In August of 2003, the FDA approved an IND application for Ion Channel Innovations, LLC to conduct the first phase 1 human trial to study the safety of gene transfer for the treatment of ED. Detailed methodology and results were published recently [6].

Following institutional review committee and biohazards committee approvals, 11 patients who had moderate to severe ED were given single-dose corpus cavernosum injection of hMaxi-K naked DNA plasmid carrying the human cDNA encoding hSlo, the gene for the α, or pore-forming, subunit of the human smooth muscle Maxi-K channel. Men 18 years or older participated in the study and had moderate to severe ED according to their International Index of Erectile Function (IIEF) scores. The ED was attributable to underlying, stable medical conditions. The men were otherwise in good health, with normal blood pressure and general and genitourinary physical examination at screening. Patients and their sexual partners signed the respective informed consents, and approved patients returned for the baseline visit 2 weeks later when gene transfer was given.

Eleven of 15 men screened qualified for entry. Three men each were treated with 500-, 1000-, or 5000-μg doses and two were given 7500 μg. The dose level selection was based on the lowest range of hMaxi-K used in preclinical studies in rodents [4]. hMaxi-K was injected into the corpus cavernosum of patients after placing a tourniquet (Actis venous flow controller; Vivus, Inc., Menlo Park, California) at the base of the penis. The tourniquet remained in place for 30 minutes to ensure that the vector was largely limited to the penis. Patients were monitored for 6 months after dosing, and annual follow-ups are planned.

The primary objective of this study was the safety and tolerability of a single injection of hMaxi-K at four escalating dose levels. This was measured by assessment of changes in clinical evaluations and laboratory tests that included general and genitourinary physical examinations, blood pressures and heart rates, ECG, general blood electrolyte and liver chemistries, hematologic parameters, endocrine tests, thyroid profiles, and urine and semen analysis. Adverse events were assessed and recorded at each visit. The DNA of semen was tested for the presence of pVAX-hSlo plasmid using reverse transcriptase polymerase chain reaction with primers specific to the plasmid [27].

Although the primary objective of this phase 1 study was safety, the key secondary study objective was assessment of the effect of hMaxi-K on ED using the erectile function (EF) domain category of the IIEF scale [33,34]. The EF domain, questions 1 through 5 and 15 of the IIEF, has been validated to assess erectile changes only [34]. Additional IIEF subdomain scores were recorded to confirm the IIEF-ED, including the mean intercourse satisfaction score—questions 6, 7, and 8—as an indicator of overall sexual satisfaction.

The study was conducted from May, 2004 to May, 2006. The mean age of the study population was 59.0 ± 10.6 years (range, 42–80 years), six subjects were white, four subjects were African American, and one subject was Hispanic. The duration of ED ranged from 1 to 20 years, the mean baseline IIEF-EF score was 6.8 ± 4.05, and 9 subjects were categorized with severe ED and 2 subjects with moderate ED according to standard classifications [34].

The initial safety question to be answered was the possible presence of detectable hMaxi-K in the semen of subjects during the 6 months after transfer. Fig. 7 shows a representative analysis of total

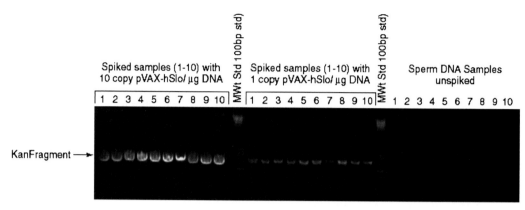

Fig. 7. Analysis of total DNA extracted from sperm for the presence of pVAX1-hSlo. Plasmid DNA was extracted from sperm, using a Qiagen (Valencia, California) total DNA extraction kit according to the manufacturer's instructions. Five milligrams of total DNA was subjected to polymerase chain reaction with primers amplifying the kanamycin (Kan) gene present in pVAX1-hSlo. In addition to unspiked samples, samples were also spiked with 1 or 10 copies of pVAX1-hSlo per milligram of total DNA as labeled above the gel. Unspiked samples gave no signal, whereas spiked samples gave a signal of the expected size for the kanamycin gene in pVAX1-hSlo. The amount of plasmid present in the sperm samples was less than the limit of detection (1 copy/µg of total DNA). Sperm DNA samples were as follows: lane 1, untreated; lanes 2–4, treated patient, samples taken on February 2, 2005 (repeat), April 19, 2005, and July 14, 2005; lanes 5–7, treated patient, samples taken on May 24, 2005, May 31, 2005, and July 12, 2005; lanes 8 and 9, patient, samples taken on March 9, 2005 and May 4, 2005; lane 10, water (negative control).

DNA extracted from sperm samples for the presence of pVAX1-hSlo plasmid. Samples spikes with 1 or 10 copies of pVAX1-hSlo per microgram provide reference comparisons for semen samples from three patients, taken at several time points. There was no detectable evidence of hMaxi-K in semen down to the 1 copy/µg of the total DNA level in any participant at any of the visits.

Table 1 is a summary of adverse events reported by patients during the study. All three patients given 500 µg, one of three patients given 1000 µg, and one of three patients given 5000 µg had adverse experiences. All the reported events occurred at least 30 days after gene transfer, and none of the events were considered related to the gene product transfer by the investigators. All three patients in the 500-µg dose group had adverse experiences; one had knee arthroscopy, one had atrial flutter with ablation reported as severe, and one had kidney stone removal by lithotripsy, also reported as severe. The atrial flutter and lithotripsy also were classified as serious adverse events. One patient given 1000 µg reported acid reflux, sciatic pain, and an upper respiratory infection, and one patient had a parasitic intestinal infection and foot edema. One patient given 5000 µg had bladder stone removal; neither patient given 7500 µg reported an adverse experience. No patients reported any discomfort from the injection, and no local physical events related to the injections were observed.

Table 1

Phase1 trial of hMaxi-K in men who have erectile dysfunction: adverse event summary by dose

Events	Dose (µg)				
	500 (n = 3)	1000 (n = 3)	5000 (n = 3)	7500 (n = 2)	Total (n = 11)
Patients reported ≥ 1 AE	3 (100%)	2 (67%)	1 (33%)	0 (0%)	6 (54.5%)
Patients with AEs related to study treatment	0 (0%)	0 (0%)	0 (0%)	0 (0%)	0 (0%)
Patients with serious AEs	2 (67%)	0 (0%)	0 (0%)	0 (0%)	2 (18.2%)
Patients with AE leading to early withdrawal	0 (0%)	0 (0%)	0 (0%)	0 (0%)	0 (0%)

Abbreviation: AE, adverse event.

No clinically significant changes were seen in the general or genitourinary physical examinations during the study. No emergent transfer-related cardiac events were noted or reported during the study, and no significant changes in ECG, as determined by shift analysis (no normal to abnormal occurrences), were observed with the exception of atrial flutter considered unrelated to treatment in one patient.

No clinically significant changes were seen in the mean blood chemistry or endocrine test values at the end of the study or at any of the interim study visits. In addition, no clinically significant changes from normal to abnormal in any blood chemistry, endocrine, hematology, or urinalysis values were seen at any visit for any patient. Mean systolic and diastolic blood pressures and heart rates did not show notable changes over time in each dose group; however, individual subject values varied from visit to visit, but no clinically significant pattern of changes was evident. No adjunctive therapies or changes in therapy were required.

The three patients given the 500-µg dose and one patient given 1000-µg of *h*Maxi-K have now completed 2-year safety follow-up safety examinations with no reported complications or adverse experiences. One patient given 1000 µg was lost to follow-up. The other patient given 1000 µg, three patients given 5000 µg, and two patients given 7500 µg doses have completed 1-year follow-up examinations with no reported complications or adverse experiences.

Examination of secondary efficacy end points indicated some suggestion of improvement in ED symptoms. Decreased IIEF-EF domain scores at each dose were observed 1 week after injection. Mean scores for the two lower dose groups (500 and 1000 µg) fluctuated around the baseline values throughout the study; however, improvements in the mean IIEF-EF scores were observed for the two higher dose groups (5000 and 7500 µg) beginning 2 weeks after transfer. Improvements were maintained in both groups through the 24 weeks of study. The positive changes from baseline for most patients were small and did not indicate improvement by IIEF scoring; however, two patients, one given 5000 µg and one given 7500 µg, showed notable improvement in IIEF-EF beginning 2 weeks after transfer and continuing improvement (from severe to mild or to no ED) at 4 weeks. The improvement was maintained through the 24-week study.

Fig. 8 displays the IIEF–mean intercourse satisfaction score for each patient at each visit. The results showed that for those men who responded to the transfers at the two higher doses there was a clinically significant increase in sexual satisfaction.

The most important finding of the study was that single injections of *h*Maxi-K at doses of 500, 1000, 5000, and 7500 µg were well-tolerated and safe, and furthermore, that no safety issues emerged during the 6 months of follow-up. No significant drug-related changes from baseline were seen in physical evaluations (general and

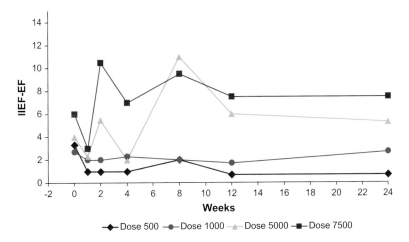

Fig. 8. *h*Maxi-K: Change in patient IIEF-MIS scores over time by dose for each Patient. MIS, mean intercourse satisfaction. (*From* Melman A, Bar-Chama N, McCullough A, et al. Plasmid-based gene transfer for treatment of erectile dysfunction and overactive bladder: results of a phase I trial. Isr Med Assoc J 2007;9:143–6; with permission.)

genitourinary), hematology, chemistry and hormone analyses, or in cardiac events evaluated by repeated ECGs (one patient who had preexisting atrial arrhythmia had a recurrence at ~1 month after dosing). No plasmid was detected in the semen of patients at any time after the injections. FDA requires that the participants in gene transfer trials, in which naked DNA is used as the vector, be followed for at least 2 years after transfer. The lack of complications or adverse experiences has now been confirmed for up to 2 years following gene transfer.

We cannot draw conclusions about efficacy from the results of phase 1 trials without randomized controlled groups. Nonetheless, efficacy measurements, made at each study visit, may provide insight into potential clinical activity. The IIEF is the standard instrument accepted as the best measure of efficacy in ED clinical trials, and patients given the two highest hMaxi-K doses had apparent sustained improvements in erectile function indicated by improved scores of the IIEF-EF domain over the length of the study. Specifically, one patient in the 5000-µg group and one in the 7500-µg group reported mostly equivalent EF improvements that approached the no ED IIEF-EF score, and they maintained the improvements for 24 weeks. Sexual satisfaction scores confirmed patient improvements.

Because the participants in this trial were not blinded to their treatments the improvement in IIEF score may have been a consequence of their belief in the effectiveness associated with the treatment; however, the preliminary results indicate that gene transfer with hMax-K has significant potential as a therapy for patients who have ED. Overall, the results suggest that further studies in a larger group of patients, with the addition of a placebo control and multiple doses, should be conducted to confirm the safety and efficacy of hMaxi-K in patients who have ED.

Summary and future directions

It remains to be confirmed in controlled clinical trials that hMaxi-K is efficacious as treatment for men who have ED. Following the promising safety outcomes at the doses of hMaxi-K in the initial phase 1 trial, cohorts of patients are being recruited to extend the observations to a series of higher doses preliminary to design of a controlled clinical trials program. The results of the first human trial of gene transfer therapy for ED suggest that gene transfer focused on ion channel therapy in the smooth muscle of organs, such as the penis and bladder, offers a promising new treatment strategy. This novel therapeutic approach may address limitations of current therapies for ED.

Preclinical studies recently reviewed [3,35] documented the important role of Maxi-K channel-mediated hyperpolarizing currents to the modulation of bladder myocyte function. Results of this work suggested that hMaxi-K gene transfer therapy also may be effective for the treatment of urinary incontinence related to bladder overactivity. In December, 2006, the FDA approved an IND for Ion Channel Innovations, LLC to conduct the first phase 1 human trial to study the safety of hMaxi-K gene transfer for the treatment of detrusor overactivity. The phase 1 trial was initiated in April, 2007.

The potential clinical advantages of a gene transfer therapy–based approach to treatment of genitourinary smooth muscle-based disorders are several: potential single therapy for restoration of normal bladder or erectile function; elimination of the need for daily medication; use in combination with other therapies to reduce dose requirements and side effects; and the development of mechanism-based, patient-specific treatment approaches. With the safe administration of hMax-K to men who have ED in the first human phase 1 trial and the initiation of the phase 1 trial of hMaxi-K for patients who have detrusor overactivity, we have entered an exciting new era in the development of safe enduring therapies for genitourinary disorders.

Acknowledgments

This trial was sponsored by Ion Channel Innovations, LLC. The author is a cofounder (along with George Christ, PhD) of Ion Channel Innovations, LLC and is grateful to Drs. Kelvin Davies, PhD and David Burkholder, PhD for assistance in the preparation of the manuscript.

References

[1] Schiff JD, Melman A. Ion channel gene therapy for smooth muscle disorders: relaxing smooth muscles to treat erectile dysfunction. Assay Drug Dev Technol 2006;4(1):89–95.
[2] Rolland A. Gene medicines: the end of the beginning? Adv Drug Deliv Rev 2005;57(5):669–73.
[3] Christ G, Hodges S, Melman A. An update on gene therapy/transfer treatments for bladder dysfunction.

Current Bladder Dysfunction Reports 2006;1(2): 119–25.

[4] Christ GJ, Day N, Santizo C, et al. Intracorporal injection of hSlo cDNA restores erectile capacity in STZ-diabetic F-344 rats in vivo. Am J Physiol Heart Circ Physiol 2004;287(4):H1544–53.

[5] Melman A. Gene transfer for the therapy of erectile dysfunction: progress in the 21st century. Int J Impot Res 2006;18(1):19–25.

[6] Melman A, Bar-Chama N, McCullough A, et al. hMaxi-K gene transfer in males with erectile dysfunction: results of the first human trial. Hum Gene Ther 2006;17(12):1165–76.

[7] Melman A, Bar-Chama N, McCullough A, et al. The first human trial for gene transfer therapy for the treatment of erectile dysfunction: preliminary results. Eur Urol 2005;48(2):314–8.

[8] Pomeranz HD, Bhavsar AR. Nonarteritic ischemic optic neuropathy developing soon after use of sildenafil (Viagra): a report of seven new cases. J Neuro-ophthalmol 2005;25(1):9–13.

[9] Rogers RS, Graziottin TM, Lin CS, et al. Intracavernosal vascular endothelial growth factor (VEGF) injection and adeno-associated virus-mediated VEGF gene therapy prevent and reverse venogenic erectile dysfunction in rats. Int J Impot Res 2003;15(1):26–37.

[10] Chancellor MB, Tirney S, Mattes CE, et al. Nitric oxide synthase gene transfer for erectile dysfunction in a rat model. BJU Int 2003;91(7):691–6.

[11] Champion HC, Bivalacqua TJ, Hyman AL, et al. Gene transfer of endothelial nitric oxide synthase to the penis augments erectile responses in the aged rat. Proc Natl Acad Sci U S A 1999; 96(20):11648–52.

[12] Garban H, Marquez D, Magee T, et al. Cloning of rat and human inducible penile nitric oxide synthase. Application for gene therapy of erectile dysfunction. Biol Reprod 1997;56(4):954–63.

[13] Magee TR, Ferrini M, Garban HJ, et al. Gene therapy of erectile dysfunction in the rat with penile neuronal nitric oxide synthase. Biol Reprod 2002;67(1): 20–8.

[14] Bivalacqua TJ, Champion HC, Abdel-Mageed AB, et al. Gene transfer of prepro-calcitonin gene-related peptide restores erectile function in the aged rat. Biol Reprod 2001;65(5):1371–7.

[15] Shen ZJ, Wang H, Lu YL, et al. Gene transfer of vasoactive intestinal polypeptide into the penis improves erectile response in the diabetic rat. BJU Int 2005;95(6):890–4.

[16] Kendirci M, Teloken PE, Champion HC, et al. Gene therapy for erectile dysfunction: fact or fiction? Eur Urol 2006;50(6):1208–22.

[17] Lau DH, Kommu SS, Siddiqui EJ, et al. Gene therapy and erectile dysfunction: the current status. Asian J Androl 2007;9(1):8–15.

[18] Benson GS, Boileau MA, et al. The penis. In: Gillenwater JY, Grayhack JT, Howards SS, editors.

Sexual function and dysfunction in adult and pediatric urology. 4th edition. New York: Lippincott Williams & Wilkins; 2002. p. 1935–74.

[19] Moreno AP, Campos de Carvalho AC, Christ G, et al. Gap junctions between human corpus cavernosum smooth muscle cells: gating properties and unitary conductance. Am J Physiol 1993;264(1 Pt 1): C80–92.

[20] Christ GJ, Brink PR, Melman A, et al. The role of gap junctions and ion channels in the modulation of electrical and chemical signals in human corpus cavernosum smooth muscle. Int J Impot Res 1993; 5(2):77–96.

[21] Nelson MT, Quayle JM. Physiological roles and properties of potassium channels in arterial smooth muscle. Am J Physiol 1995;268(4 Pt 1):C799–822.

[22] Fan SF, Brink PR, Melman A, et al. An analysis of the Maxi-K+ (KCa) channel in cultured human corporal smooth muscle cells. J Urol 1995;153(3 Pt 1): 818–25.

[23] Karicheti V, Christ GJ. Physiological roles for K+ channels and gap junctions in urogenital smooth muscle: implications for improved understanding of urogenital function, disease and therapy. Curr Drug Targets 2001;2(1):1–20.

[24] Melman A, Christ GJ. Integrative erectile biology. The effects of age and disease on gap junctions and ion channels and their potential value to the treatment of erectile dysfunction. Urol Clin North Am 2001;28(2):217–31, vii.

[25] Christ GJ, Spray DC, Brink PR. Characterization of K currents in cultured human corporal smooth muscle cells. J Androl 1993;14(5):319–28.

[26] Christ GJ, Wang HZ, Venkateswarlu K, et al. Ion channels and gap junctions: their role in erectile physiology, dysfunction, and future therapy. Mol Urol 1999;3(2):61–73.

[27] Christ GJ, Rehman J, Day N, et al. Intracorporal injection of hSlo cDNA in rats produces physiologically relevant alterations in penile function. Am J Physiol 1998;275(2 Pt 2):H600–8.

[28] Davies KP, Tar M, Rougeot C, et al. Sialorphin (the mature peptide product of Vcsa1) relaxes corporal smooth muscle tissue and increases erectile function in the ageing rat. BJU Int 2007;99(2):431–5.

[29] Davies KP, Zhao W, Tar M, et al. Diabetes-induced changes in the alternative splicing of the Slo gene in corporal tissue. Eur Urol 2007;52(4): 1229–37.

[30] Christ GJ. Gene therapy treatments for erectile and bladder dysfunction. Curr Urol Rep 2004;5(1): 52–60.

[31] Melman A, Zhao W, Davies KP, et al. The successful long-term treatment of age related erectile dysfunction with hSlo cDNA in rats in vivo. J Urol 2003;170(1):285–90.

[32] Caplan A. Commentary: improving quality of life is a morally important goal for gene therapy. Hum Gene Ther 2006;17:1164.

[33] Rosen RC, Riley A, Wagner G, et al. The international index of erectile function (IIEF): a multidimensional scale for assessment of erectile dysfunction. Urology 1997;49(6):822–30.

[34] Cappelleri JC, Rosen RC, Smith MD, et al. Diagnostic evaluation of the erectile function domain of the International Index of Erectile Function. Urology 1999;54(2):346–51.

[35] Christ G, Andersson KE, Atala A. The future of bladder research: molecular profiling, new drug targets, gene therapy, and tissue engineering. Curr Urol Rep 2007;8(2):95–9.

ELSEVIER
SAUNDERS

Urol Clin N Am 34 (2007) 631–642

UROLOGIC
CLINICS
of North America

Priapism: Current Principles and Practice

Arthur L. Burnett, MD*, Trinity J. Bivalacqua, MD, PhD

Department of Urology, The James Buchanan Brady Urological Institute,
Johns Hopkins Medical Instituitions, Baltimore, MD, USA

Priapism is defined as prolonged and persistent penile erection unassociated with sexual interest or stimulation. It constitutes a true disorder of erection physiology, associated with risks for structural damage of the penis and erectile dysfunction. The disorder is rare with an obscurity that is compounded by a limited understanding of its causes and mechanisms. The disorder remains a poorly recognized condition by many medical professionals, and for the treating urologist it implies a vexatious clinical problem generally lacking well-established corrective treatments. This article covers the current knowledge of the scientific basis of priapism and its standard clinical management.

Definition

The term "priapism" derives historically from the appellation given to the ancient Greek and Roman mythological figure Priapus, a deity of fertility and gardens. By conventional definition, priapism designates a medical term characterizing a pathologic condition of persistent penile erection in the absence of sexual excitation [1,2]. A qualifying criterion for the disorder meeting a clinical definition is that it persists beyond 4 hours [2]; however, presentations of shorter duration as well as those lasting up to months encompass the spectrum of its clinical presentations. The penis is recognized as the typically affected bodily organ, although priapism of the clitoris has been reported [3]. The corpora cavernosa typically are the structures that are uncontrollably engorged, although tumescence of the corpus spongiosum also has been observed [4,5]. Pain is a common descriptor, although this feature is not exclusively present for the diagnosis to be made.

Epidemiology

The estimation of the population risk for priapism remains largely unknown. Several epidemiologic reports have suggested that incidence rates range between 0.5 and 1 case per 100,000 person-years (the number of patients with the first episode of priapism divided by the accumulated amount of person-time in the study population) [6–8]. Pharmacologic therapies for erectile dysfunction causing prolonged erection events largely have been associated with the risk in some populations; however, specific patient populations constitute major risk categories for priapism. For instance, cohort studies involving populations with sickle cell disease demonstrated lifetime probabilities of developing priapism to be between 29% and 42% [9–12].

Clearly, epidemiologic statistics for this subject matter remain elusive. Survey studies often are limited by cases that only come to medical attention because they are significantly prolonged or painful. Further limitations are associated with diagnosis misclassifications and inaccuracies associated with retrospectively collected registry data. Thus, even representative studies may have underestimated the frequency of the problem.

Etiology

An assortment of etiologic factors have been associated with priapism (Box 1). Major etiologic categories are hematologic dyscrasias, neurologic conditions, nonhematologic malignancies, trauma,

* Corresponding author.
E-mail address: aburnett@jhmi.edu (A.L. Burnett).

doi:10.1016/j.ucl.2007.08.006

urologic.theclinics.com

Box 1. Conditions associated with priapism

Ischemic (low-flow) priapism
Sickle cell disease and other
    hemoglobinopathies
Vasoactive drugs
    Erectile dysfunction
        pharmacotherapies
    Antihypertensives (hydralazine,
        prazosin)
    Antipsychotics (chlorpromazine)
    Antidepressants (trazodone)
    Alcohol
    Cocaine
Neoplastic disease (local or metastatic)
    Penis
    Urethra
    Prostate
    Bladder
    Kidney
    Testis
    Gastrointestinal tract
Hematological dyscrasias
    Leukemia
    Polycythemia
Hyperlipidic parenteral nutrition
Hemodialysis
Heparin treatment
Fabry's disease
Neurologic conditions
    Spinal cord injury
    Anesthesia (general, regional)

Nonischemic (high-flow) priapism
Trauma
    Straddle injury
    Intracavernous injection needle
        laceration
Vasoactive drugs
Penile revascularization surgery
Neurologic conditions

erectile dysfunction pharmacotherapy, pharmacologic exposures, and idiopathic factors. It is important to recognize that these associations differ in frequency for pediatric and adult populations (Fig. 1). Conventional understanding is that adverse conditions, such as hematogenous factors or traumatic situations of the penis or perineum, alter the normal vascular rheology of the penis [13,14]. New thinking about causes of priapism

has turned to possible roles of deranged erectile mechanisms leading to uncontrolled penile erection [15–18]. These concepts may apply to such phenomena as neurogenic, "stuttering," drug-induced, and idiopathic forms of priapism.

Pathophysiology

Early understanding about the origins of priapism stemmed from the work of Frank Hinman Jr, whose studies of idiopathic priapism suggested the roles of vascular stasis in the penis and decreased venous outflow from the organ as primary pathophysiologic features [13]. Support for the proposal derived from the finding of dark, viscous blood in priapic penes after incision or aspiration of the corpora cavernosa. This finding suggested the presence of deoxygenated blood (decreased oxygen tension or increased carbon dioxide tension) indicative of ischemia. The idea of venous congestion and enhanced blood viscosity has served as a pathophysiologic basis for priapism associated with various clinical presentations, including sickle cell disease [13], assorted hematologic dyscrasias [14,19–21], parenteral hyperalimentation [22,23], hemodialysis [24], heparin-induced platelet aggregation [25], and local primary or metastatic neoplasia [26–29].

Traumatically induced priapism carries a different pathophysiologic basis. The mechanism involves excessive arterial inflow to the penis, resulting from structural injury of the arterial circulation of the organ [30–35].

New insights about the pathophysiologic basis of priapism have moved from an understanding that mechanical alterations in the rheology of the penis solely account for priapism. Molecular science of the field has evolved, much as this has occurred for erectile dysfunction more broadly in the past 2 decades. A dysregulatory hypothesis for the pathophysiology of priapism refers to dysfunctional actions of molecular factors governing corporal smooth muscle physiology [15]. In theory, the dysregulatory basis may occur at the level of the penis or at other regulatory levels of penile erection, including central or peripheral levels of the nervous system.

A leading proposal in this regard is that the nitric oxide–based signal transduction pathway, fundamental for signaling penile erection, becomes dysfunctional in association with underlying disease states [36]. Scientific evidence supports reduced nitric oxide bioactivity in the penis, which

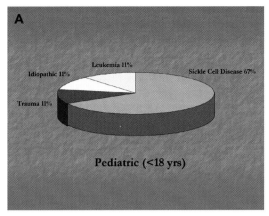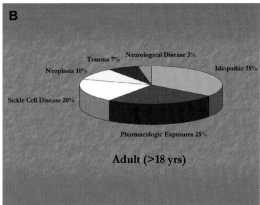

Fig. 1. Major causes of priapism and their frequencies in pediatric (*A*) and adult (*B*) populations. Data represent estimations combined from several literature sources.

leads to aberrant molecular mechanisms of the erectile response. Under these conditions, regulatory mechanisms that prevent uncontrolled penile erection are defective. Contributing features of corporal ischemia and anoxia of the penis contribute to the pathophysiology of priapism. Further, reperfusion injury results in oxidative stress and the formation of reactive oxygen species along with the release of hypoxia-induced growth factors such as transforming growth factor-β [37–42]. At the penile level, a model may be proposed by which a cycle of pathogenic factors contributes to the pathophysiology of priapism and fosters clinically observed recurrences of the disorder (Fig. 2).

Pathology

Macroscopic and microscopic changes occur in the penis in association with priapism. Recurrent

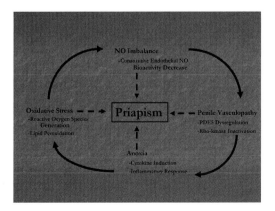

Fig. 2. Cycle of pathogenic factors. NO, nitric oxide; PDE5, phosphodiesterase type 5.

priapism of sickle cell disease results in the grossly distended and deformed megalophallus [43]. Ischemic priapism is well recognized to manifest penile tissue necrosis and progressive fibrosis as end-stage changes [13,44]. These structural changes impair the physical reactivity of the erectile tissue and its elasticity needed for physiologic blood engorgement. The metabolic factors of hypoxia, acidosis, and glucopenia contribute to impaired corpus cavernosal smooth muscle tone and contractile responses to physiologic and pharmacologic stimuli [38,45–48]. These changes have been confirmed to develop as soon as 4 hours after priapism onset, suggesting that this is the critical interval after which duration of ischemia leads to irreversible erectile tissue dysfunction [49].

Nonischemic priapism, in which there is unregulated blood entry and filling within the corpora cavernosa following trauma, displays a distinct pathology. Commonly, a fistula forms between the cavernous artery and lacunar spaces of the cavernous tissue [31,50,51]. This pathologic structure allows blood to bypass the helicine arteriolar bed, which normally serves as a vascular resistance mechanism in the penis.

Natural history

The natural course of priapism can be variable, although some specific patterns and outcomes associated with the disorder are well recognized. In general, priapism occurs and self-remits or it persists with varying pathologic consequences in the absence of proper treatment. Ischemic priapism often is manifest as a major episode of at least a few hours in duration. If untreated, it resolves eventually, although permanent damage of the penis may be expected because of the adverse consequences of the ischemia. The consequence of complete erectile dysfunction ranges from 30% [2,12] to 90% [52] in men sustaining major episodes of ischemic priapism. Ischemic priapism denoted as recurrent follows a clinical pattern of repeated events with intervening periods of tumescence [9,10,12,53]. These presentations often have been described as "stuttering" attacks, characteristically lasting less than 3 hours in duration [9]. Generally, they have not been associated with a significant extent of erectile dysfunction [9,10,53], although a recent report documented a 25% erectile dysfunction rate among patients who had sickle cell disease who had experienced only stuttering priapism [12].

Priapism also may follow a different natural course than that typically associated with ischemic events. Nonischemic priapism, which, as suggested, obviates ischemic sequelae, resolves spontaneously or persists without resolution for extended periods of time [51]. Nonischemic priapism may evolve as a variant of its primary traumatic form unassociated with a cavernosal-sinusoidal fistula in the setting of refractory ischemic priapism [54]. Common understanding holds that individuals who have nonischemic priapism generally preserve erectile ability, although evidence of erectile dysfunction has been documented in these individuals as well [50].

Classification

A classification system has been developed and widely applied to assist with practical understanding of priapism and facilitate its clinical management. The system adheres to two main divisions, ischemic and nonischemic priapism, having distinctive clinicopathologic features (Box 2). Ischemic priapism, also termed veno-occlusive or low-flow priapism, typically features little or absent intracorporal blood flow. Accordingly, it represents a true compartment syndrome involving the penis, in which there is characteristic metabolic changes and excessive intracorporal pressure increases. Nonischemic priapism, also termed arterial or high-flow priapism, features elevated vascular flow within the corpora cavernosa. It does not represent a compartment syndrome of the penis. On a practical level, ischemic priapism warrants emergency management, whereas nonischemic priapism does not carry such ramifications.

Box 2. Differentiating features in the clinical evaluation of priapism

Ischemic priapism
Idiopathic or medical disease related (commonly)
Spontaneous or precipitated by sleep or sexual activity
Painful corpora
Rigid erection
Tender penis
Dark blood (on corporal aspiration)
Abnormal cavernous blood gases (hypoxia, hypercarbia, acidosis)
Minimal or absent flow in cavernosal arteries

Nonischemic priapism
Injury related (commonly)
Precipitated by penile/perineal trauma (commonly)
Nonpainful corpora
Tumescence
Nontender penis
Bright red blood (on corporal aspiration)
Normal cavernous blood gases (consistent with normal arterial blood)
Normal to high blood flow velocities in cavernosal arteries

Diagnosis

Priapism is recognized in a generally straightforward manner owing to the physical conspicuousness of the erect penis in the absence of sexual excitation. A key principle in the evaluation is the distinction of ischemic and nonischemic priapism divisions, because the former requires emergent treatment. The initial portion of the evaluation may prompt critical management while awaiting confirmatory laboratory and radiologic study results.

History and physical examination

Generally, the clinical history should produce information such as the presence of pain, duration of priapism, role of antecedent factors, prior priapism episodes, use and success of relieving maneuvers or prior clinical treatments, existence of etiologic conditions, and erectile function status before the priapism episode. Pain typically is a differentiating feature of ischemic priapism. Inspection and palpation of the penis may indicate the extent of tumescence or rigidity, corporal body involvement (ie, whether rigidity involves only the corpora cavernosa with a soft glans penis and corpora spongiosum or all three corporal bodies), and the presence and extent of tenderness. The corpora cavernosa usually are rigid and tender to palpation with presentations of ischemic priapism, unlike that of nonischemic priapism. Abdominal, perineal, and rectal examinations may reveal signs of trauma or malignancy.

Laboratory testing

The routine evaluation of the patient who has priapism generally adheres to the application of several laboratory tests. Complete blood cell count, white blood cell differential, and platelet count may reveal the presence of acute infections or hematologic abnormalities. Reticulocyte count and hemoglobin electrophoresis may indicate the presence of sickle cell disease or trait as well as other hemoglobinopathies, and it should be administered to all men unless another cause of priapism is obvious. This recommendation is based on the fact that hemoglobinopathies are not restricted to men of African American descent; they may occur in nonobviously affected ethnic groups, including men of Mediterranean ancestry. Screening for psychoactive drugs and urine toxicology may be done to identify the pharmacologic influences of legal and illegal drugs.

Penile diagnostics

Aspirated blood from the corpus cavernosum offers an opportunity for evaluation [2,16]. The blood can be inspected visually and submitted for cavernous blood gas testing. The clinical presentation of ischemic priapism typically manifests blood that is hypoxic and, therefore, darkly colored, whereas that of nonischemic priapism commonly appears oxygenated and, therefore, bright red in color. Cavernous blood gas results provide an immediate distinction between the classic divisions of priapism. For ischemic priapism, typical findings are a Po_2 less than 30 mm Hg, Pco_2 greater than 60 mm Hg, and pH less than 7.25. For nonischemic priapism, findings are a Po_2 greater than 90 mm Hg, Pco_2 less than 40 mm, and pH of 7.40, consistent with normal arterial blood at room air conditions. Comparatively, normal flaccid penis cavernous blood gas levels are approximately equal to that of normal mixed venous blood at room air conditions (Po_2 of 40 mm Hg, Pco_2 of 50 mm Hg, and pH of 7.35).

Radiologic evaluation

Color duplex ultrasonography offers a valuable adjunct in the evaluation of the patient presenting with priapism. This diagnostic method is used instead of cavernous blood gas testing, although its use should not create a delay in management. In distinguishing ischemic from nonischemic priapism, minimal or absent blood flow is observed in the cavernosal arteries of the corpora cavernosa in the former, and normal to high blood flow velocities are observed in the cavernosal arteries with evidence of blood flow in the corpora cavernosa of the latter (Fig. 3) [51,55]. Ultrasonography also may reveal anatomic

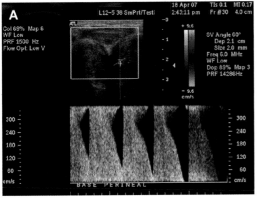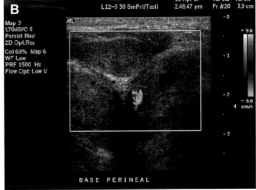

Fig. 3. Duplex scans depicting nonischemic (high-flow) priapism. (A) From the Doppler waveform, the peak systolic velocity in the cavernosal artery is elevated markedly (approximate peak systolic velocity of 300 cm/sec), and there is absence of diastolic flow. (B) A 6 × 4 × 5 mm hypoechoic focus slightly left of midline at the penile/perineal junction is compatible with a fistula/vascular formation.

abnormalities, such as a cavernous arterial fistula or pseudoaneurysm, which would confirm the diagnosis of nonischemic priapism. The study should be performed with the patient placed in lithotomy or frog leg position, to scan the perineum first and then the entire penile shaft. This important technical aspect acknowledges the possibility that an abnormality could be identified in the perineal portions of the corpora cavernosa under conditions of a straddle injury or direct scrotal trauma.

As an adjunctive study, penile arteriography may be used to identify the presence and sight of a cavernous artery fistula in the patient suspected to have nonischemic priapism [56]. This diagnostic test has a secondary role in the diagnosis of priapism and otherwise may be performed only as part of an embolization procedure. Other radiographic studies, such as penile scintigraphy and cavernosography, also have secondary roles.

Treatment

Ischemic priapism

In principle, diagnostic findings guide appropriate treatment decisions for priapism. A basic algorithm is widely supported (Fig. 4). A major episode of ischemic priapism requires immediate treatment to counteract the ischemic effects of the compartment syndrome. The insertion of a scalp vein needle (19 or 21 gauge) directly into the corpus cavernosum to aspirate blood has diagnostic and therapeutic purposes. The aspiration of

blood can be used for cavernous blood gas sampling while achieving immediate pain relief. Definitive first-line treatment of ischemic priapism consists of evacuation of blood and irrigation of the corpora cavernosa, along with intracavernous injection of an α-adrenergic sympathomimetic agent [1,2]. A dorsal nerve block or local penile shaft block may be used as a preceding penile anesthetic maneuver [1]. The technique of penile blood aspiration may vary, with techniques ranging from a transglanular intracorporal angiocatheter (16 or 18 gauge) insertion in the manner of the Winter shunt (see later discussion) to proximal corpora cavernosal needle placement for maximal corporal body irrigation [57]. Priapism resolution following aspiration with or without irrigation is approximately 30% [2].

Sympathomimetic agents are importantly applied because of their contractile effects, which may facilitate detumescence [58]. The preferred drug for this application is phenylephrine, an α_1-selective adrenergic agonist (dosed 100–200 μg every 5–10 minutes until detumescence, with 1000 μg maximally), which carries limited risks for cardiovascular side effects compared with other sympathomimetic agents having β-adrenergic activity. Monitoring for side effects using such agents is important, and blood pressure and ECG evaluation should be applied in patients with high cardiovascular risk [2]. Aspirating and irrigating with sympathomimetic injections over several hours may be necessary to achieve detumescence. Based on the medical literature, a higher resolution of ischemic priapism follows the

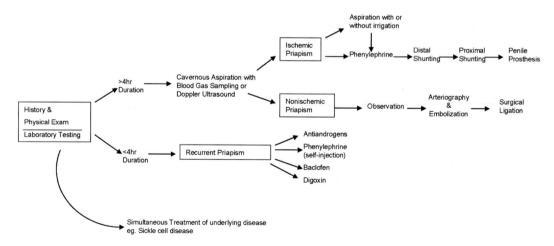

Fig. 4. Priapism treatment algorithm (*From* Burnett AL. Campbell-Walsh urology, vol. 1, 9th edition. Philadelphia: Elsevier; 2007. p. 844; with permission.)

concomitant use of sympathomimetic agents with or without irrigation (43% to 81%) than aspiration with or without irrigation alone (24% to 36%) [2]. In the absence of literature support for using oral sympathomimetic treatments (eg, terbutaline and pseudoephedrine) for ischemic priapism, these medications are omitted in current recommendations for such presentations [2].

Separate guidelines are offered for patients presenting with priapism in which an underlying etiologic disorder is identified. While intracavernous treatment of ischemic priapism is performed, concurrent management with appropriate systemic treatment should be followed as well. The recommendation applies to priapism associated with sickle cell disease as well as that associated with other hematologic diseases, metastatic neoplasia, or other etiologies in which standard treatments exist [2]. Consequently, in the example of priapism related to sickle cell disease, conventional intracavernous treatment should be performed for a prolonged episode of ischemia, even when analgesia, hydration, oxygenation, alkalinization, and even transfusion, are applied [59].

Second-line treatment, specifically surgical shunting, is instituted for priapism refractory to intracavernous treatment [1,2]. It is recognized that ischemic priapism of particularly extended durations, such as 48 to 72 hours, requires this management. The objective of surgical shunting is to facilitate blood drainage from the corpora cavernosa bypassing the veno-occlusive mechanism of these structures. Axiomatically, the least invasive surgical procedure is performed first, beginning with distal penile procedures before proceeding to more proximal ones.

A distal cavernoglanular (corporoglanular) shunt should be the first choice given its ease to perform and association with few complications [2]. Distal shunt procedures include placing a large-bore biopsy needle of a Truecut or biopty gun biopsy device (Winter shunt) [60] or a scalpel (Ebbehoj shunt) [61] percutaneously through the glans penis or excising the tunica albuginea at the tip of the corpus cavernosum (Al-Ghorab shunt) [62]. The Winter shunt often is used initially, because it can be performed at the bedside using a penile block. Variations of the Winter shunt procedure include using an angiocatheter with cut sideholes [63], a modified trocar with sideholes [64], or a Kerrison rongeur [65]. A technical maneuver of the Winter procedure is that the needle can be withdrawn beneath the glans penile skin and reinserted in different locations to create multiple

spongiosal–cavernosal communications. Once detumescence is achieved, the needle can be withdrawn completely, and the percutaneous puncture site can be closed with a single stitch of 4-0 chromic suture. Modifications have been described recently for the Ebbehoj shunt, such as the "T shunt" developed by Lue and Pescatori [66]. A simple wound closure also can be performed with this shunt procedure. The Al-Ghorab procedure is regarded to be the most effective distal shunt, although it is more invasive and, thus, commonly performed secondarily [2,67]. This procedure typically requires an operating room setting.

Proximal shunting involves creating a window between the corpus cavernosum and corpus spongiosum (Quackels or Sacher shunt) [68,69] or anastomosing the saphenous vein (Grayhack shunt) [70] or dorsal vein (Barry shunt) [71] to one of the corpora cavernosa. Serious complications have been reported following the various shunt procedures, such as urethral fistulas and purulent cavernositis following caverno-spongiosal shunts [72,73] and pulmonary embolism following the Grayhack procedure [74].

The possibility exists for erectile dysfunction to develop following performance of a shunt procedure. This may not be unexpected in some instances because the procedures involve disrupting the veno-occlusive mechanism of the penis required for maintenance of penile erection; however, if a shunt does not close in time spontaneously, shunt closure has succeeded in recovering erectile function [75]. It also may be kept in mind that erectile dysfunction may be a direct result of the prolonged priapism itself, irrespective of the shunting procedure [67].

Some investigators have advocated immediate placement of a penile prosthesis, particularly after a prolonged episode of ischemic priapism that predictably would fail to resolve with intracavernous treatment or surgical shunting [76,77]. The recommendation is based, in part, on the knowledge that performance of the surgery at a later time when significant fibrosis has developed would be extremely difficult and fraught with higher complication rates. Additionally, it has been observed that patients at this clinical juncture commonly do not respond in a satisfactory way to less invasive therapies for erectile dysfunction [52].

Nonischemic priapism

The initial management of nonischemic priapism should be observation [1,2] because spontaneous resolution occurs in up to 62% of reported cases [2]. Immediate invasive interventions, such as embolization and surgery, should be deferred unless the patient accepts the potential complication risks of such treatment and understands that there is a lack of significant adverse consequences resulting from delayed intervention [2].

Selective arterial embolization offers a secondary approach for the patient desirous of an immediate resolution [56]. Nonpermanent (eg, autologous clot, absorbable gels) and permanent (eg, coils, ethanol, polyvinyl alcohol particles, and acrylic glue) embolization materials are available; however, although all similarly achieve an approximate 75% resolution rate, nonpermanent materials produce a lesser erectile dysfunction rate (5% versus 39% with permanent substances) [2]. In addition, a complication of perineal abscess after embolization has been reported [78]. Penile exploration and direct surgical ligation of sinusoidal fistulas/pseudoaneurysms may be performed with the assistance of intraoperative color duplex ultrasonography only as an option of last resort [2]. Efficacy is noted in up to 63% of cases, although erectile dysfunction may occur in up to 50% of cases [2].

Recurrent stuttering priapism

In principle, all episodes of recurrent priapism should be treated vigorously according to recommendations for ischemic priapism [2]. Preventative strategies also have been explored to offset predictable future episodes. Such strategies have included systemic therapies, intracavernous self-injection of sympathomimetic agents, and penile prosthesis surgery. Touted systemic therapies include hormonal agents [53,79–82], baclofen [83], digoxin [84], and terbutaline [85]. Hormonal treatments (eg, gonadotropin-releasing hormone agonists, androgen receptor antagonists) have demonstrated the most consistently successful intervention, such that this therapy is supported as a primary approach [2,86]; however, such treatments do have their drawbacks. Hormonal agents should not be used in patients who have not achieved full sexual maturation and adult stature because the therapy may have a contraceptive effect and interfere with the timing of the closure of epiphyseal plates, respectively. Alternative management consists of intracavernous self-injection of phenylephrine or other sympathomimetic agents [80,87–89]. Proper instruction is required regarding injection site, dosing, potential local and systemic side effects, and duration of erection prompting treatment [2]. Phosphodiesterase type 5 (PDE5) molecular targeting has been explored recently as a novel strategy, rationally based on the discovery that PDE5 dysregulation is a mechanism of priapism [90]. A long-term scheduled PDE5 inhibitor therapeutic regimen has been described as successfully alleviating priapism in several patients [91]. It should be emphasized that the use of PDE5 inhibitors for the treatment of recurrent priapism remains investigational at present.

Risk management

Priapism carries the distinction of being one of the urologic conditions having a highly disproportionate level of medicolegal consequences. Adverse sequelae have resulted from delayed diagnosis and management, improper diagnosis, and complications from treatment. Without intervention, priapism may resolve; however, in the case of ischemic priapism, corporal fibrosis and tissue necrosis are likely and precipitate irrecoverably lost natural erectile function. Compounding the issue is the fact that many cases of priapism proceed to permanent complications because of the predisposition of the underlying condition, rather than the treatment for it.

Several recommendations are advised when dealing with priapism. Clearly, any awareness of a prolonged penile erection event should prompt proper and immediate urological attention. Diagnosis should proceed without delay and adhere to basic principles of patient evaluation and immediate penile diagnostics. Patients should be counseled regarding the adverse outcomes of priapism, including the risk for erectile dysfunction despite appropriate medical and surgical interventions. Risks of procedures should be explained carefully, and consenting for procedures should be performed and documented.

Additional clinical management challenges exist in individuals with previously treated priapism who are seeking management for erectile dysfunction. The central issue here is whether treatments for erectile dysfunction may provoke another priapism episode. The literature does provide examples of successful intervention with intracavernous pharmacotherapy [92] as well as placement of a penile prosthesis [93]. Again, thorough discussion of procedures and alternatives, and their inherent risks, should ensue.

Conceivably, all treatment modalities for erectile dysfunction may be considered, but patients should accept the potential risks for a subsequent priapism episode with their use.

For the severely affected individual, penile prosthesis surgery would seem ideal; however, because many of these patients manifest extensive corporal fibrosis, penile prosthesis surgery may be difficult [93,94]. Specialized technical maneuvers may be necessary, with which the surgeon should be familiar. The surgeon also should consider a properly selected penile prosthesis, which would function well in the fibrosed penis without exacerbating prior penile deformity. For this reason, current recommendations are to use an American Medical Systems CX device (Minnetonka, Minnesota) or Coloplast Alpha device (Minneapolis, Minnesota), avoiding devices that have unlimited girth- and length-enhancing features.

New treatment strategies

The future management of priapism can be expected to evolve over time. Immediate goals are to prevent the complications of the disorder more effectively and preserve erectile function. Fundamental to these objectives is the study and discovery of mechanism-specific therapies that address the pathogenesis of priapism and the pathophysiologic factors contributing to subsequent erectile dysfunction. Primary emphasis is given to corrective intervention for ischemic priapism, particularly for high-risk patients, such as those who have sickle cell disease and others who have already displayed recurrent priapism.

Numerous medical therapies have been brought to this clinical arena, touted to be successful based on anecdotal reports. In addition to having unclear rationales for their use, many have limited outcomes data, such that they are not endorsed by American Urological Association guidelines [2]. Currently recognized therapies having success, such as hormonal therapies and sympathomimetic self-injections, remain far from ideal.

The charge ahead for investigators and medical practitioners in this field is to bring forward therapies of improved efficacy in controlling priapism, if not therapies that are truly corrective of the disorder. Most certainly, these will be built on knowledge of the pathophysiologic mechanisms of priapism. Such understanding should translate into therapies that are proven to be efficacious using rigorous clinical trial methodology. At the present time, PDE5 molecular targeting and antifibrotic interventions seem to be the most promising as strategies for the future [95].

Summary

Although priapism may be an uncommon medical disorder affecting only a small population of male individuals, it deserves proper attention as a disorder of major significance. The disorder disproportionately affects certain populations and often leads to major complications, including permanent erectile dysfunction. Fundamental aspects of clinical management include early awareness of the problem, rigorous discernment of its ischemic and nonischemic presentations, and prompt initiation of a rational step-wise treatment plan, particularly for presentations of ischemic priapism. A true understanding of the biologic basis of the disorder has been elusive for years, with recent new insight suggesting the likelihood of improved therapies to come. In the meantime, urologists as well as the broader medical community should appreciate the importance of the disorder and be prepared to follow current principles of diagnosis and treatment to reduce or avert its complications.

References

[1] Berger R, Billups K, Brock G, et al. Report of the American Foundation for Urologic Disease (AFUD) thought leader panel for evaluation and treatment of priapism. Int J Impot Res 2001; 13(Suppl 5):S39–43.

[2] Montague DK, Jarow J, Broderick GA, et al. American Urological Association guideline on the management of priapism. J Urol 2003;170:1318–24.

[3] Monllor J, Tano F, Arteaga PR, et al. Priapism of the clitoris. Eur Urol 1996;30:521–2.

[4] Hashmat AI, Raju S, Singh I, et al. 99mTc penile scan: an investigative modality in priapism. Urol Radiol 1989;11:58–60.

[5] Sharpsteen JR Jr, Powars D, Johnson C, et al. Multisystem damage associated with tricorporal priapism in sickle cell disease. Am J Med 1993;94:289–95.

[6] Kulmala R, Lehtonen T, Tammela TL. Priapism, its incidence and seasonal distribution in Finland. Scand J Urol Nephrol 1995;29:93–6.

[7] Eland IA, Van Der Lei J, Stricker BHC, et al. Incidence of priapism in the general population. Urology 2001;57:970–2.

[8] Earle CM, Stuckey BGA, Ching HL, et al. The incidence and management of priapism in Western

Australia: a 16 year audit. Int J Impot Res 2003;15: 272–6.

[9] Emond AM, Holman R, Hayes RJ, et al. Priapism and impotence in homozygous sickle cell disease. Arch Intern Med 1980;140:1434–7.

[10] Fowler JE Jr, Koshy M, Strub M, et al. Priapism associated with the sickle cell hemoglobinopathies: prevalence, natural history and sequelae. J Urol 1991;145:65–8.

[11] Mantadakis E, Cavender JD, Rogers ZR, et al. Prevalence of priapism in children and adolescents with sickle cell anemia. J Pediatr Hematol Oncol 1999; 21:518–22.

[12] Adeyoju AB, Olujohungbe ABK, Morris J, et al. Priapism in sickle-cell disease; incidence, risk factors and complications – an international multicentre study. BJU Int 2002;90:898–902.

[13] Hinman F Jr. Priapism; reasons for failure of therapy. J Urol 1960;83:420–8.

[14] Winter CC, McDowell G. Experience with 105 patients with priapism: update review of all aspects. J Urol 1988;140:980–3.

[15] Burnett AL. Pathophysiology of priapism: dysregulatory erection physiology thesis. J Urol 2003;170: 26–34.

[16] Lue TF, Hellstrom WJG, McAninch JW, et al. Priapism: a refined approach to diagnosis and treatment. J Urol 1986;136:104–8.

[17] Levine JF, Saenz de Tejada I, Payton TR, et al. Recurrent prolonged erections and priapism as a sequela of priapism: pathophysiology and management. J Urol 1991;145:764–7.

[18] Melman A, Serels S. Priapism. Int J Impot Res 2000; 12(Suppl 4):S133–9.

[19] Pond HS. Priapism as the presenting complaint of myelogenous leukemia: case report and review of the physiology of erection and the pathophysiology and treatment of priapism. South Med J 1969;62: 465–7.

[20] Larocque MA, Cosgrove MD. Priapism: a review of 46 cases. J Urol 1974;112:770–3.

[21] Brown JA, Nehra A. Erythropoietin-induced recurrent veno-occlusive priapism associated with end-stage renal disease. Urology 1998;52:328–30.

[22] Klein EA, Montague DK, Steiger E. Priapism associated with the use of intravenous fat emulsion: case reports and postulated pathogenesis. J Urol 1985; 133:857–9.

[23] Hebuterne X, Frere AM, Bayle J, et al. Priapism in a patient treated with total parenteral nutrition. JPEN J Parenter Enteral Nutr 1992;16:171–4.

[24] Fassbinder W, Frei U, Issantier R, et al. Factors predisposing to priapism in haemodialysis patients. Proc Eur Dial Transplant Assoc 1976;12:380–6.

[25] Bschleipfer TH, Hauck EW, Diemer TH, et al. Heparin-induced priapism. Int J Impot Res 2001;13: 357–9.

[26] Chan PT, Begin LR, Arnold D, et al. Priapism secondary to penile metastasis: a report of two cases and a review of the literature. J Surg Oncol 1998; 68:51–9.

[27] Morano SG, Latagliata R, Carmosino I, et al. Treatment of long-lasting priapism in chronic myeloid leukemia at onset. Ann Hematol 2000;79:644–5.

[28] Morga Egea JP, Ferrero Doria R, Guzman Martinez-Valls PL, et al. Metastasis priapism. Report of 4 new cases and review of the literature. Arch Esp Urol 2000;53:447–52.

[29] Hettiarachchi JA, Johnson GB, Panageas E, et al. Malignant priapism associated with metastatic urethral carcinoma. Urol Int 2001;66:114–6.

[30] Burt FB, Schirmer HK, Scott WW. A new concept in the management of priapism. J Urol 1960;83:60–1.

[31] Hauri D, Spycher M, Brühlmann W. Erection and priapism: a new physiopathological concept. Urol Int 1983;38:138–45.

[32] Winter CC. Priapism. Urol Surv 1978;28:163–6.

[33] Llado J, Peterson LJ, Fair WR. Priapism of the proximal penis. J Urol 1980;123:779–80.

[34] Witt MA, Goldstein I, Saenz de Tejada I, et al. Traumatic laceration of intracavernosal arteries: the pathophysiology of nonischemic, high flow, arterial priapism. J Urol 1990;143:129–32.

[35] Ricciardi R Jr, Bhatt GM, Cynamon J, et al. Delayed high flow priapism: pathophysiology and management. J Urol 1993;149:119–21.

[36] Burnett AL, Musicki B, Bivalacqua TJ. Molecular science of priapism. Curr Sex Health Rep 2007;4: 9–14.

[37] Broderick GA, Gordon D, Hypolite J, et al. Anoxia and corporal smooth muscle dysfunction: a model for ischemic priapism. J Urol 1994;151:259–62.

[38] Saenz de Tejada I, Kim NN, Daley JT, et al. Acidosis impairs rabbit trabecular smooth muscle contractility. J Urol 1997;157:722–6.

[39] Muneer A, Cellek S, Dogan A, et al. Investigation of cavernosal smooth muscle dysfunction in low flow priapism using an in vitro model. Int J Impot Res 2005;17:10–8.

[40] Evliyaoglu Y, Kayrin L, Kaya B. Effect of allopurinol on lipid peroxidation induced in corporeal tissue by veno-occlusive priapism in a rat model. Br J Urol 1997;80:476–9.

[41] Munarriz R, Park K, Huang YH, et al. Reperfusion of ischemic corporal tissue: physiologic and biochemical changes in an animal model of ischemic priapism. Urology 2003;62:760–4.

[42] Ul-Hasan M, El-Sakka AI, Lee C, et al. Expression of TGF-β-1 mRNA and ultrastructural alterations in pharmacologically induced prolonged penile erection in a canine model. J Urol 1998;160:2263–6.

[43] Datta NS. Megalophallus in sickle cell disease. J Urol 1977;117:672–3.

[44] Spycher MA, Hauri D. The ultrastructure of the erectile tissue in priapism. J Urol 1986;135:142–7.

[45] Broderick GA, Harkaway R. Pharmacologic erection: time-dependent changes in the corporal environment. Int J Impot Res 1994;6:9–16.

[46] Kim NN, Kim JJ, Hypolite J, et al. Altered contractility of rabbit penile corpus cavernosum smooth muscle by hypoxia. J Urol 1996;155:772–8.

[47] Moon DG, Lee DS, Kim JJ. Altered contractile response of penis under hypoxia with metabolic acidosis. Int J Impot Res 1999;11:265–71.

[48] Liu SP, Mogavero LJ, Levin RM. Correlation of calcium-activated ATPase activity, lipid peroxidation, and the contractile response of rabbit corporal smooth muscle treated with in vitro ischemia. Gen Pharmacol 1999;32:345–9.

[49] Juenemann KP, Lue TF, Abozeid M, et al. Blood gas analysis in drug-induced penile erection. Urol Int 1986;41:207–11.

[50] Brock G, Breza J, Lue TF, et al. High flow priapism: a spectrum of disease. J Urol 1993;150:968–71.

[51] Hakim LS, Kulaksizoglu H, Mulligan R, et al. Evolving concepts in the diagnosis and treatment of arterial high flow priapism. J Urol 1996;155:541–8.

[52] Pryor J, Akkus E, Alter G, et al. Priapism, Peyronie's disease, penile reconstructive surgery. In: Lue TF, Basson R, Rosen R, et al, editors. Sexual medicine sexual dysfunctions in men and women. Paris: Health Publications; 2004. p. 383–408.

[53] Serjeant GR, de Ceulaer K, Maude GH. Stilboestrol and stuttering priapism in homozygous sickle-cell disease. Lancet 1985;2:1274–6.

[54] Seftel AD, Haas CA, Brown SL, et al. High flow priapism complicating veno-occlusive priapism: pathophysiology of recurrent idiopathic priapism? J Urol 1998;159:1300–1.

[55] Feldstein VA. Posttraumatic "high flow" priapism: evaluation with color flow Doppler sonography. J Ultrasound Med 1993;12:589–93.

[56] Bastuba MD, Saenz de Tejada I, Dinlenc CZ, et al. Arterial priapism: diagnosis, treatment and long-term follow-up. J Urol 1994;151:1231–7.

[57] Chung SY, Stein RJ, Cannon TW, et al. Novel technique in the management of low flow priapism. J Urol 2003;170:1952.

[58] Lee M, Cannon B, Sharifi R. Chart for preparation of dilutions of alpha-adrenergic agonists for intracavernous use in treatment of priapism. J Urol 1995; 153:1182–3.

[59] Mantadakis E, Ewalt DH, Cavender JD, et al. Outpatient penile aspiration and epinephrine irrigation for young patients with sickle cell anemia and prolonged priapism. Blood 2000;95:78–82.

[60] Winter CC. Cure of idiopathic priapism: new procedure for creating fistula between glans penis and corpora cavernosa. Urology 1976;8:389–91.

[61] Ebbehoj J. A new operation for priapism. Scand J Plast Reconstr Surg 1974;8:241–2.

[62] Ercole CJ, Pontes JE, Pierce JM Jr. Changing surgical concepts in the treatment of priapism. J Urol 1981;125:210–1.

[63] Ulman I, Avanoglu A, Herek O, et al. A simple method of treating priapism in children. Br J Urol 1996;77:460–1.

[64] Kilin M. A modified Winter's procedure for priapism treatment with a new trocar. Eur Urol 1993;24: 118–9.

[65] Goulding FJ. Modification of cavernoglandular shunt for priapism. Urology 1980;15:64.

[66] Lue TF, Pescatori ES. Distal cavernosum-glans shunts for ischemic priapism. J Sex Med 2006;3: 749–52.

[67] Nixon RG, O'Connor JL, Milam DF. Efficacy of shunt surgery for refractory low flow priapism: a report on the incidence of failed detumescence and erectile dysfunction. J Urol 2003;170:883–6.

[68] Quackels R. Treatment of a case of priapism by cavernospongious anastomosis. Acta Urol Belg 1964; 32:5–13.

[69] Sacher EC, Sayegh E, Frensilli F, et al. Cavernospongiosum shunt in the treatment of priapism. J Urol 1972;108:97–100.

[70] Grayhack JT, McCullough W, O'Connor VJ Jr, et al. Venous bypass to control priapism. Investig Urol 1964;58:509–13.

[71] Barry JM. Priapism: treatment with corpus cavernosum to dorsal vein of penis shunts. J Urol 1976;116: 754–6.

[72] Ochoa Urdangarain O, Hermida Perez JA. Priapism. Our experience. Arch Esp Urol 1998;51:269–76.

[73] De Stefani S, Savoca G, Ciampalini S, et al. Urethrocutaneous fistula as a severe complication of treatment for priapism. BJU Int 2001;88:642–3.

[74] Kandel GL, Bender LI, Grove JS. Pulmonary embolism: a complication of corpus-saphenous shunt for priapism. J Urol 1968;99:196–7.

[75] Stein RJ, Patel AS, Benoit RM. Treatment of postpriapism erectile dysfunction by closure of persistent distal glans-cavernosum fistulas 5 years after shunt creation. Urology 2005;65:592.e19–592.e20.

[76] Monga M, Broderick GA, Hellstrom WJ. Priapism in sickle cell disease: the case for early implantation of the penile prosthesis. Eur Urol 1996;30:54–9.

[77] Rees RW, Kalsi J, Minhas S, et al. The management of low-flow priapism with the immediate insertion of a penile prosthesis. BJU Int 2002;90:893–7.

[78] Sandock DS, Seftel AD, Herbener TE, et al. Perineal abscess after embolization for high-flow priapism. Urology 1996;48:308–11.

[79] Levine LA, Guss SP. Gonadotropin-releasing hormone analogues in the treatment of sickle cell anemia-associated priapism. J Urol 1993;150:475–7.

[80] Steinberg J, Eyre RC. Management of recurrent priapism with epinephrine self-injection and gonadotropin-releasing hormone analogue. J Urol 1995; 153:152–3.

[81] Dahm P, Dinesh SR, Donatucci CF. Antiandrogens in the treatment of priapism. Urology 2002;59: 138xx–138xxi.

[82] Gbadoe AD, Assimadi JK, Segbena YA. Short period of administration of diethylstilbestrol in stuttering priapism in sickle cell anemia. Am J Hematol 2002;69:297–8.

[83] Rourke KF, Fischler AH, Jordan GH. Treatment of recurrent idiopathic priapism with oral baclofen. J Urol 2002;168:2552–3.

[84] Gupta S, Salimpour P, De Tejada IS, et al. A possible mechanism for alteration of human erectile function by digoxin: inhibition of corpus cavernosum sodium/potassium adenosine triphosphatase activity. J Urol 1998;159:1529–36.

[85] Ahmed I, Shaikh NA. Treatment of intermittent idiopathic priapism with oral terbutaline. Br J Urol 1997;80:341.

[86] Levine LA, Estrada CR, Latchamsetty KC. Idiopathic ischemic priapism. Preventing recurrence. Contemp Urol 2004;16:25–34.

[87] Van Driel MF, Joosten EA, Mensink HJ. Intracorporeal self-injection with epinephrine as treatment for idiopathic recurrent priapism. Eur Urol 1990; 17:95–6.

[88] Virag R, Bachir D, Lee K, et al. Preventive treatment of priapism in sickle cell disease with oral and self-administered intracavernous injection of etilefrine. Urology 1996;47:777–81.

[89] Teloken C, Ribeiro EP, Chammas M, et al. Intracavernosal etilefrine self-injection therapy for recurrent priapism: one decade of follow-up. Urology 2005;65: 1002.

[90] Champion HC, Bivalacqua TJ, Takimoto E, et al. Phosphodiesterase-5A dysregulation in penile erectile tissue is a mechanism of priapism. Proc Natl Acad Sci USA 2005;102:1661–6.

[91] Burnett AL, Bivalacqua TJ, Champion HC, et al. Feasibility of the use of phosphodiesterase type 5 inhibitors in a pharmacologic prevention program for recurrent priapism. J Sex Med 2006;3: 1077–84.

[92] Lakin MM, Montague DK. Intracavernous injection therapy in post-priapism cavernosal fibrosis. J Urol 1988;140:828–9.

[93] Bertram RA, Carson CC, Webster GD. Implantation of penile prosthesis in patients impotent after priapism. Urology 1985;26:325–7.

[94] Kabalin JN. Corporeal fibrosis as a result of priapism prohibiting function of self-contained inflatable penile prosthesis. Urology 1994;43: 401–3.

[95] Bivalacqua TJ, Burnett AL. Priapism: new concepts in the pathophysiology and new treatment strategies. Curr Urol Rep 2006;7:497–502.

ELSEVIER
SAUNDERS

Urol Clin N Am 34 (2007) 643–649

UROLOGIC
CLINICS
of North America

Index

Note: Page numbers of article titles are in **boldface** type.

Moving?

Make sure your subscription moves with you!

To notify us of your new address, find your **Clinics Account Number** (located on your mailing label above your name), and contact customer service at:

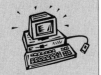

E-mail: elspcs@elsevier.com

800-654-2452 (subscribers in the U.S. & Canada)
407-345-4000 (subscribers outside of the U.S. & Canada)

Fax number: 407-363-9661

Elsevier Periodicals Customer Service
6277 Sea Harbor Drive
Orlando, FL 32887-4800

*To ensure uninterrupted delivery of your subscription, please notify us at least 4 weeks in advance of move.

United States Postal Service

Statement of Ownership, Management, and Circulation
(All Periodicals Publications Except Requestor Publications)

1. Publication Title	2. Publication Number	3. Filing Date
Urologic Clinics of North America	0 0 0 - 7 1 1 1	9/14/07

4. Issue Frequency	5. Number of Issues Published Annually	6. Annual Subscription Price
Feb, May, Aug, Nov	4	$231.00

7. Complete Mailing Address of Known Office of Publication (Not printer) (Street, city, county, state, and ZIP+4)

Elsevier Inc.
360 Park Avenue South
New York, NY 10010-1710

Contact Person
Stephen Bushing

Telephone (Include area code)
215-239-3688

8. Complete Mailing Address of Headquarters or General Business Office of Publisher (Not printer)

Elsevier Inc., 360 Park Avenue South, New York, NY 10010-1710

9. Full Names and Complete Mailing Addresses of Publisher, Editor, and Managing Editor (Do not leave blank)

Publisher (Name and complete mailing address)

John Schrefer, Elsevier, Inc., 1600 John F. Kennedy Blvd. Suite 1800, Philadelphia, PA 19103-2899

Editor (Name and complete mailing address)

Kerry Holland, Elsevier, Inc., 1600 John F. Kennedy Blvd. Suite 1800, Philadelphia, PA 19103-2899

Managing Editor (Name and complete mailing address)

Catherine Bewick, Elsevier, Inc., 1600 John F. Kennedy Blvd. Suite 1800, Philadelphia, PA 19103-2899

10. Owner (Do not leave blank. If the publication is owned by a corporation, give the name and address of the corporation immediately followed by the names and addresses of all stockholders owning or holding 1 percent or more of the total amount of stock. If not owned by a corporation, give the names and addresses of the individual owners. If owned by a partnership or other unincorporated firm, give its name and address as well as those of each individual owner. If the publication is published by a nonprofit organization, give its name and address.)

Full Name	Complete Mailing Address
Wholly owned subsidiary of	4520 East-West Highway
Reed/Elsevier, US holdings	Bethesda, MD 20814

11. Known Bondholders, Mortgagees, and Other Security Holders Owning or Holding 1 Percent or More of Total Amount of Bonds, Mortgages, or Other Securities. If none, check box. □ None

Full Name	Complete Mailing Address
N/A	

12. Tax Status (For completion by nonprofit organizations authorized to mail at nonprofit rates) (Check one)
The purpose, function, and nonprofit status of this organization and the exempt status for federal income tax purposes:
☐ Has Not Changed During Preceding 12 Months
☐ Has Changed During Preceding 12 Months (Publisher must submit explanation of change with this statement)

PS Form 3526, September 2006 (Page 1 of 3 (Instructions Page 3)) PSN 7530-01-000-9931 PRIVACY NOTICE: See our Privacy policy in www.usps.com

---

13. Publication Title	14. Issue Date for Circulation Data Below
Urologic Clinics of North America	August 2007

15. Extent and Nature of Circulation		Average No. Copies Each Issue During Preceding 12 Months	No. Copies of Single Issue Published Nearest to Filing Date
a. Total Number of Copies (Net press run)		4075	3900
b. Paid Circulation (By Mail and Outside the Mail)	(1) Mailed Outside-County Paid Subscriptions Stated on PS Form 3541. (Include paid distribution above nominal rate, advertiser's proof copies, and exchange copies)	1728	1644
	(2) Mailed In-County Paid Subscriptions Stated on PS Form 3541 (Include paid distribution above nominal rate, advertiser's proof copies, and exchange copies)		
	(3) Paid Distribution Outside the Mails Including Sales Through Dealers and Carriers, Street Vendors, Counter Sales, and Other Paid Distribution Outside USPS®	1384	1341
	(4) Paid Distribution by Other Classes Mailed Through the USPS (e.g. First-Class Mail®)		
c. Total Paid Distribution (Sum of 15b (1), (2), (3), and (4)) ▶		3112	2985
d. Free or Nominal Rate Distribution (By Mail and Outside the Mail)	(1) Free or Nominal Rate Outside-County Copies Included on PS Form 3541	114	91
	(2) Free or Nominal Rate In-County Copies Included on PS Form 3541		
	(3) Free or Nominal Rate Copies Mailed at Other Classes Mailed Through the USPS (e.g. First-Class Mail)		
	(4) Free or Nominal Rate Distribution Outside the Mail (Carriers or other means)		
e. Total Free or Nominal Rate Distribution (Sum of 15d (1), (2), (3) and (4)) ▶		114	91
f. Total Distribution (Sum of 15c and 15e) ▶		3226	3076
g. Copies not Distributed (See instructions to publishers #4 (page #3)) ▶		849	824
h. Total (Sum of 15f and g) ▶		4075	3900
i. Percent Paid (15c divided by 15f times 100)		96.47%	97.04%

16. Publication of Statement of Ownership

☐ If the publication is a general publication, publication of this statement is required. Will be printed in the November 2007 issue of this publication. ☐ Publication not required

17. Signature and Title of Editor, Publisher, Business Manager, or Owner	Date
[signature] Nanuci – Executive Director of Subscription Services	September 14, 2007

I certify that all information furnished on this form is true and complete. I understand that anyone who furnishes false or misleading information on this form or who omits material or information requested on the form may be subject to criminal sanctions (including fines and imprisonment) and/or civil sanctions (including civil penalties).

PS Form 3526, September 2006 (Page 2 of 3)